Operative Techniques in
Lower Limb Reconstruction and Amputation

Operative Techniques in Lower Limb Reconstruction and Amputation

Gordon K. Lee, MD, FACS

EDITOR

Professor of Plastic Surgery
Associate Chief of Clinical Affairs
Residency Program Director
Director of Microsurgery
Stanford University
Palo Alto, California

Kevin C. Chung, MD, MS

EDITOR-IN-CHIEF

Chief of Hand Surgery, Michigan Medicine
Director, University of Michigan Comprehensive Hand Center
Charles B. G. de Nancrede Professor of Surgery
Professor of Plastic Surgery and Orthopaedic Surgery
Assistant Dean for Faculty Affairs
Associate Director of Global REACH
University of Michigan Medical School
Ann Arbor, Michigan

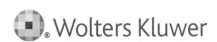

Philadelphia • Baltimore • New York • London
Buenos Aires • Hong Kong • Sydney • Tokyo

Executive Editor: Brian Brown
Development Editor: Ashley Fischer
Editorial Coordinator: John Larkin
Marketing Manager: Julie Sikora
Senior Production Project Manager: Alicia Jackson
Senior Designer: Joan Wendt
Artist/Illustrator: Body Scientific International
Senior Manufacturing Coordinator: Beth Welsh
Prepress Vendor: SPi Global

9 8 7 6 5 4 3 2 1

Printed in China

Cataloging-in-Publication Data available on request from the Publisher.
ISBN 978-1-9751-2734-3

shop.lww.com

To my wife, Yun-Ting, and my sons, Jordan and Kyle, for their love, patience, and understanding of me as a busy husband, father, and surgeon. And to my mother, Helen, and my father, Leyton, who taught me to never give up.

—GKL

To Chin-Yin and William.

—KCC

Contributors

Derek F. Amanatullah, MD, PhD
Assistant Professor
Orthopedic Surgery
Stanford Hospital and Clinics
Redwood City, California

Raffi S. Avedian, MD
Assistant Professor of Orthopaedic
  Surgery
Stanford University Medical Center
Department of Orthopaedic Surgery
Charlotte and George Schultz
Orthopaedic Tumor Center
Palo Alto, California

Joseph Baylan, MD
Resident Physician
School of Medicine
Stanford University
Palo Alto, California

Michael Bellino, MD
Assistant Professor
Department of Orthopaedic Surgery
Stanford University School of
  Medicine
Palo Alto, California

Julius Bishop, MD
Assistant Professor and Associate
  Residency Director
Department of Orthopaedic Surgery
Stanford University School of Medicine
Palo Alto, California

David W. Chang, MD, FACS
Chief of Plastic and Reconstructive
  Surgery
Director of Microsurgery Fellowship
Professor of Surgery
The University of Chicago Medicine &
  Biological Sciences
Chicago, Illinois

Vishwanath R. Chegireddy, MD
General Surgery Resident
Department of Surgery
Houston Methodist Hospital
Houston, Texas

Michael J. Chen, MD
Current Orthopaedic Resident
Department of Orthopaedic Surgery
School of Medicine
Stanford University
Stanford, California

Loretta Chou, MD
Professor of Orthopaedic Surgery
Stanford University
Redwood City, California

Catherine Curtin, MD
Associate Professor
Division of Plastic Surgery
Stanford University
Palo Alto, California

Gabrielle B. Davis, MD, MS
Resident Physician
Division of Plastic & Reconstructive
  Surgery
Department of Surgery
Stanford, California

Sahitya K. Denduluri, MD
Resident Physician
Department of Orthopaedic Surgery
Stanford University
Stanford, California

Anahita Dua, MD, MS, MBA
Vascular Surgery Fellow
Division of Vascular Surgery
Department of Surgery
Stanford Hospital and Clinics
Palo Alto, California

Anthony Echo, MD
Assistant Professor of Plastic Surgery
Houston Methodist Hospital Research
  Institute
Assistant Professor of Plastic Surgery
Weill Cornell Medicine
Assistant Clinical Professor of Surgery
Texas A&M University
Houston, Texas

**Michael W. Findlay, MBBS, PhD,
FRACS, FACS**
Program Director—Plastic Surgery
The Peter MacCallum Cancer Centre
Plastic, Reconstructive and Hand Surgeon
The Canberra Hospital Surgical Lead
Plastic, Reconstructive and Hand Surgery
Australasian Clinical Trials Network
  Director
Program for Molecular and Cellular
  Innovation in Surgery
Senior Lecturer
The University of Melbourne
Department of Surgery
Royal Melbourne Hospital
Melbourne, Australia

Deepak M. Gupta, MD
Clinical Assistant Professor of Plastic
  Surgery
Santa Clara Valley Medical Center
  and Stanford University School of
  Medicine
San Jose, California

Martin Halle, MD, PhD
Karolinska Institutet
Department of Reconstructive Plastic
  Surgery
Karolinska University Hospital
Stockholm, Sweden

Scott L. Hansen, MD
Associate Professor of Surgery
Division of Plastic and Reconstructive
  Surgery
University of California, San Francisco
Chief, Hand and Microvascular
  Surgery
University of California, San Francisco
Chief, Plastic and Reconstructive Surgery
Zuckerberg San Francisco General
  Hospital
San Francisco, California

Rachel Hein, MD
Resident
Department of Plastic Surgery
Duke University Medical Center
Durham, North Carolina

Michael C. Holland, MD
Resident Physician
Division of Plastic and Reconstructive
  Surgery
University of California, San Francisco
San Francisco, California

Scott T. Hollenbeck, MD, FACS
Associate Professor, Plastic and
  Reconstructive Surgery
Director of Microsurgery Training
Medical Student and Physician
Assistant Clerkship Director—Plastic
  Surgery
Duke University Medical Center
Durham, North Carolina

Jean-Louis Horn, MD, PhD
Professor, Anesthesiology, Regional
  Anesthesia and Acute Pain Medicine
Stanford University
Stanford, California

Patrick Horrigan, MD
Assistant Professor, University of
  Minnesota
Department of Orthopaedic Surgery
Regions Hospital
Saint Paul, Minnesota

James I. Huddleston III, MD
Associate Professor of Orthopaedic
  Surgery
Adult Reconstruction Service Chief
Department of Orthopaedic
  Surgery
Stanford University Medical
  Center
Stanford, California

Kenneth Hunt, MD
Associate Professor and Chief, Foot
  and Ankle Surgery
Department of Orthopaedic Surgery
School of Medicine
University of Colorado
Aurora, Colorado

Adam Jacoby, MD
NYU Langone Health
New York, New York

Peter Johannet, MD
Chief of Plastic Surgery
Veterans Affairs Palo Alto
Palo Alto, California
Associate Clinical Professor of Plastic
  & Reconstructive Surgery
Division of Plastic & Reconstructive
  Surgery
Stanford University
Stanford, California

Yvonne L. Karanas, MD
Chief of Plastic Surgery and
  Director
Burn Center
Santa Clara Valley Medical Center
Associate Clinical Professor
School of Medicine
Stanford University
San Jose, California

Rohit Khosla, MD
Assistant Professor of Plastic
  Surgery
Division of Plastic Surgery
Stanford University Medical Center
Palo Alto, California

So Young Kim, MD, PhD
Assistant Professor
Department of Plastic and
  Reconstructive Surgery
Inje University Sanggye Paik
  Hospital
Inje University School of Medicine
Seoul, South Korea

Michael J. A. Klebuc, MD
Associate Clinical Professor of Plastic
  and Neurosurgery
Weill Medical College
Cornell University
Director Center for Facial Reanimation
  and Functional Restoration
Houston Methodist Hospital
Houston, Texas

Ulrich Kneser, MD
Professor of Plastic and Hand Surgery
University of Heidelberg Medical
  School
Director, Department of Hand, Plastic
  and Reconstructive Surgery
Burn Unit
BG Trauma Center Ludwigshafen
Ludwigshafen, Germany

Thomas Kremer, MD
Professor of Plastic and Aesthetic
  Surgery, Hand Surgeon
Department of Plastic and Hand
  Surgery
Burn Center
Leipzig, Germany

Brock Lanier, MD
Clinical Instructor in Microsurgery
Division of Plastic and Reconstructive
  Surgery
Stanford University
Stanford, California

Kedar S. Lavingia, MD
Fellow
Division of Vascular Surgery
Stanford University
Menlo Park, California

Jason T. Lee, MD
Professor of Vascular Surgery
Director of Endovascular Surgery
Program Director, Vascular Surgery
Residency/Fellowship
Stanford University Medical Center
Stanford, California

Amber R. Leis, MD
Assistant Clinical Professor
Director of Hand Surgery
Assistant Program Director
University of California—Irvine
Orange, California

L. Scott Levin, MD, FACS
Paul B. Magnuson Professor of Bone
  and Joint Surgery
Chairman, Department of Orthopaedic
  Surgery
Professor of Surgery
Division of Plastic Surgery
University of Pennsylvania
Philadelphia, Pennsylvania

Sean S. Li, MD
Resident
Division of Plastic and Reconstructive
  Surgery
University of California, San Diego
San Diego, California

Xiangxia Liu, MD, PhD
Associate Professor and Associate Chief
Division of Plastic Surgery
First Affiliated Hospital
Sun Yat-sen University
Guangzhou, Guangdong, China

David W. Lowenberg, MD
Clinical Professor
Department of Orthopaedic Surgery
School of Medicine
Stanford University
Palo Alto, California

Andrew Lyons, MD
Clinical Instructor and Fellow
Regional Anesthesia Division
Department of Anesthesiology,
  Perioperative and Pain Medicine
Stanford University Medical Center
Palo Alto, California

Sarah Madison, MD
Anesthesiologist
Veterans Affairs Long Beach Healthcare
  System
Long Beach, California

Graeme E. McFarland, MD
Assistant Professor
Division of Vascular Surgery and
  Endovascular Therapy
Department of Surgery
University of Alabama at Birmingham
Birmingham, Alabama

Fred G. Mihm, MD
Professor
Division Chief, Critical Care Medicine
Department of Anesthesiology,
  Perioperative and Pain Medicine
Stanford University School of Medicine
Associate Medical Director, Intensive
  Care Units
Department of Anesthesiology,
  Perioperative and Pain Medicine
Stanford University Medical Center
Stanford, California

Arash Momeni, MD
Assistant Professor of Surgery
Director, Clinical Outcomes Research
Ryan-Upson Scholar in Plastic and
  Reconstructive Surgery
Division of Plastic & Reconstructive
  Surgery
Stanford University Medical Center
Palo Alto, California

Shawn Moshrefi, MD
Plastic Surgery Resident
Stanford University Medical Center
Palo Alto, California

Goo-Hyun Mun, MD, PhD
Professor
Department of Plastic Surgery
Samsung Medical Center
Sungkyunkwan University
Seoul, South Korea

Rahim Nazerali, MD, MHS, FACS
Clinical Assistant Professor of
    Surgery
Division of Plastic & Reconstructive
    Surgery
Stanford Healthcare
Palo Alto, California

Dung Nguyen, MD, PharmD
Clinical Associate Professor
Stanford University
Palo Alto, California

Hunter S. Oliver-Allen, MD
Resident Physician
Division of Plastic and Reconstructive
    Surgery
Department of Surgery
University of California, San
    Francisco
San Francisco, California

**Adrian S. H. Ooi, MBBS, MMed
(Surgery), MRCS, FAMS (Plastic
Surgery)**
Consultant Plastic Surgeon
Department of Plastic, Reconstructive
    and Aesthetic Surgery
Singapore General Hospital
SingHealth Head & Neck Disease
    Center
SingHealth
Singapore, Singapore

Paulo Piccolo, MD
Microsurgey Fellow
Division of Plastic Surgery
Department of Surgery
University of Pennsylvania
Philadelphia, Pennsylvania

Lee L. Q. Pu, MD, PhD, FACS
Professor of Surgery
Division of Plastic Surgery
University of California Davis Medical
    Center
Sacramento, California

Pierre Saadeh, MD
Vice Chair of Education
Residency Program Director
Chief of Plastic and Hand Surgery
Bellevue Hospital
Department of Plastic Surgery
School of Medicine
New York University
New York, New York

Hani Sbitany, MD, FACS
Associate Professor of Surgery
Division of Plastic and Reconstructive
    Surgery
University of California, San Francisco
San Francisco, California

Subhro K. Sen, MD
Clinical Associate Professor
Plastic and Reconstructive Surgery
Stanford University
Palo Alto, California

Michael D. Sgroi, MD
Assistant Professor of Vascular Surgery
Assistant Program Director of Vascular
    Surgery
Stanford University
Stanford, California

Ashkaun Shaterian, MD
Plastic Surgery Resident
Department of Plastic Surgery
University of California, Irvine
Orange, California

Clifford C. Sheckter, MD
Chief Resident
Division of Plastic and Reconstructive
    Surgery
Department of Surgery
Stanford University
Stanford, California

Ann-Charlott Docherty Skogh, MD, PhD
Senior Consultant in Plastic Surgery
Breast Cancer Center
Department of Surgery
Stockholm South General Hospital and
    Karolinska Institute
Stockholm, Sweden

Rachel C. Steckelberg, MD, MPH
Clinical Instructor
Regional Anesthesia Fellow
Department of Anesthesiology,
    Perioperative, and Pain Medicine
Stanford University Hospital
Palo Alto, California

Robert J. Steffner, MD
Assistant Clinical Professor
Musculoskeletal Tumor Surgery
Department of Orthopaedic Surgery
School of Medicine
Stanford University
Redwood City, California

John T. Stranix, MD
Chief Resident
Hansjörg Wyss Department of Plastic
    Surgery
NYU Langone Health
New York, New York

Ahmed Suliman, MD
Associate Professor, University of
    California San Diego, California
Section Chief, Veterans Healthcare
    Administration
Division of Plastic & Reconstructive
    Surgery
University of California San Diego
Section of Plastic & Reconstructive
    Surgery
Veterans Healthcare Administration
University of California, San Diego
    Medical Center
Veterans Healthcare Administration,
    San Diego
San Diego, California

Alex Wong, MD, FACS
Associate Professor of Surgery
Director, Basic, Translational, and
    Clinical Research
Director, Microsurgery Fellowship and
    Medical Student Education
Division of Plastic and Reconstructive
    Surgery
Keck School of Medicine of USC
Los Angeles, California

Kyong-Je Woo, MD, PhD
Assistant Professor
Department of Plastic Surgery
College of Medicine
Ewha Womans University
Ewha Womans University Medical
    Center
Seoul, Korea

Ming Zhuo-Stine, MD
Clinical Instructor and Fellow
Department of Anesthesiology
Stanford University Hospitals
Stanford, California

Preface

Lower extremity reconstruction leverages the expertise of various specialties in the total care of patients with diseases and trauma afflicting the lower extremity. These conditions can include traumatic injuries that require bone, nerve, muscle, tendon, and flap coverage. Similarly, the oncologic consideration mandates a comprehensive collaborative approach among various specialties for not only the resection of the tumor but also vascular reconstruction and possible soft tissue coverage.

This book on lower extremity reconstruction and amputation incorporates the expertise of orthopedic surgery, vascular surgery, and plastic surgery in the care of the lower extremities. The organization of the textbook is technique based to illustrate various possibilities of reconstructive options as well as time-honored procedures that have proven to be effective. As the Editor-in-Chief, I have read every word in this volume to impart my personal guidance. This book is not geared to a particular specialty but is inclusive of all needs in the care of lower extremities so that a holistic approach can yield the most elegant and definitive treatment for the whole spectrum of lower extremity problems. I applaud the leadership of LWW for their commitment to education in promoting this textbook, and I very much appreciate the readers for continuing to embrace these operative technique textbooks that strive to provide expedient guidance in the care of patients with lower extremity injuries and conditions.

Kevin C. Chung, MD, MS
Chief of Hand Surgery, Michigan Medicine
Director, University of Michigan Comprehensive Hand Center
Charles B. G. de Nancrede Professor of Surgery
Professor of Plastic Surgery and Orthopaedic Surgery
Assistant Dean for Faculty Affairs
Associate Director of Global REACH
University of Michigan Medical School
Ann Arbor, Michigan

Contents

Video Clips

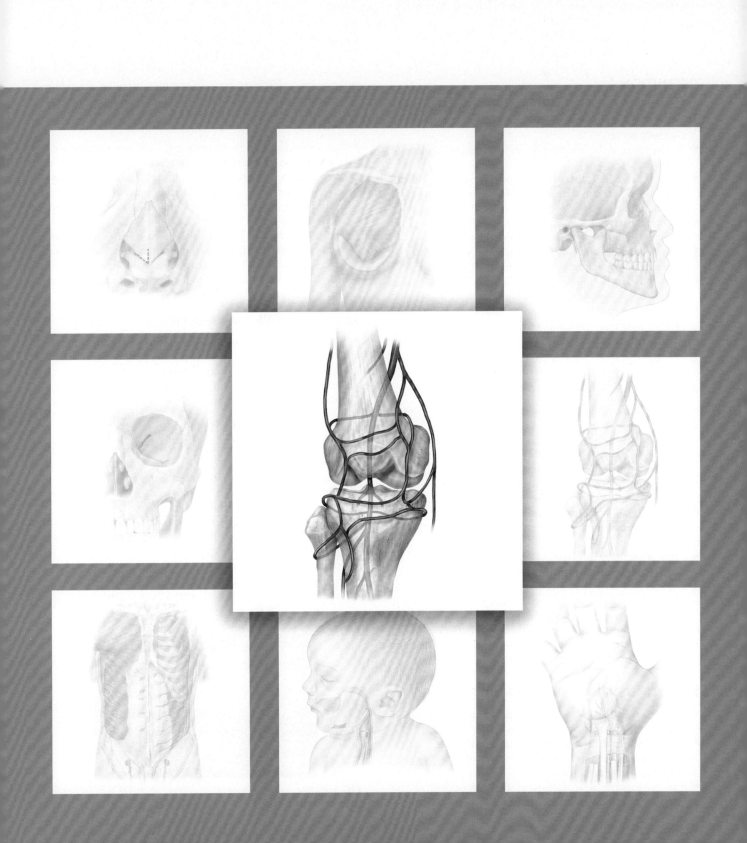

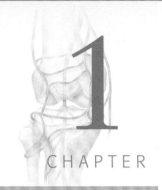

Section I: Anesthesia and Emergency Procedures
Femoral and Adductor Canal Blocks

CHAPTER 1

Sarah Madison and Jean-Louis Horn

DEFINITION

- A peripheral nerve block is an analgesic technique in which local anesthetics are injected percutaneously in proximity to a sensory nerve.
- The location of the injection determines the distribution of analgesia.
- Femoral nerve block may be used for postoperative analgesia for procedures on the anterior thigh, knee, medial leg, or medial ankle.
- Adductor canal block may be used for postoperative analgesia for procedures on the knee or medial leg.
- A continuous infusion of local anesthetic via a perineural catheter can provide analgesia for several days after surgery.
- Nerve blocks are often part of a multimodal regimen that also includes systemic medications.
- Nerve blocks can reduce pain and opioid consumption and enhance satisfaction and recovery.[1]
- Depending on the location and extent of surgery, nerve blocks may be used for surgical anesthesia.

ANATOMY

- The femoral nerve arises from the lumbar plexus and is formed by the ventral rami of L2-L4.
- In the area of the femoral triangle, the femoral nerve lies deep to the fascia iliaca, lateral to the femoral artery, and superficial to the iliacus muscle.
- The femoral nerve divides into anterior and posterior divisions and descends as the saphenous nerve to the medial leg.
- The posterior branch provides motor innervation to the quadriceps muscles as well as sensory articular branches to the knee joint.
- The saphenous nerve, obturator nerve (posterior division), and the nerve to the vastus medialis lie within the adductor canal.
- The adductor canal is bounded by the sartorius and the vasto-adductor membrane medially, the vastus medialis anteriorly, and adductor longus and magnus muscles posteriorly.
- The adductor canal also contains the femoral artery and vein.
- The saphenous nerve and the nerve to the vastus medialis supply sensory branches to the knee.[2]

PATIENT HISTORY AND PHYSICAL FINDINGS

- A preoperative history and physical must be performed prior to any anesthetic technique.
- A thorough history and physical exam will include anesthetic history, exercise tolerance, cardiopulmonary examination, and airway examination.
- Any pre-existing neuropathies in the distribution of the block should be defined and documented.

- Any local infections, masses, previous surgeries, or other irregularities at the site of injection should be identified.

IMAGING

- Ultrasound imaging confers efficiency and increases the success rate of most peripheral nerve blocks.
- Using a high-frequency linear transducer, scan in a transverse orientation at the level of the inguinal crease. The femoral artery and femoral nerve should be easily identified in cross-section (**FIG 1**).
- The adductor canal block is often performed in a location that is proximal to the true adductor canal, near the point at which the sartorius muscle covers the femoral vessels. The nerve can be visualized next to the femoral artery, just deep to the sartorius muscle (**FIG 2**).

NONOPERATIVE MANAGEMENT

- The balance of risks and benefits must be considered before any nerve block. Sometimes, it is more appropriate to only employ systemic medications for pain control.
- Opioids and nonopioid adjuvant medications may be used when medically appropriate, with or without a nerve block.

SURGICAL MANAGEMENT

- Femoral nerve block is indicated for postoperative analgesia of the anterior thigh, knee, medial leg, or medial ankle, or for surgical anesthesia of the anterior thigh.
  - When combined with a sciatic block, it can be used for surgical anesthesia of the foot/ankle.
- Local anesthetics will affect both motor and sensory nerves. Blocking the femoral nerve at the level of the inguinal crease results in quadriceps weakness.
- Adductor canal block is indicated for postoperative analgesia of the knee, medial leg, or medial ankle.
  - It can be used as a surgical anesthetic in conjunction with a sciatic block for procedures on the foot/ankle.

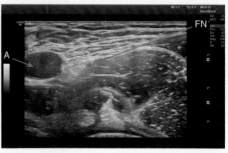

FIG 1 • Ultrasound image of femoral nerve block. FN, femoral nerve; A, femoral artery.

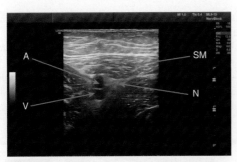

FIG 2 • Ultrasound image of adductor canal block. SN, saphenous nerve; SM, sartorius muscle; A, femoral artery; V, femoral vein.

- A nerve block in the adductor canal is less likely to cause quadriceps weakness than a femoral nerve block; however, local anesthetic may spread proximally and affect motor nerves.
  - The nerve to the vastus medialis is reliably anesthetized with an adductor canal block, but the overall effect on quadriceps function is minimal.[3]

Preoperative Planning

- Surgical site, extent of incision, anticipated degree of pain, and any pre-existing conditions that increase risk of complications should be considered before offering the patient a nerve block.
- Postoperative ambulatory status should be determined to optimize dosing.

- Crutch training, if appropriate, should take place prior to surgery.
- Inpatients should be labeled as a "fall risk" and should not get out of bed without assistance.
- Femoral nerve blocks for outpatients should be carefully considered and only performed with close follow-up and an otherwise low risk of falls.
- The use of crutches and a knee immobilizer may attenuate fall risk with ambulation after a femoral nerve block.

Positioning

- The patient should be positioned supine with the operative leg slightly externally rotated.
- The bed should be flat with hips extended.
- The patient's ipsilateral hand may be kept out of the sterile field by lightly taping it to the chest.
- The operator should stand on the side to be blocked, with the ultrasound machine on the other side of the patient.

Approach

- With the use of ultrasound, the nerve may be approached either in-plane (needle parallel to transducer surface) or out-of-plane (needle perpendicular to transducer surface) with the ultrasound probe placed in a transverse orientation.
- When a nerve stimulator technique is used, the needle approach is generally *with* the long axis of the nerve, at a 45-degree angle to the skin.

■ Femoral Block: Ultrasound-Guided Technique

- Position the patient as described above, with ASA (American Society of Anesthesiologists) standard monitors and supplemental oxygen applied.
- IV sedation, usually with fentanyl and midazolam, may be titrated to patient comfort.
- Using a high-frequency linear transducer, scan at the level of the inguinal crease in a transverse orientation to visualize the femoral artery and nerve in cross-section.
  - The best image may be obtained in a location proximal to the bifurcation of the femoral artery where the neurovascular bundle is closest to the skin.
  - Identify the fascia lata, fascia iliaca, femoral nerve, and iliacus muscle.
  - Slowly tilt the ultrasound transducer to optimize nerve imaging.
- Estimate the depth of the nerve in the ultrasound image.
- After sterile skin preparation, place a skin wheal just lateral to the ultrasound probe.
  - The depth of the nerve should guide the insertion site; start closer to the probe for more superficial targets, and farther away if the target is deeper.
- Insert the block needle in the plane of the ultrasound image, visualizing the tip of the needle in real-time as the target is approached (**TECH FIG 1**).
  - The needle should pass through the fascia iliaca just lateral to the nerve.
  - Tactile feedback through the needle may include a "pop" as the needle traverses fascial layers.

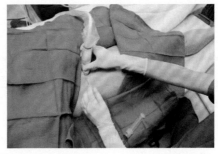

TECH FIG 1 • Positioning and approach for ultrasound-guided in-plane femoral nerve block.

- Take care to avoid the lateral edge of the nerve. The patient may experience a paresthesia if the nerve is contacted directly.
- The lateral circumflex femoral artery or one of its branches may be in the needle path or pass through the nerve, and should be avoided.
- After careful aspiration, inject a small amount of local anesthetic.
  - Local anesthetic spread should appear as hypoechoic fluid filling the space deep to fascia iliaca and surrounding the nerve.
  - The needle may be advanced closer to the nerve as a local anesthetic pocket is formed (hydrodissection); this reduces the risk of needle-nerve contact.
  - When the needle is positioned in close proximity to the nerve, and local anesthetic spread is confirmed around the nerve, an additional 10 to 15 mL of local anesthetic can be injected.

- Local anesthetic selection and volume of injection depend on the goals of the block.
  - For a surgical block, use 20 to 30 mL of 1.5% mepivacaine, 2% lidocaine, 0.5% bupivacaine, or 0.5% ropivacaine.
  - For an analgesic block, use 15 to 20 mL of 0.25% bupivacaine or 0.25% ropivacaine.
- A catheter may be placed for continuous local anesthetic infusion.
  - Use 0.2% ropivacaine or 0.125% of bupivacaine at 4 to 6 mL/h for continuous infusion, with a patient-controlled bolus of 2 to 4 mL every 30 minutes.
  - Infusions are generally continued for 2 to 3 days following surgery.

■ Femoral Block: Nerve Stimulator Technique

- Following patient positioning and preparation described above, identify and mark the inguinal crease.
- Standing near the patient's hip and facing the head, palpate the femoral pulse along the crease.
- After sterile prep, place a local anesthetic skin wheal 2 cm lateral to the femoral artery pulse.
- Insert a stimulating block needle at a 45 to 60 degree angle to the skin in a cephalad direction (**TECH FIG 2**).
  - A quadriceps twitch ("patellar snap") should be elicited at a current of 0.2 to 0.5 mA. Redirect the needle until the appropriate stimulation is observed.
  - Sartorius contraction indicates a needle placement on the anterior division of the femoral nerve. Further advancement of the needle toward the posterior division of the nerve will usually solve this.
  - Aspiration of blood indicates intravascular placement. Reposition the needle.
  - Muscle contraction at a current of greater than 0.5 mA usually indicates inadequate needle-nerve proximity and may result in an incomplete or failed block.

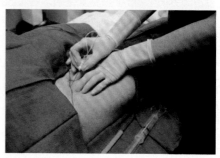

TECH FIG 2 • Positioning and approach for stimulator-guided femoral nerve block.

- Muscle contraction at a current of less than 0.2 mA may indicate intraneural needle placement. Withdraw the needle slightly before injecting, carefully noting injection pressure.
- Avoid high-pressure injection (greater than 15 psi), indicative of an intraneural needle placement.
- Once an acceptable motor response is elicited, inject local anesthetic as above. The motor response should terminate with injection (Raj test).

■ Adductor Canal Block: Ultrasound-Guided Technique

- Position and prepare the patient as for a femoral block. Externally rotating the leg may facilitate access to the adductor canal.
- Place a high-frequency linear transducer in a transverse orientation over the medial thigh at the midpoint between ASIS and the superior pole of the patella.
  - Identify the sartorius, vastus medialis, and adductor longus muscles.
  - The femoral artery and vein lie within the adductor canal.
  - The saphenous nerve may be visualized just lateral to the artery, beneath the sartorius muscle and the vasto-adductor membrane.
- Estimate the depth of the nerve in the ultrasound image.
- After sterile skin preparation, place a skin wheal just lateral to the ultrasound probe.
  - The depth of the nerve should guide the insertion site.
- Insert the block needle in the plane of the ultrasound image, visualizing the tip of the needle in real-time as the target is approached (**TECH FIG 3**).
  - Traverse the sartorius muscle to position the needle tip just lateral to the femoral artery.
  - A "pop" may be felt as the needle passes through fascial layers.

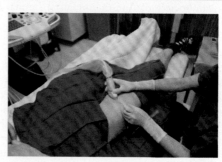

TECH FIG 3 • Positioning and approach for ultrasound-guided adductor canal block.

- Take care to avoid the femoral vein, which often lies deep and lateral to the artery, and may not be visible when pressure is applied to the ultrasound transducer.
- After careful aspiration, inject a small amount of local anesthetic.
  - Observe local anesthetic spread in the ultrasound image. This should appear as hypoechoic fluid filling the space deep to sartorius and lateral to femoral artery.
  - Ensure that local anesthetic is not tracking back along the sartorius muscle, but rather staying contained in the adductor canal while partially surrounding the femoral artery.

- The needle should be advanced beyond the subsartorial fascia.
- When the needle is positioned in close proximity to the nerve, and local anesthetic spread is confirmed around the nerve, an additional 10 to 15 mL of local anesthetic can be injected.
- The adductor canal block can be used as an analgesic block or as a surgical block in combination with sciatic block for surgery below the knee.
  - For a surgical block, use 15 to 20 mL of 1.5% mepivacaine, 2% lidocaine, 0.5% bupivacaine, or 0.5% ropivacaine.
- For an analgesic block, use 10 to 15 mL of 0.25% bupivacaine or 0.25% ropivacaine.
- A catheter may be placed for continuous local anesthetic infusion.
  - Use 0.2% ropivacaine or 0.125% bupivacaine at 4 to 6 mL/h for continuous infusion, with a patient-controlled bolus of 2 to 4 mL every 30 minutes.
  - Infusions are generally continued for 2 to 3 days following surgery.

PEARLS AND PITFALLS

Positioning	▪ In obese patients, retracting and taping the abdominal pannus helps optimize ultrasound imaging.
Sterility	▪ For catheter placement, nerve blocks should be performed under strict sterile conditions.
Paresthesias	▪ Avoid needle-to-nerve contact if possible. Use hydrodissection to achieve proper needle placement.
Vascular puncture	▪ The femoral and adductor canal blocks involve needle placement in close proximity to vascular structures. To avoid vascular puncture, always visualize the needle tip in the ultrasound image while advancing.
Local anesthetic toxicity	▪ Even with acceptable needle visualization, vascular puncture can occur. Always aspirate before injection, inject slowly, and visualize local anesthetic spread in the ultrasound image. Epinephrine may be used at a low concentration (1:400 000) as a vascular marker. Do not exceed the maximum safe dose of local anesthetics.
Catheter placement	▪ Once a catheter is placed, its position should be confirmed with ultrasound imaging. Inject a small volume of local anesthetic through the catheter to ensure appropriate spread around the nerve.
Dressing	▪ Catheters should be secured with a clear occlusive dressing. An anchoring device may be used as well and should be secured away from the surgical field or tourniquet site.
Block assessment	▪ Quadriceps weakness is an early sign of successful femoral nerve block. Femoral and adductor canal nerve blocks are reliably assessed with testing the skin over the medial malleolus.

POSTOPERATIVE CARE

- Following a nerve block procedure, patients should be monitored for at least 30 minutes for any signs of local anesthetic toxicity.
- Patients should be contacted every day until the block wears off or the catheter is removed.
- Leakage from the catheter site is normal and expected but can be minimized with the application of surgical glue at the insertion site.
- Patients should be educated on expected weakness and fall risk.
  - Crutches and a knee immobilizer should be provided when appropriate.
  - Careful consideration should be given to using continuous femoral blocks for outpatients.
- Patients should be encouraged to use their systemic analgesics as needed.
  - Perioperative use of multimodal analgesia may include acetaminophen, NSAIDs, and/or gabapentinoids around the clock to improve pain management and decrease opioid usage.

- Systemic analgesics should be initiated prior to the block wearing off.
- Dressings should be left alone until the catheter is removed.
  - Dressing changes are not necessary and may increase the risk of infection or catheter dislodgement.

OUTCOMES

- Peripheral nerve blocks provide better pain control than traditional medications; they reduce opioid consumption and its associated side effects.
- Patient satisfaction is higher when peripheral nerve blocks are used for perioperative pain control.
- Pain management strategies that include a peripheral nerve block may reduce the systemic inflammatory response and reduce persistent pain that is associated with surgery.[4]

COMPLICATIONS

- Peripheral nerve blocks have a low complication rate.
- Short-term complications may include prolonged numbness, weakness, or paresthesias.

- Long-term numbness, weakness, or paresthesias are rare.
  - In a multicenter, international clinical registry of regional anesthetics, the all-cause 60-day rate of neurological sequelae is 8.3/10 000.[5]
  - Local anesthetic systemic toxicity (LAST) is a rare but potentially deadly complication.
  - A LAST protocol should be in place in institutions where nerve blocks are performed.
    - LAST checklist and resuscitation guidelines should be posted in the block area (https://www.asra.com/content/documents/asra_last_checklist.2011.pdf).
    - Resuscitation medications (including Intralipid) and equipment should be available in the block area.
    - Access to cardiopulmonary bypass should be available in case of refractory cardiovascular collapse.

REFERENCES

1. Kessler J, et al. Peripheral regional anaesthesia and outcome: lessons learned from the last 10 years. *Br J Anaesth*. 2015;114(5):728-745.
2. Burckett-St Laurant D, et al. The nerves of the adductor canal and the innervation of the knee: an anatomic study. *Reg Anesth Pain Med*. 2016;41(3):321-327.
3. Grevstad U, et al. The effect of local anesthetic volume within the adductor canal on quadriceps femoris function evaluated by electromyography: a randomized, observer- and subject-blinded, placebo-controlled study in volunteers. *Anesth Analg*. 2016;123(2):493-500.
4. He Y, Li Z, Zuo YX. Nerve blockage attenuates postoperative inflammation in hippocampus of young rat model with surgical trauma. *Mediators Inflamm*. 2015;2015:460125.
5. Sites BD, Barrington MJ, Davis M. Using an international clinical registry of regional anesthesia to identify targets for quality improvement. *Reg Anesth Pain Med*. 2014;39(6):487-495.

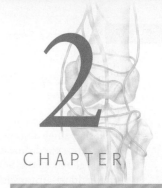

Popliteal Nerve Blocks

Ming Zhuo-Stine and Sarah Madison

DEFINITION

- The popliteal nerve block targets the sciatic nerve in the popliteal fossa proximal to its bifurcation into the common peroneal and tibial nerves.
- It is a commonly used block for surgeries involving the lower leg, ankle, and foot.
- The nerve block can provide surgical anesthesia or postoperative analgesia. The duration of the block varies based on the choice of local anesthetic and the choice of single injection versus continuous catheter technique. For painful surgeries, the continuous catheter technique can provide several days of excellent postoperative pain control.[1]
- The popliteal nerve block spares the medial aspect of the lower leg, an area that is innervated by the saphenous nerve. A femoral or saphenous nerve block must be performed in conjunction with a popliteal block for full sensory blockade of the lower leg (**FIG 1**).

ANATOMY

- The sciatic nerve consists of two distinct nerves, the tibial and common peroneal nerves, which provide motor and sensory innervation to the majority of the lower leg. The

two nerves have their own epineurium and are encased in an additional layer of connective tissue.[2,3]
- Within the popliteal fossa, the branches of the sciatic nerve usually lie lateral and posterior to the popliteal vessels. More proximally, the nerve can be found between the biceps femoris, and semitendinosus and semimembranosus tendons.
- 2 to 10 cm proximal to the popliteal fossa crease, the sciatic nerve bifurcates into the tibial and common peroneal nerves. The common peroneal nerve then travels laterally around the head and neck of the fibula, whereas the large tibial nerve continues caudally with the popliteal vessels.
- The popliteal nerve block is often performed proximal to the point of bifurcation or at the point of bifurcation, with injection of local anesthetic in or around the common connective tissue sheath described by some as the "paraneural sheath."[4,5]

PATIENT HISTORY AND PHYSICAL FINDINGS

- Assess patient's pain history and proposed surgery to determine if a popliteal nerve block is appropriate for the procedure.
- Examine patient for preexisting neuropathy and weakness.
- Assess for contraindications or increased risk of complications with regional anesthesia:
  - Patient refusal
  - Allergy to local anesthetic
  - Infection at site of nerve block or systemic infection
  - Coagulopathy
  - Preexisting neuropathy
  - Increased risk of compartment syndrome
- The patient's surgeon and primary anesthesia team should agree with placement of block.
- Determine if a single injection nerve block or perineural catheter is indicated depending on the requirements for surgical anesthesia and postoperative analgesia. If a prolonged block is preferred for outpatient surgery, ensure that the patient will be able to care for an insensate limb at home and can be contacted for follow-up.
- Prior to starting the nerve block, ensure that the patient will be able to proceed with surgery and anesthesia (consents completed, appropriately NPO, etc.).

SURGICAL MANAGEMENT

Preoperative Planning

- Patient preparation:
  - Surgical and anesthesia consents signed
  - Monitors—blood pressure cuff, ECG, pulse oximeter, capnography
  - Supplemental oxygen via nasal cannula or facemask
  - Pillows, blankets, or tables to aid positioning

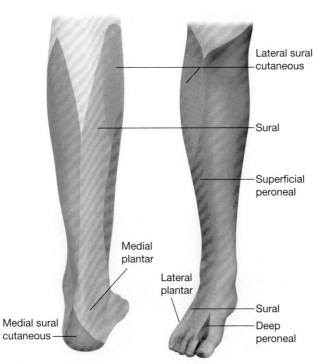

Lateral sural cutaneous

Sural

Superficial peroneal

Medial plantar

Lateral plantar

Sural

Deep peroneal

Medial sural cutaneous

FIG 1 • Sensory distribution of the leg.

- Skin marker to mark the site laterality and surface landmarks
- Sedation to optimize patient comfort—typically midazolam and fentanyl
- Rescue drugs and emergency airway equipment available
- Supplies for single injection technique:
  - Antiseptic skin disinfectant
  - Sterile gloves, mask, hat
  - Sterile drapes or towels
  - 50- to 100-mm 20- to 22-gauge short-bevel insulated stimulating needle
  - Small syringe and small gauge needle with lidocaine for skin infiltration
  - 30 mL local anesthetic of choice
  - Nerve stimulator and/or ultrasound machine with high-frequency linear probe, sterile ultrasound probe cover, and ultrasound gel
- Supplies for continuous catheter technique:
  - Antiseptic skin disinfectant
  - Sterile gloves, gown, mask, hat
  - Ultrasound machine with high-frequency linear probe or nerve stimulator
  - 30 mL local anesthetic of choice
  - Sterile regional anesthesia tray:
    - Drapes or towels
    - Gauze
    - A 100-mm block needle, often a 17- or 18-gauge Tuohy needle
    - A flexible nerve block catheter with connector (may use stimulating catheter with nerve stimulator technique)
    - 10- to 20-mL syringe
    - Local anesthetic or saline for injection through needle
    - Extension tubing
    - Small syringe and small gauge needle with lidocaine for skin infiltration
    - Surgical skin glue
    - Transparent dressing
    - Catheter stabilization device
    - Ultrasound probe cover with ultrasound gel

Approach

- **Ultrasound-Guidance Versus Nerve Stimulation**
  - Nerve localization can be achieved using peripheral nerve stimulators and/or ultrasound guidance.
  - Over the past decade, ultrasound-guided nerve blocks have rapidly gained popularity because they provide several advantages compared to the nerve stimulator technique. The use of ultrasound provides direct, real-time visualization of target nerves, needle advancement, and spread of local anesthetic in the desired location.[6] With continuous catheter techniques, the precise location of the catheter tip can be visualized. Blood vessels and smaller peripheral nerves can be identified and avoided. Research suggests that ultrasound guidance provides an improvement in time required to perform the block, block onset, and block success.[7-10]
  - For the popliteal sciatic block, ultrasound allows visualization of the precise point where the sciatic nerve bifurcates, which is variable between patients. Identifying this location is helpful in blocking both components of the sciatic nerve.
  - For these reasons, although this chapter briefly covers nerve stimulator approaches, the focus will be on ultrasound-guided techniques, which have become routinely used in regional anesthesia.

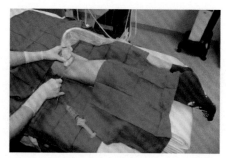

FIG 2 • In-plane approach to popliteal sciatic nerve block.

- Ultrasound in-plane versus out-of-plane needle insertion approaches
  - With the in-plane approach, the needle is inserted at the side of the transducer, in line with the ultrasound beam (**FIG 2**). Because the needle is within the plane of imaging, the entire needle shaft and tip should be seen as echogenic line. In-plane approach is often used due to superior visualization of the entire needle as it is advanced toward the target.
  - With the out-of-plane approach, the needle is introduced perpendicular to the transducer (**FIG 3**). The needle crosses the plane of the ultrasound beam such that the needle shaft and tip are seen as an echogenic dot on ultrasound. Needle tip localization is more difficult with this approach. Techniques to help locate the needle tip include looking for tissue displacement, scanning for the needle tip, and injection of fluid to separate tissue planes (hydrodissection). One advantage of using the out-of-plane approach is that the needle traverses only skin and adipose tissue, avoiding muscle.
- Approaches related to patient positioning
  - A wide range of positions can be used during popliteal sciatic nerve blockade. Each is discussed and illustrated in further detail in the following section.
  - Choice of positioning is typically dictated by a combination of patient comfort, patient mobility, operator ergonomics, and the operator's personal preference. Body habitus, pain, or the presence of external fixation devices may limit the ability of the patient to assume a lateral or prone position.
  - Patients may be positioned supine or prone for nerve stimulator techniques.
  - Patients may be positioned supine, lateral, or prone for ultrasound-guided nerve blocks. Regardless of the position, the ultrasound image is identical. If the out-of-plane needle insertion approach is desired, prone or lateral positioning provides better access.

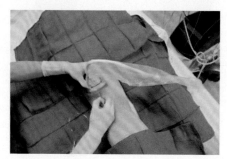

FIG 3 • Out-of-plane approach to popliteal sciatic nerve block.

■ Nerve Stimulator, Lateral Approach

- The patient is positioned supine with leg slightly elevated to visualize foot movement. This is best achieved by placing the leg on a small stack of blankets such that the foot and heel protrude beyond the blankets.

- Main landmarks are the popliteal fossa crease and the muscular groove between the biceps femoris and vastus lateralis muscles. The site of needle insertion is within the muscular groove, about 7 to 8 cm cephalad to the popliteal crease; the muscular groove may be accentuated by having the patient lift their leg off of the plane of the table. Use a skin marker to denote landmarks.

- Prepare the skin with an antiseptic solution and infiltrate the proposed needle insertion point with local anesthetic via a small gauge needle. Connect the peripheral nerve stimulator to a 100-mm 20- to 22-gauge short-bevel insulated stimulating needle. Using sterile technique, insert the needle perpendicular to the skin and advance in a horizontal plane between the vastus lateralis and biceps femoris muscles until femur is contacted; bony contact provides a reference point for nerve localization.

The sciatic nerve is typically 1 to 2 cm beyond the skin-to-femur distance and located posterior to the femur (**TECH FIG 1**).

- With the nerve stimulator set to 1.5 mA, withdraw needle almost to the skin and redirect at a 30-degree angle posteriorly until foot twitch is seen, typically at a depth of 5 to 7 cm. Stimulation of the common peroneal nerve causes dorsiflexion and foot eversion. Stimulation of the tibial nerve, which is more medial, results in plantar flexion and foot inversion. Tibial stimulation is preferred because it may result in a higher rate of complete sciatic nerve block.[11] Local twitches of the biceps femoris muscle or vastus lateralis muscle indicates that the needle is located too superficial or anterior, respectively.

- If a motor response is not elicited, withdraw needle to skin and redirect 5 to 10 degrees more posterior.

- Once sciatic nerve stimulation is obtained, make small needle adjustments until twitches are obtained at 0.3 to 0.5 mA.

- Check for intravascular placement with gentle aspiration and then slowly inject 30 to 40 mL of local anesthetic.

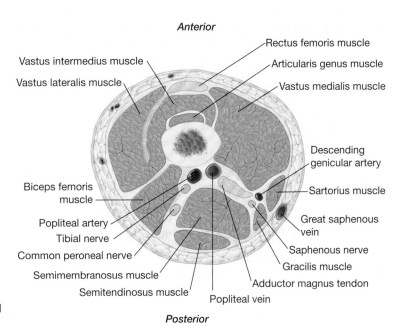

TECH FIG 1 • Cross-sectional anatomy of the distal thigh (right leg 8 cm above knee).

■ Nerve Stimulator, Posterior Approach

- Position the patient prone with the leg to be blocked protruding from the end of the bed or slightly elevated on a blanket to allow for visualization of foot movement.

- Primary landmarks are the popliteal fossa crease, tendon of the biceps femoris laterally, and tendons of the semitendinosus and semimembranosus muscles medially. Knee flexion against resistance can help accentuate the tendons and identify the knee crease. The needle insertion point is about 7 cm above the popliteal fossa crease 1 cm lateral and 1 cm caudal to the apex of the popliteal fossa. Use a skin marker to denote landmarks (**TECH FIG 2**).

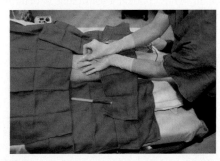

TECH FIG 2 • Positioning and landmarks for stimulator-guided popliteal block.

- Prepare the skin with an antiseptic solution and infiltrate the proposed needle insertion point with local anesthetic via a small-gauge needle. Connect the peripheral nerve stimulator set at 1.5 mA to a 50-mm 20- to 22-gauge short-bevel insulated stimulating needle.
- Using sterile technique, insert the needle 45 to 60 degrees to the skin, then advance the needle until foot twitches are obtained. Typical depth is 3 to 5 cm from the skin. Stimulation of the common peroneal nerve causes dorsiflexion and foot eversion. Stimulation of the tibial nerve, which is more medial, results in plantar flexion and foot inversion. Tibial stimulation is preferred because it may result in a higher rate of complete sciatic nerve block.[11]
- If a motor response is not elicited, withdraw the needle to the skin and redirect 5 to 15 degrees laterally. If there is continued difficulty localizing the sciatic nerve, withdraw needle to skin and reinsert 1 cm laterally in incremental steps.
- Once sciatic nerve stimulation is obtained, make small adjustments to the needle position to obtain foot twitches at 0.3 to 0.5 mA.
- Check for intravascular placement with gentle aspiration, and then slowly inject 30 to 40 mL of local anesthetic.

■ Nerve Stimulator, Continuous Catheter Technique

- Use the same procedure as for single injection nerve stimulator technique described above, but with a larger insulated stimulating Tuohy needle to allow for passage of a catheter. An in situ catheter allows for continued dosing of local anesthetic to provide prolonged anesthesia and analgesia. Either a stimulating or nonstimulating catheter can be used:
  - Nonstimulating catheter:
    - After localizing the sciatic nerve with motor response at 0.3 to 0.5 mA, inject local anesthetic to open up space for the catheter.
    - Insert a catheter through the Tuohy needle and advance 3 cm past the tip of the needle. If catheter insertion is difficult, slight adjustment of the needle or direction may facilitate catheter advancement.
    - Carefully withdraw needle while simultaneously advancing the catheter. Aspirate the catheter to check for inadvertent intravascular placement and secure using a catheter stabilization device and clear dressing.
  - Stimulating catheter:
    - Localize the sciatic nerve with a motor response around 0.5 mA. Do not inject local anesthetic or saline through the needle or the motor response will be lost. D5W can be used if necessary.
    - Insert a stimulating catheter with the nerve stimulator now attached to the catheter. Advance the catheter 3 to 5 cm past the needle tip while maintaining a motor response. If motor response is lost, withdraw and readvance the catheter. If catheter insertion is difficult, withdraw the catheter and adjust the needle slightly to facilitate catheter advancement.
    - Once the catheter is in a satisfactory position, the needle can then be carefully withdrawn while advancing the catheter simultaneously. Feed additional catheter under the skin to minimize premature dislodgment. Aspirate the catheter to check for inadvertent intravascular placement and secure.

■ Ultrasound-Guided, In-Plane Needle Insertion Approach

- Of the various approaches described, this is the most commonly used approach due to ease of needle and target visualization.
- Positioning—Patients may be positioned supine, lateral decubitus, or prone (**TECH FIG 3**). Regardless of the position selected, ultrasound imaging and needling are similar. Thus, patient positioning is determined by a combination of patient comfort, patient mobility, and operator ergonomics and preference.
  - Supine position
    - Position the patient supine with the operative leg elevated using blankets, pillows, or a table to accommodate an ultrasound probe beneath the thigh.
    - The operator is positioned on the side to be blocked with the ultrasound screen on the opposite side of the patient.
  - Lateral decubitus position
    - Position patient lateral with the procedural leg on top, knee extended. The dependent leg can be bent at the knee to enhance stability.
    - Operators may choose to stand in front of the patient, facing the anterior thigh with the ultrasound probe directed toward themselves or stand behind the patient, facing the posterior aspect of the thigh, pointing the probe away from themselves.
  - Prone position
    - Position the patient prone with the operative leg slightly abducted. A blanket folded under the lower leg may help relax the hamstring tendons to facilitate ultrasound transducer placement.
    - The operator is positioned on the side to be blocked with the ultrasound screen on the opposite side of the patient.
- Imaging
  - Disinfect the skin with an antiseptic solution, drape the procedural area, and cover the ultrasound probe with a sterile ultrasound sheath and gel.
  - Place the transducer in a transverse orientation in the popliteal fossa to obtain a short-axis view of the nerves.
  - Perform a systematic survey of the surrounding structures. Identify the femur. The pulsatile popliteal artery and the accompanying vein are located posterior to the

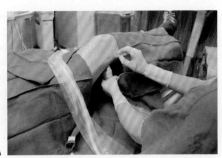 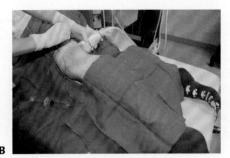

TECH FIG 3 • Supine, lateral decubitus **(A)**, and prone positioning **(B)** for in-plane ultrasound-guided popliteal block.

femur. The sciatic nerve appears as a hyperechoic oval structure with a honeycomb pattern that is posterior and lateral to the artery, medial to the biceps femoris muscle, and lateral to the semitendinosus and semimembranosus muscles.

- Optimize the ultrasound image by adjusting variables especially frequency, gain, depth, and focal zones. Tilting the ultrasound transducer to direct the beam caudally may enhance the visualization of the nerve by bringing the ultrasound plane more perpendicular to the nerve.
- Scan proximally and distally along the sciatic nerve to identify the bifurcation point of the common peroneal and tibial nerves. This division usually occurs 2 to 7 cm proximal to the popliteal crease and at a depth of 2 to 4 cm.
- Choose a location just proximal to the bifurcation, where the peroneal and tibial nerves are still enclosed in a common connective tissue sheath (**TECH FIG 4**).

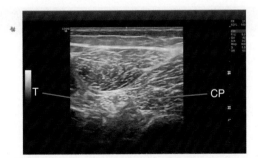

TECH FIG 4 • Ultrasound image of the sciatic nerve at its bifurcation. T, tibial nerve; CP, common peroneal nerve.

- Needling
  - Determine the optimal needle path. Identify small vessels that should be avoided. The needle insertion point will be near the lateral aspect of the transducer.
    - Choose an insertion point lateral to the transducer. The needle will traverse the biceps femoris muscle.
    - Choose an insertion point close to the transducer to decrease the amount of muscle tissue along the needle path.
  - Infiltrate the skin with local anesthetic at the insertion site. Use a 20- to 22-gauge 100-mm block needle. Flush the tubing and syringe to remove air since air will obscure the ultrasound image.
  - Introduce the block needle in the same plane as the ultrasound beam with the bevel of the needle facing the probe. The needle shaft and tip should always be visualized during needle advancement.
  - Carefully advance needle under direct visualization toward the nerve sheath, taking care to bring the needle close to the edge of the nerve, to avoid puncturing the nerve.
  - Aspirate, then inject 1 to 2 mL of local anesthetic. Never inject or advance needle if patient complains of pain or if high pressure (greater than 15 psi) is met on injection or if the nerve is swelling. These signs dictate an immediate repositioning of the needle tip.
  - If in the correct location, the hypoechoic fluid should surround the nerve completely.
  - If fluid spread is not ideal, reposition needle to achieve adequate circumferential spread with a total of 20 to 30 cc local anesthetic.

■ Ultrasound-Guided, Out-of-Plane Needle Insertion Approach

- Needle localization is more difficult with an out-of-plane approach in comparison to an in-plane approach. Because the needle crosses the plane of the ultrasound beam, the needle shaft and tip are seen only as an echogenic dot. The advantage is that the needle traverses only skin and adipose tissue, avoiding muscle.

- Positioning—Patients may be positioned lateral decubitus or prone for out-of-plane needling. Regardless of the position selected, ultrasound imaging and needling are identical. Choose the best position based on patient comfort and operator preference.
- Imaging
  - Disinfect and prepare the site as described above.
  - Place the transducer in the transverse orientation in the popliteal fossa to obtain a short-axis view of the sciatic nerve.

- Follow the same steps for imaging as with the in-plane ultrasound approach.
- Needling
  - Align the sciatic nerve in the center of the ultrasound screen and place a wheal of local anesthetic in the center of the probe, close to the probe.
  - Insert a block needle through the skin wheal directed approximately 60 to 80 degrees cephalad. Aim to place the needle tip to the side of the nerve to avoid nerve trauma.
  - As the needle crosses the plane of the ultrasound beam, it will appear in cross-section as an echogenic dot. Because both the needle shaft and tip have a similar appearance, track the tip with the probe as the needle is advanced. If not directly visualized, the needle tip may be inferred by tissue displacement along the needle path as well as hydrolocation.
  - Aspirate, and then slowly inject local anesthetic while observing the fluid spread. Ideally, hypoechoic fluid should be seen spreading circumferentially around the hyperechoic nerve. Inject 20 to 30 mL of local anesthetic.

■ Ultrasound-Guided Continuous Catheter Technique

- Catheter placement provides a continuous infusion or additional boluses of local anesthetic to provide prolonged anesthesia or pain control.
- Strict aseptic technique is crucial for prevention of infectious complications.
- Both in-plane and out-of-plane ultrasound-guided approaches can be utilized.
- Catheter placement utilizes the same needle placement procedure as described above but requires a larger needle for passage of a perineural catheter. After the needle is confirmed to be the correct location, an additional 5 to 10 mL bolus of saline or local anesthetic solution is injected to facilitate catheter advancement.
- Carefully advance the catheter about 3 to 5 cm past the needle tip. If catheter insertion is difficult, withdraw the catheter and try small adjustments of the needle. Before or after needle removal, confirm catheter tip location with injection through the catheter, watching for appropriate spread.
- Carefully withdraw the needle while simultaneously advancing the catheter in different tissues. Overfeeding additional catheter under the skin may help prevent accidental dislodgment.
- Carefully secure the catheter in place with an anchoring device and clear dressing. Use a total of 20 to 30 mL of local anesthetic.

PEARLS AND PITFALLS

Identification of nerve and structures	■ Knowledge of both surface anatomy and ultrasound anatomy is essential. ■ Tilt the transducer beam caudally toward the foot to direct ultrasound waves perpendicular to the nerve and enhance visualization. ■ Asking the patient to plantar flex and extend their foot causes the tibial and common peroneal nerves to slide against each other, known as the *"seesaw sign."*[12] ■ At the popliteal crease, the vessels are immediately anterior to the tibial nerve. Reduce transducer pressure to visualize the popliteal vein. Trace the nerve proximally to where the common peroneal joins to form the sciatic nerve.
Nerve block coverage	■ In combination with a saphenous nerve block, popliteal block provides complete sensory blockade below the knee. ■ Popliteal block does not cover thigh tourniquet pain. The patient may require general anesthesia or a femoral nerve block instead of a selected saphenous when a thigh tourniquet is used.
Approach	■ Ultrasound imaging allows for various patient positions and needle approaches. Choice of approach depends on patient and operator comfort.
Catheter placement	■ For a continuous technique, once the needle is in optimal position, inject a small amount of saline or local anesthetic to facilitate catheter advancement. ■ Check the catheter tip location by injecting a small volume of saline or local anesthetic with ultrasound visualization. ■ Feed additional catheter in the muscle or subcutaneous tissue to prevent inadvertent catheter dislodgment.
Postblock safety	■ Always counsel patients on fall risk and injury risk to a numb extremity. Providing a boot will improve stability. Patients must not weight bear until the block has fully resolved. ■ Both thorough preoperative counseling and clarification of patient expectations are essential to the successful management of the block.

POSTOPERATIVE CARE

- Block onset time varies dramatically from 10 to 45 minutes depending on patient, medication selection, and proximity of the injectate to the nerve.
- Thorough patient education is essential for the successful function and safety of the nerve block.
- All patients should be followed postoperatively for block resolution and to detect complications.
- All patients with nerve block catheters should be evaluated daily while in the hospital or contacted by phone if receiving nerve block infusion at home.
- Catheter leakage at the site of insertion and catheter dislodgment may occur. Patients should have additional analgesics available for breakthrough pain or in the event of catheter dislodgment.

COMPLICATIONS

- Injuries as a result of an insensate limb—Instruct patient, nurses, and caregivers on proper care of an insensate extremity including fall precautions and positioning. Avoid nerve blocks in patients who have a high risk of compartment syndrome.
- Infection—Use strict aseptic technique, avoid perineural catheter placement in patients with active infections, and limit duration of perineural catheter use.
- Hematoma formation—Ultrasound imaging and avoidance of vascular trauma or multiple needle passes may minimize risk.
- Nerve injury—Rare complication from direct needle trauma or intraneural injection; usually resolves in weeks to months. Risk may be increased in patients with preexisting nerve injury. More common causes of nerve injury include surgical, ischemic, and compressive nerve injuries. Avoid tourniquet placement over nerve block site to decrease ischemic nerve injury. Avoid needle advancement or injection if the patient complains of pain or paresthesias or if increased pressure (greater than 15 psi) is felt during injection. Avoid needle advancement during an ultrasound-guided procedure if the target or needle tip is poorly visualized.

- Local anesthetic toxicity—Avoid intravascular injection by aspirating prior to injection and aspirating frequently during injection. Patients should be monitored following the nerve block. Have rescue medications, such as lipid emulsion, and emergency airway equipment readily available.

REFERENCES

1. Singelyn FJ, Aye F, Gouverneur JM. Continuous popliteal sciatic nerve block: an original technique to provide postoperative analgesia after foot surgery. *Anesth Analg.* 1997;84(2):383-386.
2. Andersen HL, Andersen SL, Tranum-Jensen J. Injection inside the paraneural sheath of the sciatic nerve: direct comparison among ultrasound imaging, macroscopic anatomy, and histologic analysis. *Reg Anesth Pain Med.* 2012;37(4):410-414.
3. Franco CD. Connective tissues associated with peripheral nerves. *Reg Anesth Pain Med.* 2012;37(4):363-365.
4. Perlas A, et al. Ultrasound-guided popliteal block through a common paraneural sheath versus conventional injection: a prospective, randomized, double-blind study. *Reg Anesth Pain Med.* 2013;38(3):218-225.
5. Karmakar MK, et al. High-definition ultrasound imaging defines the paraneural sheath and the fascial compartments surrounding the sciatic nerve at the popliteal fossa. *Reg Anesth Pain Med.* 2013;38(5):447-451.
6. Sinha A, Chan VW. Ultrasound imaging for popliteal sciatic nerve block. *Reg Anesth Pain Med.* 2004;29(2):130-134.
7. Liu SS. Evidence basis for ultrasound-guided block characteristics onset, quality, and duration. *Reg Anesth Pain Med.* 2016;41(2):205-220.
8. Salinas FV. Evidence basis for ultrasound guidance for lower-extremity peripheral nerve block: update 2016. *Reg Anesth Pain Med.* 2016;41(2):261-274.
9. Perlas A, et al. Ultrasound guidance improves the success of sciatic nerve block at the popliteal fossa. *Reg Anesth Pain Med.* 2008;33(3):259-265.
10. Abrahams MS, et al. Ultrasound guidance compared with electrical neurostimulation for peripheral nerve block: a systematic review and meta-analysis of randomized controlled trials. *Br J Anaesth.* 2009;102(3):408-417.
11. Taboada Muniz M, et al. Lateral approach to the sciatic nerve block in the popliteal fossa: correlation between evoked motor response and sensory block. *Reg Anesth Pain Med.* 2003;28(5):450-455.
12. Schafhalter-Zoppoth I, et al. The "seesaw" sign: improved sonographic identification of the sciatic nerve. *Anesthesiology.* 2004;101(3):808-809.

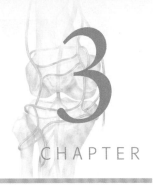

Ankle Block

Andrew Lyons and Fred G. Mihm

DEFINITION

- Ankle block is a highly effective peripheral nerve block that results in anesthesia of the entire foot. This block has been shown to reduce both postoperative pain and opioid consumption following foot surgery.[1,2]
- Though a number of injections are required, a low total volume of local anesthetic injectate is required to successfully perform an ankle block.
- The ankle block can be useful due to its relatively low-risk profile, technical ease, and efficacy.
- Typical plastic surgery procedures that utilize this block include tendon repair and distal foot or toe amputation.

ANATOMY

- An ankle block is the selective blockade of both the saphenous nerve and the four terminal branches—deep and superficial peroneal, tibial, and sural nerves—of the sciatic nerve.
- Ankle block is considered to be an easy block to perform because the terminal nerves of interest are generally superficial and are reliably located next to readily identifiable surface landmarks.

POSITIONING AND PREPARATION

- Ankle block is most commonly performed with the patient in the supine position.
- Elevation of the foot by bolstering the calf with a pillow will facilitate access to the ankle (**FIG 1**).
- It is helpful to have an assistant available to gently place the leg in either internal or external rotation.

MATERIALS

- Topical disinfectant (chlorhexidine, betadine, or equivalent)
- Sterile gloves
- Ultrasound with a small, high-frequency linear probe
- 20-mL sterile syringe
- 22-gauge short-bevel block needle
- Non-epinephrine containing local anesthetic

GENERAL CONSIDERATIONS

- The goal of the ankle block is to deliver local anesthetic adjacent to the five nerves that innervate the foot.
- Needle insertion can be either in-plane or out-of-plane for each of the terminal nerve blocks that comprise an ankle block.
- 3 to 5 mL of local anesthetic per nerve is required for a successful block.
- The tibial nerve should be addressed before blocking the other nerves because of its relatively larger size and resultant resistance to the effects of local anesthetics.
- The use of ultrasound guidance augments the clinical efficacy of an ankle block, especially for the tibial and deep peroneal nerves, which are relatively deep.[3–6]
- A small high-frequency linear ultrasound transducer is recommended.

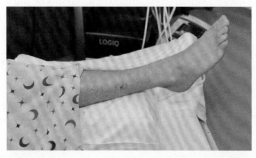

FIG 1 • Proper positioning of the foot is essential when performing an ankle block. The patient is placed supine and a pillow is used to facilitate access to the ankle.

Tibial Nerve

- Landmark technique: Inject 3 to 5 mL of local anesthetic in the deep tissue of the ankle posterior to the medial malleolus and the posterior tibial artery. The injection is typically performed after the needle contacts the underlying bone (tibia) and is withdrawn 0.5 to 1 cm.
- Unlike the other nerve blocks that comprise an ankle block, a nerve stimulator can be used as an adjunct for nerve block; plantar flexion of the toes indicates proper needle placement with tibial nerve stimulation.
- Ultrasound-guided technique: Place the ultrasound probe horizontally just superior and posterior to the medial malleolus to visualize the tibial nerve (**TECH FIG 1A**).
  - The tibial nerve is superficial to both the belly and the tendon of the flexor hallucis longus.
  - The tibial nerve lies immediately posterior to the posterior tibial vessels of the ankle; at this level, the nerve and vessels may be easily mistaken for one another. Sometimes, a fascia separates the nerve from the vessels, placing the nerve deeper and partially behind the vessels (**TECH FIG 1B**).
  - Color Doppler imaging may be helpful in distinguishing the posterior tibial artery from surrounding structures.

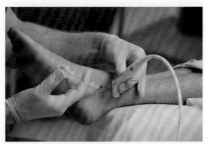 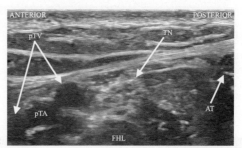

TECH FIG 1 • A. Tibial nerve block is performed by injecting local anesthetic into the deep tissue of the ankle. **B.** Ultrasound image of a tibial nerve block demonstrating the nerve (*TN*) in the deep tissue of the ankle just posterior to the vascular complex formed by both the posterior tibial artery (*pTA*) and the posterior tibial vein (*pTV*). Note the flexor hallucis longus (*FHL*) is found deep to the nerve. The Achilles tendon (*AT*) serves as the most posterior boundary of the image.

Deep Peroneal Nerve

- Landmark technique: Identify the extensor hallucis longus tendon and the dorsalis pedis pulse on the dorsal aspect of the ankle. Insert the block needle between these two landmarks perpendicular to the skin and inject 3 to 5 mL of local anesthetic into the deep tissue.

- Ultrasound-guided technique: Place the ultrasound probe in a transverse orientation over the anterior foot just above the line joining the malleoli (**TECH FIG 2A**) to visualize the deep peroneal nerve adjacent to the dorsalis pedis artery (**TEHC FIG 2B**).

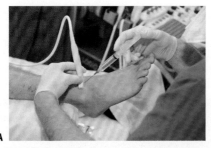 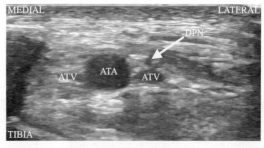

TECH FIG 2 • A. Deep peroneal nerve block is performed by injecting local anesthetic into the deep tissue of the anterior ankle. **B.** Ultrasound image of a deep peroneal nerve block demonstrating the deep peroneal nerve (*DPN*) located lateral to the distal-most branch of anterior tibial artery (*ATA*), also known as the dorsalis pedis artery. Branching of the anterior tibial vein (*ATV*) is common at this location.

Superficial Peroneal Nerve

- Landmark technique: Identify the line between the injection point for the deep peroneal nerve block and the lateral malleolus. Inject 3 to 5 mL subcutaneously along this line.

- Ultrasound-guided technique: Place the ultrasound probe in a transverse orientation just lateral to the deep peroneal nerve (**TECH FIG 3A**) to allow for visualization of the superficial peroneal nerve (**TECH FIG 3B**).

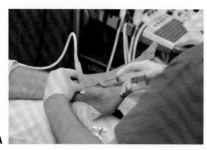
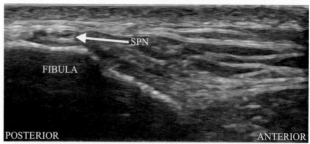

TECH FIG 3 • A. Superficial peroneal nerve block is performed by injecting local anesthetic into the subcutaneous tissue of the ankle just lateral to the location of deep peroneal nerve block. **B.** Ultrasound image of a superficial peroneal nerve block demonstrating the superficial peroneal nerve (*SPN*) in the subcutaneous tissue along the line between the location of the deep peroneal nerve and the lateral malleolus. This nerve is sometimes difficult to visualize using an ultrasound.

■ Sural Nerve

■ Landmark technique: Inject 3 to 5 mL of local anesthetic in the subcutaneous plane along the line formed between the lateral malleolus and the Achilles tendon.

■ Ultrasound-guided technique: Place the ultrasound probe just posterior to the lateral malleolus to visualize the sural nerve (**TECH FIG 4A**).
　■ The sural nerve lies adjacent to the short saphenous vein in the groove between the Achilles tendon and the peroneus brevis muscle (**TECH FIG 4B**).

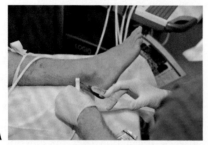
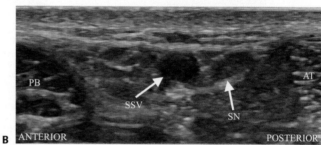

TECH FIG 4 • A. Sural nerve block is performed by injecting local anesthetic into the subcutaneous tissue of the groove between the lateral malleolus and the Achilles tendon. A calf tourniquet may facilitate the ultrasound imaging of this block by enlarging the short saphenous vein. **B.** Ultrasound image of a sural nerve block demonstrating the sural nerve (*SN*) in the groove between the Achilles tendon (*AT*) and the peroneus brevis (*PB*) muscle. The short saphenous vein (*SSV*) is anterior to the sural nerve.

■ Saphenous Nerve

■ Landmark technique: Inject 3 to 5 mL of local anesthetic in the superficial tissue of the ankle 1 cm anterior to the medial malleolus.

■ Ultrasound-guided technique: Place the ultrasound probe in a transverse orientation, just anterior to the medial malleolus (**TECH FIG 5A**) to visualize the saphenous nerve traveling lateral to the great saphenous vein (**TECH FIG 5B**).

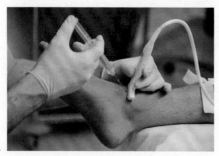
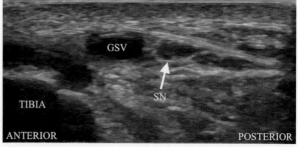

TECH FIG 5 • A. Saphenous nerve block is performed by injecting local anesthetic into the subcutaneous tissue of the ankle just anterior to the medial malleolus. A calf tourniquet may facilitate the ultrasound imaging of this block by enlarging the great saphenous vein. **B.** Ultrasound image of a saphenous nerve block demonstrating the saphenous nerve (*SN*) just posterior to the great saphenous vein (*GSV*).

■ Complications

- ■ Multiple injections about the ankle may result in significant patient discomfort. IV sedation can be used to enhance patient comfort during the procedure.
- ■ Intravascular injection is uncommon and the risk for local anesthetic toxicity is low, as small volumes of local anesthetic are generally used. The absence of epinephrine from the local anesthetic solution eliminates the risk of intravenous epinephrine toxicity and reduces risk of ischemia of the anesthetized foot.
- ■ Induration of the superficial tissues around injection sites is not uncommon.
- ■ Ankle hematoma as a result of vascular injury may also occur, but is usually self-limited.

TECHNIQUES

REFERENCES

1. Tryba M. Ankle block: a safe and simple technique for foot surgery. *Curr Opin Anaesthesiol.* 1997;10(5):361-365.
2. Vadivelu N, et al. Role of regional anesthesia in foot and ankle surgery. *Foot Ankle Spec.* 2015;8(3):212-219.
3. Chin KJ, et al. Ultrasound-guided versus anatomic landmark-guided ankle blocks: a 6-year retrospective review. *Reg Anesth Pain Med.* 2011;36(6):611-618.
4. Fredrickson MJ. Ultrasound-guided ankle block. *Anaesth Intensive Care.* 2009;37(1):143-144.
5. Redborg KE, et al. Ultrasound improves the success rate of a tibial nerve block at the ankle. *Reg Anesth Pain Med.* 2009;34(3):256-260.
6. Redborg KE, et al. Ultrasound improves the success rate of a sural nerve block at the ankle. *Reg Anesth Pain Med.* 2009;34(1):24-28.

Epidural Anesthesia

Rachel C. Steckelberg, Jean-Louis Horn, and Sarah Madison

DEFINITION

- Neuraxial anesthesia is a type of regional anesthesia technique in which anesthesia medication is injected into the tissue surrounding the nerve roots as they exit the spine (eg, epidural anesthesia) and/or directly into the cerebrospinal fluid (eg, spinal anesthesia or subarachnoid anesthesia).
- Continuous epidural anesthesia is a neuraxial anesthetic technique that may be used for postoperative analgesia, surgical anesthesia, and obstetric analgesia.
- Epidural anesthesia may be used to provide anesthesia at any level below the chin, either alone or in combination with general anesthesia.
- Epidural anesthesia may be administered as a single injection or as a continuous infusion via a catheter.
- The location of the epidural placement determines the distribution of analgesia. An epidural block may be performed at the cervical, thoracic, lumbar, or sacral (eg, caudal) levels.
- A continuous infusion of local anesthesia and/or opioid pain medication may provide postoperative pain control for several days after surgery.
- Motor block with an epidural may range from none to complete, depending on the choice of drug, concentration, dosage, and/or level of administration.
- Epidural analgesia is often part of a multimodal regimen that also includes systemic medications.

ANATOMY

- The epidural space surrounds the spinal meninges (eg, dura mater) and the spinal nerve roots as they course outward to become peripheral nerves. It also contains venous plexuses, lymphatics, and fat tissue.
- Knowledge of surface anatomy landmarks is essential for safe and reliable epidural placement (Table 1).

- In the cervical area, the most prominent spinous process is usually C7.
- The inferior angle of the scapula can be used to estimate the level of the T7 spinous process with the arms located at the side.
- The spinal cord terminates at level L1 in adults. The dural sac terminates at S2.
- The body of L4 and/or the interspace between L4 and L5 spinous processes typically can be found by drawing a line between the highest points of both the iliac crests (Tuffier line).
- The line connecting the posterior superior iliac spine (PSIS) crosses at the level of the S2 posterior foramina.
- The sacral hiatus is located by palpating for a depression (eg, the sacral hiatus) just above or between the gluteal clefts and above the coccyx. This is the point of entry for caudal epidural blocks.
- By counting up or down from these surface anatomy reference points, other spinal levels can be identified.
- Epidural anesthesia may be performed at any level of the spinal cord. However, each epidural location (cervical, thoracic, and lumbar) has unique anatomic features (Table 2).
- The angle of the spinous processes become progressively less angled closest to the base of the spine. For example, the spinous processes of the cervical and lumbar spine are more horizontal than the spinous processes in the thoracic spine, which are typically slanted in a more caudad direction and can overlap significantly. Thus, the technique for placement of the epidural needle varies considerably depending on the level selected.
- The ideal location of epidural placement is at the same dermatome of the surgical incision.

Table 1 Anatomic Landmarks for Identifying Vertebral Levels for Epidural Injection

Anatomic Landmark	Features
C7	Vertebral prominence (most prominent spinous process in neck)
T3	Root of spine of scapula
T7	Inferior angle of scapula
L4	Line between iliac crests
S2	Line between posterior inferior iliac spines
Sacral hiatus	Depression or groove above or between gluteal clefts directly above the coccyx

Table 2 Anatomic Features of Cervical, Thoracic, and Lumbar Spine Regions

Anatomic Feature	Cervical	Thoracic	Lumbar
Size	Small	Larger	Largest
Spinous process	Slender, often bifid (C2-C6)	Long and thick, project inferiorly	Short and blunt, project posteriorly
Transverse process	Small	Large	Large and blunt
Size of intervertebral discs	Thick (compared to vertebral bodies)	Thin (compared to vertebral bodies)	Very large

PATIENT HISTORY AND PHYSICAL FINDINGS

- A preoperative history and physical must be performed prior to epidural placement. Particular attention should be paid to anesthetic history, preexisting neuropathies, history of bleeding diatheses, medication history (especially any use of blood thinning medications), medication allergies, a history of prior neuraxial anesthesia and/or spine surgery (including spinal fusion surgery), and any history of spine disorders (including spina bifida and/or scoliosis). If imaging of the spine is available and would be useful for epidural placement, it should be reviewed.
- Physical exam should pay particular attention to any localized infections, masses, or other irregularities at the site of the planned epidural placement or surrounding areas.
- Contraindications to epidural anesthesia include patient refusal, bleeding disorders, severe hypovolemia, elevated intracranial pressure, infection at the site of epidural needle placement, flow-limiting cardiac lesions such as mitral or aortic valve stenosis, and local spinal pathology.

IMAGING

- When available, previous imaging of the spine should be reviewed, but routine imaging is not typically required prior to epidural placement.
- Preinsertion ultrasound will assist in accurate identification of the vertebral level of interest, the midline, and the depth of the epidural space (**FIG 1**).[1-3]

NONOPERATIVE MANAGEMENT

- The balance of risks and benefits must be considered for every interventional technique, including epidural anesthesia. Depending on a number of factors (including patient history, anatomy, surgery type, etc.), it may be more appropriate to employ alternative methods of analgesia, including peripheral nerve blocks and/or systemic medications for pain control.
- Careful attention must be paid to the maximum dose of additional opioid or other local anesthetic medications used for pain control when an epidural is in place.
- Nonopioid pain medications can also be useful adjuncts to epidural anesthesia/analgesia.

SURGICAL MANAGEMENT

- Epidural anesthesia is indicated for postoperative analgesia of any surgical procedure below the level of the neck.
- Thoracic epidurals are rarely used for primary surgical anesthesia, but more commonly for intraoperative and postoperative analgesia.

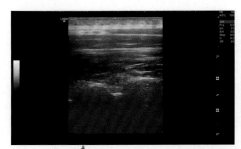

FIG 1 • Ultrasound of the lumbar and thoracic spine for epidural placement.

- Single injection or catheter techniques are useful for chronic pain management.
- Infusions via an epidural catheter are helpful in providing prolonged analgesia and may enhance postoperative ventilation in patients with underlying lung pathology following thoracic or chest wall surgery.
- Local anesthetic via epidural administration will block sympathetic, sensory, and motor nerves. The effects are dependent on the volume, concentration, and type of medication administered via the epidural.

Preoperative Planning

- Surgical site, extent of incision, anticipated degree of postoperative pain, and/or any preexisting conditions (bleeding disorders, preexisting neuropathies, etc.) that may increase the risk of complications should be discussed among the care team prior to epidural placement.
- If an epidural anesthetic is under consideration, the risks and benefits should be discussed with the patient. The patient must be informed and prepared for neuraxial anesthesia and the epidural must be an appropriate anesthetic technique for the type of surgery.
- Epidural anesthesia is rarely considered an appropriate mode of analgesia for outpatient procedures.
- Neuraxial anesthetic techniques, such as epidural anesthesia, should only be performed in facilities that have the equipment and drugs needed for intubation, resuscitation, and general anesthesia available.

Positioning

- The most common patient positions for epidural placement are sitting and lateral.
- In very obese patients, it may be easier to appreciate the anatomic midline with the patient in the upright (eg, sitting) position.
- In the sitting position, the patient should rest the elbows on his or her thighs or a table, or should hug a pillow. The bed should be flat and the patient's hips level to the bed.
- The patient should be instructed to arch his/her back to provide spinal flexion.
- Arching the back like a "mad cat" maximizes the area between the adjacent spinous processes and brings the spine closer to the skin surface (**FIG 2A**).
- Alternatively, the lateral decubitus position may be considered for epidural placement. In this position, the patient lies on his or her side with knees flexed into the chest and pulled high, assuming the "fetal" position (**FIG 2B**). An assistant should help the patient hold this position.

Approach for Lumbar and Thoracic epidurals

- Depending on the level of desired epidural placement, the epidural space may be approached either medially (more common for lumbar epidurals) or paramedially (more common for thoracic epidurals).
- Midline Approach: The patient should be positioned with the back plane perpendicular to the floor, so that as the epidural needle passes through the back tissues into deeper tissues, it will stay midline. The needle entry site should be between two spinous processes at the level of interest.
- Paramedian Approach: The paramedian approach is preferred for thoracic epidurals, or when the placement is difficult (due to severe arthritis, kyphoscoliosis, and/or prior spine surgery, etc.).

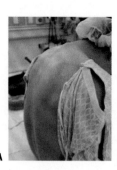 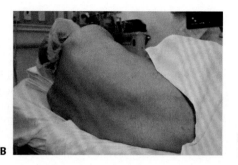

FIG 2 • A. Positioning for epidural placement (Sitting). **B.** Positioning for epidural placement (Lateral).

TECHNIQUES

■ Preparation

- Position the patient as described above and apply standard monitors: blood pressure, ECG (electrocardiogram), end tidal CO_2 (carbon dioxide), and pulse oximetry.
- Intravenous sedation (such as midazolam and/or fentanyl) may be administered for patient comfort.

- The spinous processes are typically palpable and can be used to identify the midline and the desired site of epidural needle placement, as described above.
- A sterile field is obtained by cleansing the area with chlorhexidine or similar solution before placing a fenestrated drape.

■ Epidural Placement

- After sterile skin preparation, a skin wheal is placed using a small gauge needle (such as 27 gauge) to inject local anesthetic at the desired site of epidural needle placement.
- A 17- or 18-gauge Tuohy needle is generally used for epidural catheter placement in adults.
- When using a midline approach, the needle is introduced at the midline and directed slightly cephalad (**TECH FIG 1A**).
- When using a paramedian approach, the needle is introduced approximately 2 cm lateral to the inferior aspect of the superior spinous process of the desired level. The needle is then advanced at a 10- to 30-degree angle toward the midline (**TECH FIG 1B**).
- When performing a lumbar or cervical epidural block, the needle is directed only slightly cephalad. When performing a thoracic epidural block, the needle must be directed more acutely to access the epidural space.
- The initial subcutaneous tissues offer little resistance initially to the needle passage. Note: if the paramedian approach is utilized, often the needle is lateral to most of the interspinous ligaments and penetrates the paraspinous muscles; it may encounter little resistance initially.

- As the needle passes deeper, it will pass through supraspinous and interspinous ligaments, and resistance will begin to increase.
- Using the loss-of-resistance technique during epidural placement, a syringe with a freely moveable plunger is attached to the epidural needle and filled with either saline or air.
- If the needle is correctly positioned in the ligament, the plunger will meet with resistance. However, once the needle passes into the epidural space, there will be a sudden loss of resistance, and the air or saline will freely inject with no rebound.
- Thus, the epidural space is located by the passage of a needle from an area of high resistance (ligamentum flavum) to an area of low resistance (the epidural space).
- Once the epidural space is located, a flexible epidural catheter is fed through the needle into the epidural space to the desired depth, typically 3 to 5 cm.
- After the epidural catheter is in place and secured, aspiration is recommended to ensure no CSF or blood can be aspirated.
- A test dose (typically 3 mL of lidocaine 1.5% with 5 µg/mL epinephrine) is injected via the catheter, and the patient is observed for signs and symptoms of intravascular, subdural, or subarachnoid injection.

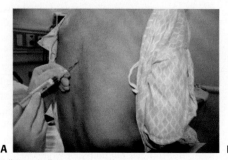 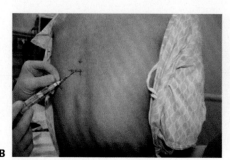

TECH FIG 1 • A. Midline needle insertion technique for epidural placement. **B.** Paramedian needle insertion technique for epidural placement.

■ Anesthetic Administration

- Local anesthetic (with or without opioid) is then slowly titrated by bolus or continuous infusion through the catheter to provide analgesia.
- Local anesthetic selection is based on the desired speed of onset, degree of motor blockade, and duration of anesthesia. Chloroprocaine, lidocaine, and mepivacaine are short-acting local anesthetics commonly used for surgical anesthesia. Longer-acting agents include ropivacaine and bupivacaine.
- Local anesthetic dose may be estimated by using 1 to 1.5 mL local anesthetic per desired dermatomal level of blockade. Once the initial blockade has regressed 1 to 2 dermatomal levels, a second dose of approximately 50% of the initial dose should maintain the original level of anesthesia. A continuous infusion can also maintain anesthesia. The rate of infusion depends on the concentration and type of local anesthetic chosen, the use of adjuvant medications in the infusate, and patient-specific factors. Typically, a rate of 6 to 8 mL/h is adequate.

- Dilute formulations of local anesthetics may be used in combination with fentanyl and/or hydromorphone to provide postoperative analgesia.
- Ropivacaine may produce less motor block than a similar concentration of bupivacaine while maintaining a satisfactory sensory block.
- The dose of epidural medication may need to be decreased in parturient, obese, and elderly patients. This may be due to several factors, including a potential for reduced CSF and/or a decrease in total epidural space in these patient populations. In addition, hormonal factors in the parturient patient population have been proposed to make neural endings more sensitive to local anesthetics.
- The addition of epinephrine to epidurally administered lidocaine may prolong the duration of nerve block by up to 50%. The prolongation of blockade with epinephrine added is less dramatic when using other local anesthetics, such as bupivacaine and/or etidocaine.
- Infusions are generally continued for 2 to 5 days following the surgery, depending on patient characteristics and the nature of the surgical procedure for which it was placed.

PEARLS AND PITFALLS

Sterility	■ Sterile conditions must be maintained at all times when placing an epidural.
Locating the epidural space	■ Placement of the needle should be done logically, based on 3D understanding of the anatomy. Needle redirection should not be random. Systematic small angle needle changes should be made.
Intravascular or intra-neural injection/local anesthetic toxicity (LAST)	■ Aspiration for detection of blood or CSF is recommended prior to injection through the needle or catheter to avoid toxic side effects if epidural medication is injected intrathecally or intravascularly. Test dosing may be helpful to avoid accidental intrathecal or intravascular bolus.
Segmental block	■ May be due to septations within the epidural space. Spread of medication within the epidural space is gravity dependent. A patchy block may be corrected by injecting additional local anesthetic with the patient positioned to optimize coverage of the areas that are spared. Sacral sparing may occur due to the large size of the L5, S1, and S2 nerve roots.
Unilateral block	■ May occur if medication is delivered via a catheter that has either exited the epidural space and/or coursed laterally.
Failed epidural blocks	■ The loss of resistance technique is somewhat subjective. Local anesthetic injection may be misplaced between ligaments or paraspinous muscles. The paramedian approach can be more challenging since the needle travels through softer tissues with false loss of resistance. Epidural space anatomy may be variable, making the spread of local anesthetics less predictable.
Block assessment	■ The extent of sensory blockade may be assessed using a blunt needle tip, cold, and/or other stimulus.

POSTOPERATIVE CARE

- Following placement of an epidural, patients should continue to be monitored for local anesthetic toxicity as long as the epidural medication is infusing. Typically, this is done by clinical exam. Early signs and symptoms of local anesthetic toxicity include tinnitus, blurred vision, dizziness, tongue paresthesias, and/or perioral numbness. Symptoms may progress to seizures and/or cardiac arrest if toxicity is severe and/or not treated early.

- Maximum recommended dose(s) for some commonly used local anesthetics: chloroprocaine and procaine 12 mg/kg; lidocaine and mepivacaine 4 to 5 mg/kg (7 mg/kg with epinephrine); bupivacaine and ropivacaine 3 mg/kg.
- The dermatomal level of sensory blockade may be assessed to determine the level of sympathectomy.
- Patients should be assessed at least once daily until the epidural is removed. This includes an evaluation of epidural function, query on side effects, determination of patient-

controlled epidural analgesia (PCEA) usage, degree of motor block, and a check of the insertion site and dressing.

- Depending on the epidural medication in use, patients should be educated on possible weakness and fall risk and should be tested for muscle strength before ambulation.
- Patients should be encouraged to supplement their epidural analgesia with nonopioid systemic analgesics as needed.
- Routine dressing changes are not necessary and may increase the risk of infection or catheter dislodgement. The dressing covering the epidural insertion site should be left alone until the epidural catheter is removed.
- Patients should be continually monitored by nursing staff for signs and symptoms of epidural hematoma and/or epidural abscess, including back pain, fever, and numbness or weakness that is progressive or in excess of what is expected. These symptoms should prompt immediate evaluation by the anesthesia team. If epidural hematoma or abscess is suspected, imaging and neurosurgical consultation for surgical decompression should occur within hours of the onset of symptoms to reduce the risk of permanent complications.

OUTCOMES

- In addition to providing excellent postoperative anesthesia, epidural anesthesia has been shown to be an important factor in the survival rate of flaps in breast reconstruction plastic surgery cases due to the effects on the distribution of direct blood flow to the microcirculation.[4]
- A continuous thoracic epidural infusion is associated with reduced bleeding due to hypotension during combined plastic surgeries involving breast, abdomen, gluteus, and liposuction.[5]
- Pain management strategies that include epidural anesthesia may be associated with reduced morbidity and cost savings in abdominal wall reconstruction surgeries.[6]
- Epidural use is also associated with shortened length of hospital stay.[6]

COMPLICATIONS

- In general, the use of epidural anesthesia is associated with a very low rate of severe or disabling neurologic complications.
- Overall, long-term complications (neurologic or otherwise) are very rare with epidural placement. The incidence of serious complications following regional anesthesia (including epidural, as well as spinal anesthesia, peripheral nerve blocks, and intravenous regional anesthesia) is estimated to be 0.01%.[7]
- Undiagnosed spinal stenosis has been identified as a risk factor for cauda equina syndrome and paraparesis.[8]
- Postdural puncture headache (PDPH) is a potential complication of epidural placement that may occur after a "wet tap," in which the epidural needle passes through the epidural space and into the subarachnoid space. Subarachnoid placement of the epidural needle is often made immediately apparent by the free flow of CSF. Occasionally, however, the findings are subtler, and subarachnoid placement of the epidural catheter is detected by aspiration of CSF or by induction of a dense block with the test dose. Typically, PDPH is described as bilateral, frontal, or retro-orbital, with extension into the neck. It is characterized by symptom

alleviation in the supine position, and worsening when upright ("postural headache"). PDPH is postulated to be due to leakage of CSF from a defect in the dura and intracranial hypotension. Initial treatment is conservative and includes administration of IV fluids, recumbent positioning, analgesics, and caffeine. Epidural blood patch may also be considered if conservative treatment fails, although many PDPH are self-limited.

- Neuropathies from epidural placement are rare. Epidural abscess and/or hematoma must be ruled out immediately (see below). Prolonged neuropathy related to epidural placement may be associated with paresthesias from the needle or catheter during placement, multiple attempts at block placement, and/or a technically difficult block. Peripheral neuropathies may be due to direct trauma to the nerve roots. Not all neurological deficits following regional anesthetic are always due to the block.[8]
- Epidural abscess is a rare complication of epidural placement and is a medical and surgical emergency. Symptoms of an epidural abscess are often insidious and delayed and progress from unexplained back or vertebral pain, to nerve root or radicular pain, then motor or sensory deficits, and finally paraplegia and/or paralysis. Prognosis is strongly related to the stage at the time of diagnosis. If suspected, catheter should be removed, antibiotics started, and neurosurgery consulted.[8]
- Epidural hematoma is another rare complication of epidural placement. Risk factors include a pre-existing bleeding diathesis or use of anticoagulation medication(s). The American Society of Regional Anesthesia (ASRA) guidelines should inform timing of epidural placement/removal and dosing of anticoagulation when such medications are indicated. Symptoms of hematoma include severe, sharp back and/or leg pain with motor weakness, and/or sphincter dysfunction. Surgical decompression must occur within 24 hours, and as soon as possible to maximize the chance of recovery.
- Local anesthetic systemic toxicity (LAST) is a rare but potentially deadly complication. Minimize risks with careful dose calculation.

REFERENCES

1. Arzola C, Davies S, Rofaeel A, et al. Ultrasound using the transverse approach to the lumbar spine provides reliable landmarks for labor epidurals. *Anesth Analg.* 2007;104:1188.
2. Chin KJ, Karmakar M, Peng P. Ultrasonography imaging facilitates spinal anesthesia in adults with difficult surface anatomic landmarks. *Anesthesiology.* 2011;115:94.
3. Tran D, et al., Preinsertion paramedian ultrasound guidance for epidural anesthesia. *Anesth Analg.* 2009;109(2):661-667.
4. de la Parra M, Camacho M, de la Garza J. DIEP flap for breast reconstruction using epidural anesthesia with the patient awake. *Plast Reconstr Surg Glob Open.* 2016;4(5):e724.
5. Nociti JR, et al. Thoracic epidural anesthesia with ropivacaine for plastic surgery. *Rev Bras Anesthesiol.* 2002;52(2):156-165.
6. Fischer JP, et al. The use of epidurals in abdominal wall reconstruction: an analysis of outcomes and cost. *Plast Reconstr Surg.* 2014;133(3):687-699.
7. Auroy Y, Narchi P, Messiah A, et al. Serious complications related to regional anesthesia: results of a prospective survey in France. *Anesthesiology.* 1997;87(3):479-486.
8. Moen V, Dahlgren N, Irestedt L. Severe neurological complications after central neuraxial blockades in Sweden 1990-1999. *Anesthesiology.* 2004;101(4):950-959.

Fasciotomy of the Thigh, Lower Leg, and Foot

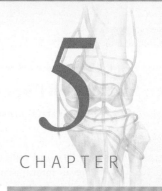

Graeme E. McFarland and Jason T. Lee

CHAPTER 5

DEFINITION

- Fasciotomy is indicated to treat compartment syndrome and prevent nerve injury and myonecrosis.
- Compartment syndrome most often occurs in the setting of reperfusion of an acutely ischemic limb or in severe limb trauma.
- Compartment syndrome can also occur in the setting of occlusive deep vein thrombosis (DVT) of the iliofemoral veins resulting in phlegmasia.
- Fasciotomy is indicated for treatment of active compartment syndrome, prophylactically for patients at high risk for compartment syndrome, or for those in which a reliable exam is difficult to obtain (ie, head trauma) and heightened concern for compartment syndrome.
- Isolated compartment syndrome of the thigh is rare and often due to femur fracture. The anterior compartment of the thigh is most commonly involved.[1]

ANATOMY

- There are three fascial compartments of the thigh all surrounded by the strong fascia lata.
  - Anterior:
    - Muscles: Sartorius, articularis genus, rectus femoris, vastus lateralis, vastus intermedius, and the vastus medialis
    - Neurovascular: Femoral nerve
  - Medial (adductor):
    - Muscles: Adductor longus/brevis/minimus, gracilis, pectineus, and external obturator
    - Neurovascular: Obturator nerve
  - Posterior:
    - Muscles: Adductor magnus, biceps femoris, semitendinosus, and semimembranosus
    - Neurovascular: Sciatic nerve
- There are four fascial compartments of the lower leg.
  - Anterior:
    - Muscles: Tibialis anterior, extensor hallucis longus, extensor digitorum longus, and the peroneus tertius
    - Neurovascular: Anterior tibial artery and vein and the deep peroneal nerve
  - Lateral:
    - Muscles: Fibularis longus/brevis
    - Neurovascular: Superficial peroneal nerve

  - Superficial posterior:
    - Muscles: Gastrocnemius, soleus, plantaris
    - Neurovascular: Tibial nerve
  - Deep posterior compartment:
    - Muscles: Tibialis posterior, flexor hallucis longus, flexor digitorum longus, and popliteus
    - Neurovascular: Tibial nerve, posterior tibial artery and veins, and the peroneal artery and veins
- There are technically nine compartments of the foot.
  - Medial compartment:
    - Muscles: Abductor hallucis and flexor hallucis brevis
  - Lateral compartment:
    - Muscles: Flexor digiti minimi brevis and abductor digiti minimi
  - Superficial central compartment:
    - Muscles: Flexor digitorum brevis
  - Central central compartment
    - Muscles: Quadratus plantae
  - Deep central compartment
    - Muscles: Adductor hallucis compartment
  - Intrinsic compartment:
    - Muscles: Four intrinsic muscles (compartments) between the 1st and 5th metatarsals

DIAGNOSIS

- Compartment syndrome can be diagnosed by directly measuring the compartment pressures with a Stryker monitor set or with an arterial line transducer system.
- Compartment pressures greater than 30 mm Hg are indicative of compartment syndrome.
- The "6 P's" of the compartment syndrome exam are pain, paresthesia, paresis, pallor, pulselessness, and poikilothermia.
- "Pain out of proportion to examination" and pain with passive flexion are the most consistent signs of compartment syndrome.
- A clinical suspicion for compartment syndrome warrants surgical intervention regardless of compartment pressure measurement.
- Paresthesias and paresis are late signs of compartment syndrome and are indicative of poor functional outcomes.
- Severe pain of the foot along with dorsal swelling can indicate compartment syndrome of the foot.[2]

■ Thigh Fasciotomy (**TECH FIG 1**)

- Anterolateral incision is made along the mid portion of the thigh for the length of the thigh.
- Make a straight longitudinal incision through the fascia lata and reflect the vastus lateralis medially off the lateral intermuscular septum to release the anterior compartment.

- Make a small 2-cm incision in the lateral intermuscular septum and extend proximally and distally for the length of the incision to release the posterior compartment.
- To release the medial or adductor compartment, make a medial incision longitudinally for the length of the thigh. Incise the fascia lata for the length of the incision.

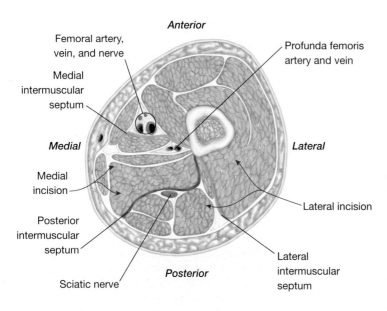

Labels on figure:
Anterior
Femoral artery, vein, and nerve
Medial intermuscular septum
Medial
Medial incision
Posterior intermuscular septum
Sciatic nerve
Posterior
Profunda femoris artery and vein
Lateral
Lateral incision
Lateral intermuscular septum

TECH FIG 1 • Thigh Fasciotomy. This figure demonstrates the two-incision approach for fasciotomy of the thigh. The medial incision carried deep through the fascia lata releases the adductor compartment. The lateral incision carried deep through the fascia lata releases the anterior compartment. The lateral intermuscular septum is then incised to open the posterior compartment. All important neurovascular bundles should not be exposed with this approach.

■ Lower Leg Fasciotomy

- Anterior and lateral compartments are released through a lateral incision made approximately 6 to 8 cm lateral to the anterior shaft of the tibia (**TECH FIG 2A**).
- The incision is carried from approximately 3 to 4 cm distal to the lateral tibial tuberosity to approximately 2 to 3 cm proximal to the lateral malleolus.
- Subcutaneous dissection is carried deep to expose the underlying fascia.
- The anterior compartment is released by making an incision in the fascia 2 cm lateral to the tibia. The fascia is then cut for the length of the incision.
- Identify the intermuscular septum between the anterior and lateral compartments. Make an incision through the fascia 1 cm posterior to the septum and then carry proxi-

mally and distally for the length of the incision, taking care to protect the common peroneal nerve proximally which lies behind the head of the fibula.
- To release the superficial and deep posterior compartments, a longitudinal incision is made medially 2 cm posterior to the medial border of the tibia for the same length as the lateral incision (**TECH FIG 2B**).
- Expose the underlying fascia and make the incision 2 to 3 cm posterior to the tibia successfully releasing the superficial posterior compartment.
- The deep posterior compartment is released by taking down the soleus muscle from its attachment to the posterior aspect of the tibia and the interosseous membrane. This needs to be carried for the length of the incision (**TECH FIG 2C**).[3]

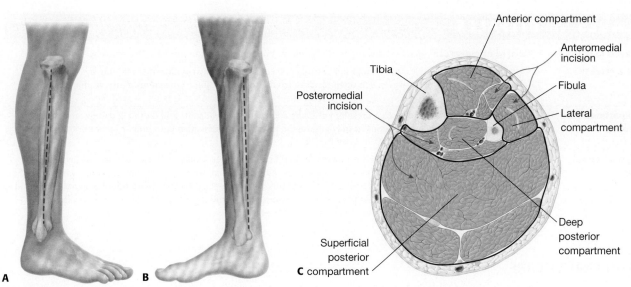

TECH FIG 2 • Lower leg fasciotomy. This figure demonstrates the two-incision approach to a four compartment fasciotomy of the lower leg. **A.** Lateral incision is made 6 to 8 cm lateral to the anterior shaft of the tibia and carried proximally 3 cm distal to the tibial tuberosity and distally to 2 cm proximal to the medial malleolus. **B.** The medial incision is created 2 cm posterior to the medial aspect of the tibia and carried for the same length of the lateral incision. **C.** The anterior compartment is released by cutting the fascia anterior to the intermuscular septum and carried for the length of the incision. The lateral compartment is released in similar fashion through the fascia lateral to the intermuscular septum. The superficial posterior compartment is released by incising the fascia just deep to the medial incision. The deep posterior compartment is then released by freeing the soleus from its attachments to the tibia.

■ Foot Fasciotomy

- Dual dorsal incisions are used for release of all nine compartments.
- A dorsal medial incision is made over the 2nd metatarsal and carried medial and lateral to the 2nd metatarsal releasing the 1st and 2nd interosseous compartments. Blunt dissection is carried deep to release the central compartments and medial to release the medial compart-

ment, if possible, posterior to the 1st metatarsal (**TECH FIG 3A**).
- A second dorsal incision is made over the 4th metatarsal and carried medially and laterally to the 4th metatarsal releasing the 3rd and 4th interosseous compartments. This can be carried laterally, posterior to the 5th metatarsal to release the lateral compartment (**TECH FIG 3B**).
- Occasionally, a medial incision is required to successfully release the medial and central compartments.

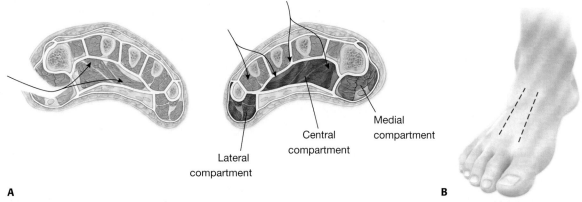

TECH FIG 3 • Foot fasciotomy. **A.** Occasionally, a medial incision is required to release the medial and central compartments. This is created along the medial border of the 1st metatarsal and carried through the medial compartment into the central compartment. **B.** Typically, a two-incision approach on the dorsal surface of the foot is all that is required. The first incision is made over the 2nd metatarsal and carried deep to the medial side to open the 1st interosseous compartment and then posterior to the 1st metatarsal to open the medial compartment. The incision is then carried deep to the lateral side of the 2nd metatarsal to open the 2nd interosseous compartment and the central compartment. The second incision is made over the 4th metatarsal. In a similar fashion, this is carried medial to open the 3rd interosseous compartment and deep to further open the central compartment. Finally, the incision is carried deep laterally to the 4th metatarsal to open the 4th interosseous compartment and then deep to the 5th metatarsal to open the lateral compartment.

PEARLS AND PITFALLS

Delayed diagnosis	■ Delayed diagnosis can often be catastrophic and result in functional losses, if not limb loss entirely.
Fascia release	■ Often the fascia can be released through smaller subcutaneous incisions by running scissors "blindly" along the fascia, superficially. This, however, can often result in troublesome bleeding from venous injury, or injury to the deep peroneal nerve.
Compartment release	■ Inadequate compartment release can result in ongoing compartment syndrome and disabling complications. Often, extending the subcutaneous incisions to fully expose the fascia and ensure adequate compartment release is the safest practice.
Nerve or vessel injury	■ Iatrogenic nerve or vessel injury can lead to certain disabling conditions similar to those in which the fasciotomy was initially indicated to prevent. The common peroneal and superficial peroneal nerve are the most commonly injured during lateral compartment release. To prevent this, terminate the proximal incision in the fascia 5 cm distal to the fibular head to prevent injury to the common peroneal nerve, and distally direct the incision towards the lateral malleolus to avoid injuring the superficial peroneal nerve.

POSTOPERATIVE CARE

- Patients require frequent neurovascular check every 1 to 2 hours for the initial postoperative period.
- Critical care monitoring and adequate IV fluid resuscitation are essential for renal protection in the setting of myoglobin release.
- Typically, fasciotomy wounds are initially dressed with wet to dry dressings that are changed 2 to 3 times daily to allow frequent evaluation of the underlying muscle.
- After the initial 24- to 48-hour period following compartment release, a wound vacuum dressing can be used to decrease the frequency of dressing changes and promote healing.
- Occasionally, if the limb is not too edematous, the fasciotomy incisions can be closed several days after the procedure to heal by tertiary intention.
- Frequently, skin grafting is required to ultimately heal the incision.

OUTCOMES

- Functional outcomes following fasciotomy depend mainly on the underlying injury, as well as time to procedure and adequacy of compartment release.
- Appropriate timing of fasciotomy is essential for improved outcomes. For fasciotomies delayed greater than 12 hours from the onset of compartment syndrome, limb loss is as high as 50%, with only approximately 8% maintaining normal limb function.
- Fasciotomy wound closure can be attempted during the same hospitalization if the swelling allows for tension-free closure of the skin. Occasionally, skin graft closure is required.

REFERENCES

1. Ojike NI, Robers CS, Giannoudis P. Compartment syndrome of the thigh: a systematic review. *Injury.* 2010;41(2):133-136.
2. Frink M, Hildebrand F, et al. Compartment syndrome of the lower leg and foot. *Clin Orthop Relat Res.* 2010;468(4):940-950.
3. Sheridan GW, Matsen FA. Fasciotomy in the treatment of the acute compartment syndrome. *J Bone Joint Surg Am.* 1976;58(1):112.

Drainage of Abscesses of Lower Leg and Foot

Michael C. Holland and Scott L. Hansen

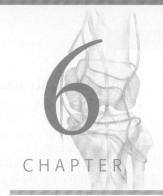

DEFINITION

- Infections of the foot, ankle, and lower leg range in severity from minor local cellulitis to rapidly progressive necrotizing fasciitis.
- Abscesses are a result of infection leading to inflammation and cell death, whereby a cavity is created that is filled with a mixture of bacteria, inflammatory cells, and necrotic tissue.
- Painful areas of fluctuance can be identified on physical exam and are most commonly surrounded by signs of inflammation (redness, warmth, pain, and swelling) but may also be found in isolation.
- Abscesses of the lower extremity and foot are frequently the result of trauma creating a break in the skin's natural barrier, allowing for colonizing or environmental pathogens to proliferate in the skin and deeper subcutaneous tissues.

ANATOMY

- The lower leg, ankle, and foot are comprised of 28 bones.
- Soft tissues include the overlying skin and subcutaneous tissue as well as muscles that are divided into anatomically distinct compartments in both the lower leg as well as the foot.
  - The four compartments of the lower leg include the anterior, lateral, superficial posterior, and deep posterior divided by fascia.
  - The nine compartments of the foot include the calcaneal—communicating with the deep posterior compartment of the leg, superficial, medial, lateral, adductor, and four interosseous.
- The primary neurovascular structures include the anterior tibial, peroneal, and posterior tibial arteries and paired veins; superficial peroneal, deep peroneal (fibular), tibial, saphenous, and sural nerves; and greater and lesser saphenous veins in the superficial tissues (**FIG 1**).

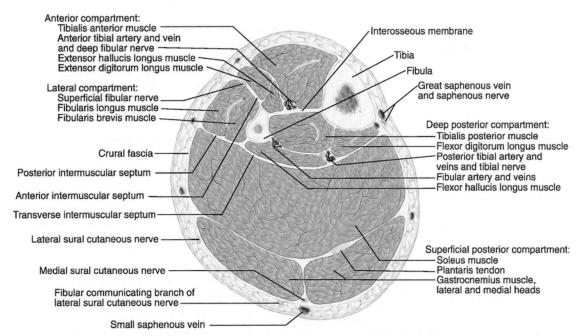

FIG 1 • Cross section of lower leg demonstrating four compartments separated by intramuscular septae, neurovascular structures, and soft tissue. (From Pansky B, Gest TR. Lower limbs. In: *Lippincott's Concise Illustrated Anatomy: Back, Upper Limb, and Lower Limb*. Vol. 1. Baltimore, MD: Wolters Kluwer; 2012:198.)

PATIENT HISTORY AND PHYSICAL FINDINGS

- The patient's initial complaint is typically of pain and swelling at the site of infection. They may also notice changes in skin color and drainage of fluid. There may be a history of antecedent trauma.
- Systemic symptoms such as fevers, chills, malaise may not be present early in the disease.
- Past medical history of diabetes mellitus, vascular disease, immunodeficiency, injection drug use prior fracture, and prior surgery may predispose to infection and abscess formation.
- Physical exam may reveal erythema, swelling, tenderness, warmth, fluctuance, visible drainage, and eschar. Many times, erythema and tenderness will be the only physical exam findings, so a high index of suspicion for underlying fluid collection is necessary.

IMAGING

- Despite its inability to well characterize fluid collections, standard multiple view radiographs are the first initial test to identify any bony injury or radiopaque foreign bodies as well as gas from anaerobic bacteria. Subtle soft tissue changes may also be demonstrated but are harder to appreciate by the untrained examiner.
- Ultrasonography may show cobble stoning of the subcutaneous tissues, which is indicative of edema. Discrete, hypoechoic fluid collections may also be identified.
- When multiple abscesses are suspected or ultrasound findings are equivocal, CT with IV contrast of the lower extremity can be extremely valuable.
- MRI is similar to CT in its ability to diagnose soft tissue infections; however, its use is limited by cost and time required to obtain the study.

DIFFERENTIAL DIAGNOSIS

- Cellulitis
- Abscess
- Septic arthritis
- Necrotizing fasciitis
- Plantar fasciitis
- Seroma
- Hematoma
- Gout
- Cyst
- Tumor

NONOPERATIVE MANAGEMENT

- Antibiotic therapy alone is often insufficient to manage abscesses, and drainage is the primary treatment strategy.

SURGICAL MANAGEMENT

Preoperative Planning

- In patients who are hemodynamically unstable, antibiotic therapy should not be withheld while awaiting cultures.
- In patients who are otherwise stable, consider deferring antibiotics until cultures have been obtained.
- If hardware is present, consider need for removal with orthopedic surgery consultation, as well as need for bony debridement.
- Ensure medical comorbidities are addressed.
- Ensure appropriate laboratory investigations are obtained including complete blood count, basic metabolic panel, C-reactive protein, sedimentation rate, and blood cultures.
- Antibiotic selection should cover gram-positive organisms with methicillin-resistant *Staphylococcus aureus* (MRSA) coverage, and due to prevalence of gram-negative organisms in foot infections, gram-negative coverage should also be provided while awaiting culture results.

Positioning

- Supine position is sufficient for exposure.

Approach

- The goal is to completely drain the abscess cavity, remove any debris or dead tissue, thoroughly irrigate, and allow wound to heal by secondary intention.

TECHNIQUES

■ Abscess Drainage

- Identify abscess cavity by palpation of fluctuance and correlate to previous imaging (**TECH FIG 1A**).
- A linear incision is designed over the most fluctuant area, attempting to avoid making the incision over weight-bearing area or known neurovascular structures or tendons.
- An incision is made through the skin with a no. 15 scalpel. If the incision was designed immediately over the cavity, abscess fluid will be released immediately.
  - Ensure the incision is opened up sufficiently in a proximal and distal direction (**TECH FIG 1B**).
- Obtain microbiology cultures, including bacterial cultures (aerobic, anaerobic) as they are most common. If there is clinical suspicion of other rare pathogens, send those as indicated such as fungal, yeast, mycobacteria, etc.

- Using a curved hemostat or Kelly clamp, spread gently throughout the abscess cavity for complete drainage.
- Gently probe the extent of the cavity in all directions to ensure that the cavity has been completely opened through the incision and that there are no residual fluid collections or loculations.
- Visualize cavity to ensure no necrotic tissues remaining. Adequately debride all necrotic tissues (**TECH FIG 1C,D**).
- If necrotic tissue, especially muscle, is encountered beyond the extent of abscess cavity, consider diagnosis of necrotizing soft tissue infection or necrotizing fasciitis, need for wide excision of all necrotic tissue, and addition of protein synthesis inhibiting antibiotics (eg, clindamycin).
- Irrigate the cavity with at least 3 L of saline.
- Pack the cavity with surgical packing, ensuring to apply enough packing to prevent the wound from closing prematurely.

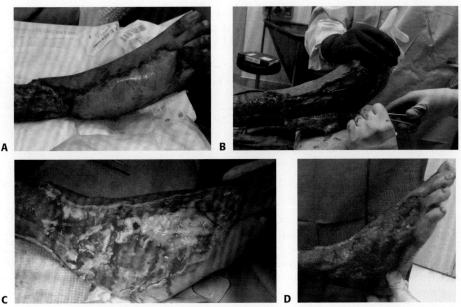

TECH FIG 1 • **A.** Necrotic right lateral foot wound with underlying abscess. **B.** Sharp debridement and drainage of wound and abscess. **C.** Wound after debridement and drainage of abscess with continued necrotic tissue. **D.** Granulating wound prior to split-thickness skin grafting.

PEARLS AND PITFALLS

Preoperative workup	▪ Failure to get bacterial cultures
Technique	▪ Incomplete drainage: ensure that entirety of abscess cavity is explored and septations are taken down ▪ Ensure incision is large enough ▪ Use copious (generally at least 3 L of irrigation)
Postoperative care	▪ Failure to ensure glycemic control
Dressings	▪ Applying an occlusive dressing can result in reaccumulation of abscess and inability to monitor wound. Do not apply negative pressure wound therapy on grossly infected wound ▪ Ensure enough packing is used to prevent wound from closing prematurely
Wound hazards	▪ Do not probe wound with digit, as you may injure yourself with potential foreign body

POSTOPERATIVE CARE

▪ Surgical management with drainage alone has been recommended for small (less than 5 cm abscesses) without associated cellulitis or systemic signs of infection.

▪ However, a recent randomized control trial (RCT) has demonstrated superior cure rates for patients who received post drainage antibiotics for 7 to 14 days, even in uncomplicated cases.[1]

▪ Patients require at least twice daily dressing changes until wound heals by secondary intention.

▪ Negative pressure wound therapy e.g. Wound VAC may be considered for abscesses that result in large open wounds, however, should not be placed at time of initial debridement and should be placed only after wound appears healthy and without signs of residual infection.

▪ Blood sugar control
▪ Smoking cessation
▪ Early range of motion should be encouraged to prevent stiffness and contracture.

COMPLICATIONS

▪ Persistent infection
▪ Missed diagnosis of necrotizing infection
▪ Injury to neurovascular structures
▪ Hematoma

REFERENCE

1. Talan DA, Mower WR, Krishnadasan A, et al. Trimethoprim-sulfamethoxazole versus placebo for uncomplicated skin abscess. *N Engl J Med*. 2016;374(9):823-832.

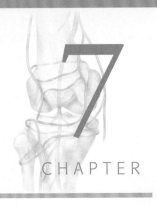

Excision of Soft Tissue Tumors of the Foot and Ankle

CHAPTER 7

Raffi S. Avedian, Robert J. Steffner, and Subhro K. Sen

DEFINITION

- Soft tissue tumors of the ankle may be benign or malignant (soft tissue sarcoma) and exhibit a variable natural history ranging from latency to rapid growth.
- Tumors located entirely above the muscle, fascia, or tendon are considered superficial, whereas tumors involving the fascia or located deep to it are considered deep.

ANATOMY

- The ankle is a synovial joint involving the tibia, talus, and fibula. Tendons of the leg muscles travel around the ankle in discrete groups each contained in a retinaculum (**FIG 1**).
- The anterior tibial artery and deep peroneal nerve travel anterior to the ankle joint just lateral to the anterior tibialis tendon.
- The posterior tibial artery and tibial nerve travel along the medial aspect of the lower leg, in the fascial plane between the deep and superficial compartments. At the ankle, they course posterior to the posterior tibial tendon along the medial malleolus.
- The tendons of the peroneus muscles travel along the posterior aspect of the lateral malleolus to their attachments in the foot.

PATHOGENESIS

- The mechanism for soft tissue tumor formation is not known.
- Risk factors for sarcoma development include radiation exposure, radiotherapy, pesticide exposure, and hereditary conditions including Li-Fraumeni syndrome and retinoblastoma gene mutation.

NATURAL HISTORY

- All soft tissue sarcomas have the potential for local recurrence and metastasis.
- Soft tissue sarcomas exhibit a spectrum of natural history from slow-growing low-grade tumors with low risk of metastasis to high-grade sarcoma that may grow rapidly and pose a high risk of metastasis.
- Lungs are the most common site of metastasis. Lymph node involvement is rare.
- Angiosarcoma, clear cell sarcoma, epithelioid sarcoma, rhabdomyosarcoma, myxofibrosarcoma, and synovial sarcoma are associated with increased risk of lymph node spread compared to other sarcomas.
- Benign tumors by definition do not have metastatic potential but can grow to large sizes and cause symptoms.

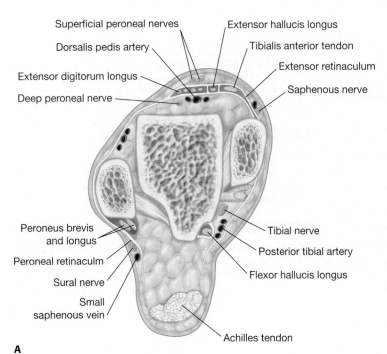

FIG 1 • A. Cross-sectional anatomy of the ankle. Notice that the tendons are contained within a retinacular layer.

A

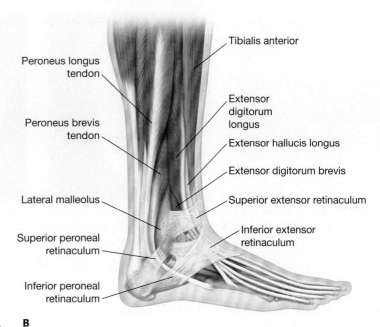

FIG 1 (Continued) • **B.** Oblique view of the ankle anatomy.   **B**

PATIENT HISTORY AND PHYSICAL FINDINGS

- Conducting a thorough history and examination is important to assess duration of symptoms, comorbidities, physical dysfunction, organ involvement, overall health, and patient expectations in order to best tailor treatment strategy for the individual patient.
- Many sarcomas may be asymptomatic with the only patient complaint being the presence of a mass.
- Neurovascular examination is mandatory for any extremity tumor.

IMAGING

- Magnetic resonance imaging is the principal imaging modality used to characterize tumors, formulate differential diagnosis, define local tissue infiltration, and devise a surgical plan.
- Plain radiographs are used if there is concern for bone involvement or to demonstrate mineralization within a tumor such as vascular malformations.
- Staging for soft tissue sarcomas consists primarily of lung imaging.

DIFFERENTIAL DIAGNOSIS

- The differential diagnosis for a soft tissue tumor includes benign tumors, sarcomas, lymphoma, infection, and inflammatory lesions (eg, rheumatoid nodules).
- There are over 50 sarcoma subtypes. Common histologies include pleomorphic undifferentiated sarcoma, synovial sarcoma, leiomyosarcoma, malignant peripheral nerve sheath tumor, and liposarcoma.

SURGICAL MANAGEMENT

- The appropriate treatment for any musculoskeletal tumor is based on its diagnosis and natural history.
- Biopsy incisions are considered contaminated and must be resected at the time of definitive surgery. Care should be taken to place the biopsy in a location that does not interfere with the final surgical plan.

- Simple marginal excision is appropriate for most benign tumors, whereas wide resection with a clean margin is performed for soft tissue sarcomas.
- Given the relatively low volume of tissue in the lower leg and ankle, soft tissue reconstruction with local or free flaps is often needed.

Preoperative Planning

- A patient is considered ready for surgery after completion of staging and multidisciplinary review of pertinent imaging, pathology, and treatment strategy.
- The retinacula and tendon sheaths around the ankle are robust tissues that act as barriers to tumor penetration. Careful assessment of preoperative imaging is needed; however, these tissues often can be used as a margin around the tumor (see **FIG 1**).
- When tumor abuts, but does not encase blood vessels or nerves, they can be dissected free by leaving adventitia and epineurium on the tumor as the margin.
- The surgical plan is created by thorough study of the preoperative MRI scan. Fluid-sensitive sequences and fat-suppressed contrast images show the extent of disease that must be accounted for in the excision. T1 fat-sensitive images show the normal anatomy best including fat planes between tumor and critical structures such as nerves and vessels (**FIG 2**).

Positioning

- Patient positioning is based on the surgeon's assessment of the critical anatomy of the surgery and how best to visualize it during surgery. Supine and lateral positions are most common.
- If a flap is to be used, the harvest must be performed using a separate back table and instruments and the surgical sites completely isolated to avoid contamination.

Approach

- The surgical approach varies based on location of the tumor.
- Previous biopsy and surgical scars are considered contaminated and must be excised en bloc with the tumor.

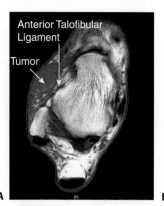 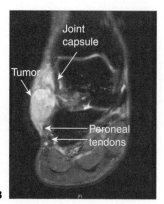

FIG 2 • A. Axial T1 MRI of a 57-year-old man with a myxofibrosarcoma on the lateral aspect of the ankle. Note that the tumor sits on the joint capsule and anterior talofibular ligament. **B.** Coronal MRI highlighting the tumor and its relationship to the surrounding anatomy. Notice that the joint capsule and retinaculum around the peroneal tendons act as a barrier to tumor penetration.

TECHNIQUES

■ Excision of Soft Tissue Tumor of the Ankle

- Tourniquet is used at discretion of surgeon using gravity exsanguination rather than Esmarch to avoid tumor compression.
- A margin of normal skin is marked around previous biopsy incisions and incorporated into the surgical approach (**TECH FIG 1A**).
- The dissection is beveled away from the sarcoma through the subcutaneous tissue to the deep fascia or retinacular layer at a point that is clear away (ideally 1–2 cm if possible) from palpable tumor or tumor visualized on preoperative MRI.

- The deep fascia and retinacula are cut and used as the deep margin. Occasionally, the joint capsule may have to be included in the deep margin.
- Cutaneous nerves often are involved in the tumor. They should be cut away from the tumor and buried in the deep layers to minimize risk of symptomatic neuroma formation.
- If the tumor partially encases the tendons, the retinaculum or tendon sheath may be incised on the uninvolved side of the tendon and lifted off as the margin on the tumor preserving the tendon (**TECH FIG 1B**).
- An assessment of joint stability is performed, and ligament reconstruction or augmentation is performed if indicated.
- Free tissue transfer is performed to reconstruct soft tissue defects.

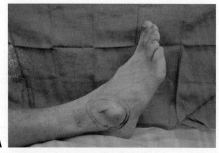 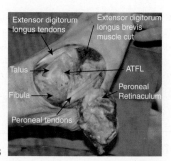

TECH FIG 1 • A. Photograph showing planned incision that includes wide excision of previous biopsy incision. Because the tumor is superficial, which is often the case for ankle tumors, a large paddle of skin is removed as the margin on top of the tumor. **B.** Photograph illustrating the deep dissection. The tumor was abutting the joint and partially encasing the peroneal tendons. The retinacular tissues around the tendons were opened and peeled off the tendons allowing the tumor to be removed safely while preserving the tendons. Similarly, the joint capsule, retinaculum of the extensor digitorum longus, and periosteum of the fibula serve as deep margin for the more anterior portion of the tumor.

PEARLS AND PITFALLS

Wound breakdown	▪ Soft tissue reconstruction should be without tension.
	▪ Patients should be counseled about the importance of leg elevation and activity modification.
Positive margins (sarcoma excision)	▪ Appropriate preoperative planning is important to minimize risk of unplanned positive margins.
	▪ Inability to primarily close a wound should not interfere with the decision to remove a tumor with a clean margin. Plan on soft tissue reconstruction.
	▪ Planned positive margins around critical structures such as nerves and vessels may be appropriate in certain settings.

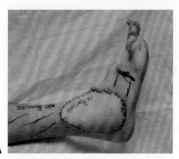 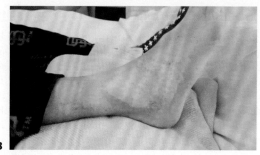

FIG 3 • **A.** Photograph immediately after completion of free anterolateral thigh flap. **B.** 5 years after surgery.

POSTOPERATIVE CARE

- The ankle is splinted ideally in the neutral extended position.
- Weight bearing may begin once soft tissues including flaps and ligament reconstructions, if performed, have healed sufficiently, typically 6 weeks after surgery.
- Extremity elevation is recommended while patient is in bed.
- Antibiotics may be administered while drains are in place.

OUTCOMES (FIG 3)

- Oncological outcomes include local recurrence and metastasis. Surveillance for recurrence should be managed by a multidisciplinary sarcoma team. Local recurrence is higher when margins are positive.
- Functional outcomes depend on the extent of tissue resection and patient overall health status. Most patients will experience some form of disability that is proportional to the volume of soft tissue resection. Estrella et al. reported on a small series of six patients who underwent resection of foot and ankle sarcoma followed by free flap coverage. The average Revised Musculoskeletal Tumor Society (Enneking) functional score was 92.8% at average 49-month follow-up.[1]

COMPLICATIONS

- Local recurrence occurs in a minority of patients with sarcoma and is more common in patients with positive margins.
- Deep infection can occur at any time after surgery and requires aggressive therapy including surgical debridement and antibiotic therapy to achieve limb salvage.
- Wound breakdown

REFERENCE

1. Estrella EP, Wang EHM, Caro LDD, Castillo VG. Functional outcomes of reconstruction for soft tissue sarcomas of the foot and ankle. *Foot Ankle Online J.* 2001;2(3):2.

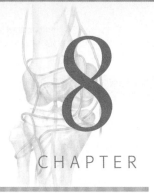

8 CHAPTER

Ankle and Foot Bone Tumors

Robert J. Steffner, Raffi S. Avedian, and Sahitya K. Denduluri

DEFINITION

- Bone tumors of the foot and ankle are usually primary tumors. Metastatic bone cancer to sites below the knee is rare but not impossible.
- Primary bone tumors can be benign, low-grade malignant, or high-grade malignant.
- Surgery is considered for benign tumors with progressive growth or those producing symptoms. Malignant bone tumors are generally operative in both a curative and palliative setting.

ANATOMY

- There is minimal soft tissue coverage in the ankle and foot. Surgical resections requiring skin excision and/or placement of bulk cortical allograft should consider the need for soft tissue coverage to minimize the risk of infection and nonunion.
- When functional deficit and donor site morbidity for free tissue transfer are anticipated, consideration should be given to below-knee amputation. Patients may recover faster and have better long-term function with a prosthesis.[1]

PATIENT HISTORY AND PHYSICAL FINDINGS

- It is important to ask patients about prior trauma and infections at the site of concern.
- A clinical history focusing on the duration of symptoms, presence of night pain, and systemic symptoms can help delineate benign from malignant etiologies.
- Physical exam focuses on the presence of prior incisions, skin mobility over the tumor, and neurovascular status distal to the site of tumor involvement.

IMAGING

- Obtain plain radiographs of the involved site.
- Perform an MRI scan with and without contrast to assess the extent of tumor and involvement of critical structures such as tendons, nerves, and vessels. Also perform a whole bone MRI to demonstrate the extent of intramedullary involvement of tumor and look for skip lesions.
- Make every effort to obtain any prior imaging for comparison.
- Quality of imaging and the interpretation of imaging are vital for surgical planning.
- Upon diagnosis of a primary bone malignancy, staging studies are performed to assess for regional or distant metastatic disease. This generally requires a chest CT and whole body bone scan.

DIFFERENTIAL DIAGNOSIS

- Benign and malignant bone tumors can be found in the foot and ankle. Distinguishing between benign and malignant guides the extent of surgical management.
- Benign tumors include simple cyst, intraosseous ganglion, and enchondroma.
- Benign but active tumors include aneurysmal bone cyst (primary or secondary), giant cell tumor, osteoid osteoma, and, in pediatric patients, chondroblastoma.
- Malignant bone tumors include osteosarcoma, chondrosarcoma, Ewing sarcoma, primary lymphoma of bone, and metastatic carcinoma.

NONOPERATIVE MANAGEMENT

- Benign-appearing lesions that are not causing symptoms can be followed with serial imaging. Stable appearance on serial imaging studies supports nonsurgical management.

SURGICAL MANAGEMENT

- Symptomatic benign bone tumors and benign but active bone tumors are most often treated with intralesional curettage or marginal excision.
- Malignant bone tumors may require multidisciplinary management with the possible need for chemotherapy and/or radiation in addition to surgery.
- In nonmetastatic or oligometastatic primary bone cancer, the goal of surgery is resection with negative margins.

Preoperative Planning

- If needed, size-matched fresh-frozen allografts should be coordinated from an appropriate vendor well ahead of time. The surgeon should assure that the graft has been delivered to the hospital. It is wise to have a back-up allograft available.
- Bone cuts are planned off T1-sequences from the first MRI scan. It is important to appreciate any soft tissue extensions and to look for fat planes around neurovascular structures to make sure they are free from tumor. Determination of appropriate margins is based on the specific diagnosis and the type of tissue at the level of resection.

Positioning

- Positioning depends on tumor location. Please see the "Techniques" section below.

Approach

- An oncologic approach allows for a limited tissue biopsy while maintaining the possibility of wide resection in the setting of a malignant diagnosis. If oncologic principles are followed, the majority of patients will be eligible for limb salvage.[2]

■ Benign Bone Tumor of the Talus (TECH FIG 1A,B)

- Patient positioned supine with an ipsilateral hip bump on a radiolucent table
- Tourniquet used after gravity exsanguination
- Localize tumor with intraoperative fluoroscopy
- To access talar body, an oblique osteotomy of the medial malleolus or distal fibula is often required. The surgeon may predrill bone in a lag-by-technique fashion before the osteotomy. This facilitates repair at the end of the surgery.
- A cortical window or cartilage flap is created with a curette or high-speed bur to access the bone tumor (**TECH FIG 1C**).
- Tissue is removed and sent for frozen section. If the pathology report is consistent with a benign tumor and matches the patient's clinical history and imaging, the surgery proceeds.

- The cortical window is expanded to adequately visualize and remove the tumor through intralesional curettage.
- Tumor margins are extended with use of a high-speed bur to smooth out the internal cavity of the cyst. Adjuvant treatments such as cryosurgery (liquid nitrogen) and argon beam coagulation can penetrate bone and further the zone of tumor kill. These measures lower the risk of local tumor recurrence.[3]
- Care should be taken near cartilage and growth plates to avoid damage to these structures. It is appropriate to accept a higher risk of local tumor recurrence in order to avoid injury to these structures.
- The resultant bone defect is filled with a substance of the surgeon's choice. In general, we use allograft in young patients; artificial bone void filler in young adults (mixture of calcium phosphate and calcium sulfate) and cement in older individuals.
- Supplementary internal fixation may be needed in weight-bearing locations and large defects (**TECH FIG 1D**).

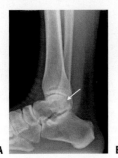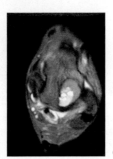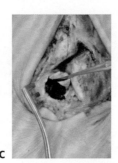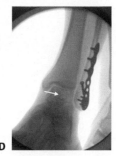

TECH FIG 1 • A. Lateral radiograph of a secondary Aneurysmal Bone Cyst of the talar body (*arrow*). **B.** Axial Fat-suppressed T2 MRI image demonstrating fluid-fluid levels. **C.** Photo after oblique osteotomy of the distal fibula to access the talar body. A cartilage flap is made to access the bone tumor. **D.** Fluoroscopic image demonstrating cancellous allograft filler in the talar body and internal fixation of the distal fibular osteotomy (*arrow*).

■ Malignant Bone Tumors of the Foot and Ankle

General Principles

- Use separate instruments for tumor resection and bone defect reconstruction.
- Obtain a thorough preoperative neurovascular exam.
- Consider an epidural catheter that can be test-dosed before surgery and used once a postoperative nerve exam is obtained.
- Use a thigh tourniquet and gravity to exsanguinate the leg.
- Hold paralytic medications if a nerve dissection is needed.
- Ellipse biopsy tract and keep in continuity with the resected tumor.
- Generally work from normal anatomy to abnormal anatomy.
- Clip or tie any arteries or veins that could be used for microvascular anastomosis.
- Measure bone cuts several times before cutting.
- After the bone cut, send a marrow margin for frozen section from the nonresection side.

- Orient resected specimens before sending to pathology.
- Fresh-frozen allografts are opened when frozen sections are negative. The allograft should be cultured and then placed in warm water bath with antibiotics for thirty minutes before use.

Distal Fibula Resection

- Lateral position on a beanbag. Straight lateral incision (**TECH FIG 2A**).
- Anteriorly, assess relationship of tumor with extensor digitorium longus and peroneus tertius.
- Posteriorly, assess relationship of tumor with peroneus longus and brevis and flexor hallucis longus (FHL).
- At the ankle joint, release the tibiofibular ligaments, talofibular ligaments, and calcaneofibular ligament.
- Make proximal bone cut early and roll fibula to expose the intraosseous membrane (**TECH FIG 2B,C**).
- Deep to FHL is the peroneal artery and vein; the latter may need to be ligated.
- Remove the tumor and send a marrow margin for frozen section.
- No bony reconstruction is necessary.

- Use a medium suture anchor to create a soft tissue sleeve for the peroneal tendons. This maintains length-tension relationships and avoids tendon subluxation (**TECH FIG 2D**).
- If possible, use absorbable suture to approximate the extensor digitorium longus muscle belly to the peroneus brevis.

- Immobilize for 6 weeks in a short leg splint with a mold in dorsiflexion and eversion.
- Obtain recovery room radiograph to check for any tibiotalar tilt. If present, the splint will need to be changed.
- Partial progressive weight-bearing begins at 6 weeks. Long-term, the patient may need a custom ankle brace.

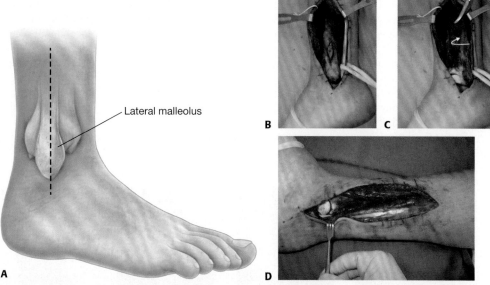

A

Lateral malleolus

B   **C**

D

TECH FIG 2 • A. Illustration of the straight lateral approach for a distal fibula bone tumor. **B.** Anterior and posterior dissection with ellipse of biopsy tract. Notice the margin of normal tissue left with the malignant bone tumor. **C.** External rotation of the distal fibula after proximal bone cut (*arrow*). This exposes the intraosseous membrane and posterior ligamentous structures. **D.** Use of remaining soft tissues to create a sling for gliding of the peroneal tendons. This also prevents tendon subluxation.

First Metatarsal (**TECH FIG 3A,B**).

- Supine position with a small contralateral hip bump.
- Dorsal incision that is just medial to the extensor hallucis longus (EHL) tendon. The tarsometatarsal (TMT) joint serves as the proximal extent of the incision (**TECH FIG 3C**).
- Ellipse circumferentially around the base of the great toe. If away from tumor, the skin around the great toe can be used for soft tissue coverage.
- Proximally, release the EHL tendon.
- Medially, dissect over the fascia of the abductor hallucis, leaving the muscle with tumor.
- Laterally, transect the extensor hallucis brevis.
- Come through the TMT joint proximally. The lateral aspect of the joint is close to the deep peroneal nerve and the deep plantar branch of the dorsalis pedis artery. Disarticulate and lift. Release the anterior tibialis tendon from the base of the first metatarsal and tag with suture.

- From plantar direction release the adductor hallucis and flexor hallucis brevis off the sesamoids. Transect the FHL tendon.
- Try to preserve the medial plantar artery and nerve.
- Release the intermetatarsal ligament and remove the resected specimen (**TECH FIG 3D**).
- Frozen section should be sent if there are any areas concerning for a positive margin.
- Scuff the medial cuneiform and attach the anterior tibialis tendon to this area with a suture anchor (**TECH FIG 3E**).
- Place a short leg splint for 2 weeks then allow heel weight bearing for the next 4 weeks.
- Once swelling is reduced, the patient is fit for a custom insert to go inside the shoe.
- Monitor postoperatively for lesser toe ulcers, flat foot deformity, and imbalance.

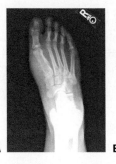
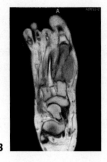

A   **B**

TECH FIG 3 • A. AP foot radiograph demonstrating an aggressive bone tumor of the first metatarsal. **B.** T1 coronal MRI showing Ewing sarcoma of the first metatarsal.

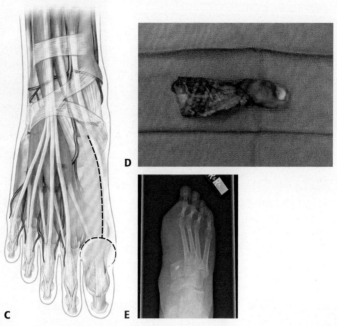

TECH FIG 3 (Continued) • **C.** Illustration of the dorsal incision with circular ellipse around the great toe used for first metatarsal resection. **D.** Resected specimen after oncologic amputation of the first metatarsal. **E.** AP foot radiograph after surgery demonstrating suture anchor repair of the anterior tibialis tendon into the medial cuneiform.

Calcaneus

- Patient is positioned lateral on a beanbag. Blankets are used to create a platform for the top leg. Make sure the down leg will not obscure intraoperative fluoroscopic images.
- If there is concern for a postoperative equinus contracture, a gastrocnemius recession can be done before tumor resection.
- A lateral approach is made (**TECH FIG 4A**). Identify the peroneal tendons and sural nerve (**TECH FIG 4B**). Tumor extent will dictate the ability to salvage these structures. *As able, try to preserve the tenosynovium over the peroneal tendons.*
- A geometric tumor resection can utilize CT-guidance. To use this technology, a preoperative CT scan with *fiducials* or an intraoperative scan with an O-arm machine is needed. In the operating room, an array is placed close to the surgical site and points are cross-referenced between the CT scan and the patient's intraoperative position (**TECH FIG 4C**). This allows simultaneous localization in the axial, coronal, and sagittal planes.
- The angle of Gissane and posterior facet provide orientation.
- Using measurements from the preoperative MRI scans, use a sterile marker to draw the geometric cuts. If available, use CT guidance to confirm that the proposed geometric cuts are free from tumor.
- Use a microsaw to cut bone up to the opposite cortex. Use an osteotome to complete the resection. This

will minimize risk to the medial plantar artery. Roll the resected bone and release the remaining soft tissue attachments (**TECH FIG 4D**).
- Perform frozen sections from the cut margins of the remaining bone as needed. Once frozen sections are negative, establish a new clean field and open reconstruction equipment.
- Use wax paper from surgical gloves to draw the bone defect.
- A fresh frozen femoral head allograft is opened and prepared as noted in "General Principles."
- Fashion the allograft with a microsaw to fit the wax paper template. Maintain the subchondral bone of the femoral head for the plantar surface of the allograft (**TECH FIG 4E**).
- Place cancellous allograft at the femoral head allograft-host bone junction.
- Temporarily stabilize with k-wires.
- Using fluoroscopic views of the lateral foot and Harris axial, navigate percutaneous screws from the heel into the anterior process of the Calcaneus. Try to minimize the number of drill holes through the allograft (**TECH FIG 4F**).
- Soft tissue closure may be primary or require flap reconstruction.
- In general, a short leg splint is applied for 6 weeks. Front foot weight bearing is then allowed until 3 months postoperatively. Partial progressive weight bearing is then initiated.

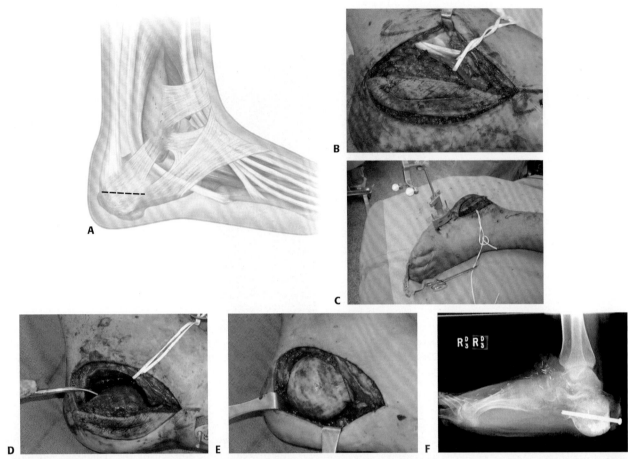

TECH FIG 4 • A. Illustration of the lateral approach to the calcaneus used for tumor resection. **B.** Ellipse of the biopsy tract with identification of the peroneal tendons, which were amenable to preservation. **C.** Placement of the array into the fifth metatarsal. The array is used to couple the patient's intraoperative anatomy to a CT scan to facilitate localization during the geometric resection of tumor. **D.** The tumor is gently rolled out, and soft tissue attachments from the medial side are released to remove the tumor. **E.** Placement of the fashioned fresh-frozen allograft femoral head into the calcaneal defect. The subchondral surface is used on the plantar aspect of the foot. **F.** Follow-up lateral radiograph of the femoral head allograft stabilized with two percutaneous 2.7-mm screws. The host-allograft junctions appear healed. This patient required free tissue transfer for soft tissue coverage.

Distal Tibia

- Supine position without a hip bump.
- Incision is along the anteromedial tibia (**TECH FIG 5A**).
- Save the saphenous vein and nerve if possible.
- Release the posterior compartment fascia, identify and protect the tibial nerve and posterior tibial artery, which is found between the flexor digitorum longus and FHL muscles.
- Release the anterior compartment fascia, identify and protect the deep peroneal nerve and anterior tibial artery, which is found between the tibialis anterior and EHL muscles.
- The neurovascular bundle at the anterior ankle goes from medial to lateral relative to the EHL tendon.
- Measure resection lengths off the medial malleolus.
- Mark rotation on the nontumor side both proximal and distal to the bone cuts.
- Use retractors to protect the soft tissues around the tibia. Use the microsaw to cut bone while irrigating to prevent bone necrosis from heat.
- Roll the resected segment and release the intraosseous membrane.

- Check marrow margins from the intramedullary canal of the remaining bone at the proximal and distal ends (**TECH FIG 5B**).
- Measure the length of the resected specimen (**TECH FIG 5C**).
- Prepare the fresh-frozen allograft as described in the "General Principles" section. Start by making the allograft longer than the resected specimen.
- Make small cuts and recheck fit of the allograft.
- Check plain radiographs of the entire tibia in the operating room to assure proper fit of the allograft and confirm that a deformity is not being created.
- Select a plate that spans the intercalary defect and gets multiple points of fixation on both sides.
- Try to avoid open growth plates. If possible, consider compression plating across the host-allograft junctions. Be careful, too much compression and placement of cortical screws through a poorly contoured plate can lead to a fractured allograft.
- Hybrid fixation with locking screws is beneficial in short segments. Locking screws are also preferred on the allograft side as it minimizes risk of fracture (**TECH FIG 5D**).

TECHNIQUES

- Only use enough screws on the allograft side to eliminate gross motion at the host-allograft junction. Too many screws can weaken the allograft.[4]
- A small second plate can be used to improve rotational strength if that is a concern.

- Closure is often primary. If there is notable skin loss, free tissue transfer may be needed.
- Patients are placed in a short leg splint. They are usually nonweight bearing for approximately six months. Partial progressive weight bearing is then started.

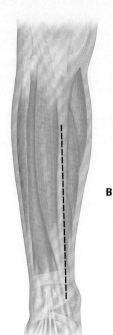
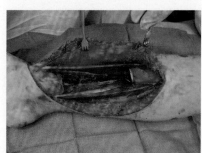
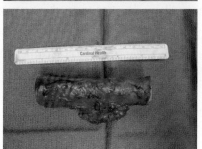
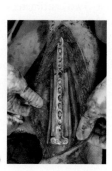

TECH FIG 5 • A. Illustration of the antero-medial incision for intercalary resection of the distal tibial diaphysis. **B.** Bone defect after resection of the distal tibia bone tumor. **C.** Length measurement of the resected segment of distal tibia. **D.** Spanning plate with hybrid internal fixation across the fresh-frozen intercalary allograft used to reconstruct the bone defect after tumor resection.

PEARLS AND PITFALLS

Imaging	▪ MRI scans are performed with and without contrast and done as a "tumor protocol." Tumor protocol at our institution represents T1 axial, T2 fat-suppressed, and T1 fat-suppressed pre- and postcontrast images.
Localization	▪ There are many small bones and joints in the foot and ankle. It is helpful to use intraoperative fluoroscopy to assure incisions are appropriately placed.
Biopsy	▪ The oncologic approach to biopsy should be in-line with the incision necessary to perform a wide resection of the tumor.
Frozen section	▪ Bone is too hard for frozen section processing. If sending a bone sample for frozen section, ask the pathologist to do a "touch prep" to examine cells inside the bone sample.
Implant selection	▪ Future imaging will be needed to assess healing and look for recurrent tumor. Use of titanium implants can limit artifact on future MRI and CT scans. This benefit should be weighed against the need for a durable implant. New carbon implants may provide both strength and limited artifact on imaging.
Healing	▪ Healing at the host-allograft junction can be augmented by step-cuts that increase the surface contact area between the two sides. Using microsurgery, vascularized bone, most commonly the fibula, can be set at the junction to aid healing and improve bone strength.

POSTOPERATIVE CARE

- Please see individual sections under "Techniques."
- In all cases, patients are initially placed in a short leg splint and instructed to elevate the lower extremity at or above heart level for soft tissue rest.

- Structural fresh-frozen allograft used to fill defects in the lower extremity generally needs 6 months of nonweight bearing followed by partial progressive weight bearing to achieve full weight bearing over 4 to 6 weeks.
- Radiographs are done at 6 weeks and 3 months after surgery and then every 3 months for the first 2 years.

- Any mention of acutely worsened pain should trigger an assessment for infection and fracture.

OUTCOMES

- Very few studies have looked at outcomes of tumors about the foot and ankle, likely due to their rare incidence.
- Benign bone tumors of the foot and ankle are 3 to 4 times more frequently encountered than malignant bone tumors.[5,6]
- In patients with malignant bone tumors of the foot, one center reported that half were treated with some form of amputation.[5]
- A single-institution study found that the overall and disease-free survival rate at 9 years was 65% and 40%, respectively, for both benign and malignant bone and soft tissue tumors of the foot and ankle.[6]

COMPLICATIONS

- Leg length discrepancy: May develop from early physeal arrest. Two centimeters or less is well tolerated with a shoe lift. Anticipating this problem allows the surgeon to shut down the contralateral physis.
- Fracture: Fresh-frozen cortical allograft does not fully vascularize. The implant spanning the allograft will be needed for load-sharing forever and should not be removed. It is wise to restrict cutting and pivoting sports and activities.
- Nonunion: Allograft-host bone junctions can be slow to heal, especially at diaphyseal-diaphyseal junctions.

Additional surgery to place cancellous autograft at the junction may be needed.

- Infection: Poor soft tissue coverage and lack of blood supply to bulk cortical allografts puts the surgical site at risk of infection. Generally, patients are maintained on oral antibiotics for three months after surgery. Infected allograft needs to be removed to clear the infection.
- Local recurrence: The surgeon should follow the patient for 5 years for high-grade and 10 years for low-grade malignancies to assess for local recurrence. MRI is generally the imaging modality of choice. The first postoperative scan is performed 3 months after surgery and serves as a baseline for future comparison.

REFERENCES

1. Pinzur MS, et al. Controversies in lower-extremity amputation. *J Bone Joint Surg Am.* 2007;89(5):1118-1127.
2. Hogendoorn PC, et al. Bone sarcomas: ESMO Clinical Practice Guidelines for diagnosis, treatment and follow-up. *Ann Oncol.* 2010;21(suppl 5):v204-v213.
3. Giacomo GD, et al. Local adjuvants in surgical management of bone lesions. *J Cancer Ther.* 2015;6(6):9.
4. Kuchinad RA, et al. The use of structural allograft in primary and revision knee arthroplasty with bone loss. *Adv Orthop.* 2011;2011: 578952.
5. Ruggieri P, et al. Review of foot tumors seen in a university tumor institute. *J Foot Ankle Surg.* 2014;53(3):282-285.
6. Azevedo CP, et al. Tumors of the foot and ankle: a single-institution experience. *J Foot Ankle Surg.* 2013;52(2):147-152.

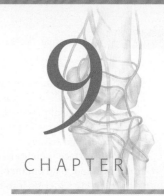

Debridement of Soft Tissue Infections of the Foot and Ankle

9

Hunter S. Oliver-Allen, Michael C. Holland, and Scott L. Hansen

DEFINITION

- Soft tissue infections of the lower leg and foot include a spectrum of severity from superficial cellulitis to rapidly progressive necrotizing fasciitis.
- Soft tissue infections of the foot and ankle can involve skin, subcutaneous tissue, fascia, muscle, ligaments, tendons, joints, and around the nails.
- Secondary infections can be due to peripheral vascular disease (PVD), diabetes, metabolic conditions, and immunocompromised patients.
- Infections of the foot and ankle are often categorized into three groups: soft tissue infections, bone infections, and diabetic infections.
- Infections can be further characterized into nonpurulent (cellulitis and erysipelas), purulent (abscess), necrotizing soft tissue infections (NSTI) (including necrotizing cellulitis, myositis, and fasciitis) as well as tendonitis and septic arthritis.
- Immediate goal is to treat and control the infection.
- Long-term goal is for limb salvage, preserve limb function, and decrease risk for amputation.

- Infections are most commonly caused by bacteria, however can also be due to viral, fungal, or mycobacteria.
- Some may respond to treatment with topical, oral, or intravenous antibiotics alone, while others will require surgical debridement of devitalized tissue.
- Typically present as painful lesions with skin changes invariably present, with or without involvement of deeper tissues.

ANATOMY

- The lower leg, ankle, and foot comprise 28 bones.
- Soft tissues include muscles that are divided into anatomically distinct compartments in both the lower leg and the foot (**FIG 1**).
  - The four compartments of the lower leg include the anterior, lateral, superficial posterior, and deep posterior divided by fascia.
  - The nine compartments of the foot include the calcaneal—communicating with the deep posterior compartment of the leg, superficial, medial, lateral, adductor, and four interosseous.

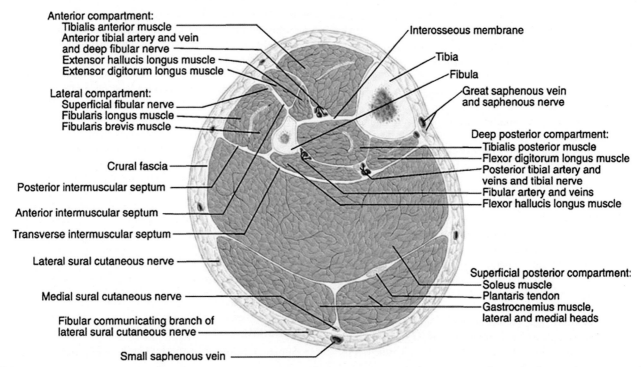

Anterior compartment:
 Tibialis anterior muscle
 Anterior tibial artery and vein
 and deep fibular nerve
 Extensor hallucis longus muscle
 Extensor digitorum longus muscle

Lateral compartment:
 Superficial fibular nerve
 Fibularis longus muscle
 Fibularis brevis muscle

Crural fascia

Posterior intermuscular septum

Anterior intermuscular septum

Transverse intermuscular septum

Lateral sural cutaneous nerve

Medial sural cutaneous nerve

Fibular communicating branch of
lateral sural cutaneous nerve

Small saphenous vein

Interosseous membrane

Tibia

Fibula

Great saphenous vein
and saphenous nerve

Deep posterior compartment:
 Tibialis posterior muscle
 Flexor digitorum longus muscle
 Posterior tibial artery and
 veins and tibial nerve
 Fibular artery and veins
 Flexor hallucis longus muscle

Superficial posterior compartment:
 Soleus muscle
 Plantaris tendon
 Gastrocnemius muscle,
 lateral and medial heads

FIG 1 • Cross section of the leg showing the compartments. (From Pansky B, Gest TR. Lower limbs. In: *Lippincott's Concise Illustrated Anatomy: Back, Upper Limb, and Lower Limb*. Vol. 1. Baltimore, MD: Wolters Kluwer; 2012:198.)

- The primary neurovascular structures include the anterior tibial, peroneal, and posterior tibial arteries and paired veins; superficial peroneal, deep peroneal, tibial, saphenous, and sural nerves; and greater and lesser saphenous veins in the superficial tissues.
- Plantar surface is composed of thick glabrous epidermis and dermis, and a subcutaneous layer with vertical fibrous septae, densely adhering it to the plantar fascia and periosteum.

PATHOGENESIS

- Infections result from breakdown of natural defenses in skin such as with trauma or open wound and invasion of resident skin flora or environmental pathogens.[1]
- Patients with neuropathy and vascular disease and are immunocompromised have increased risk of infection.[1]
- Group A beta-hemolytic streptococcus is the most common and second most common is *Staphylococcus aureus*.
- Infections are also commonly polymicrobial, especially in diabetic patients.
- NSTI result from bacterial invasion and subsequent angiothrombosis decreasing blood supply causing tissue necrosis They are classified into two groups:[2]
  - Type I is a polymicrobial infection consisting of anaerobic bacteria and aerobic bacteria.
  - Type II is monomicrobial infections typically of group A streptococcus or other beta-hemolytic streptococcus alone or with other pathogens.

PATIENT HISTORY AND PHYSICAL FINDINGS

- The patient's initial complaint is typically of pain and swelling at site of infection. They may also notice changes in skin color and drainage of fluid. There may be a history of antecedent trauma.
- Systemic symptoms such as fevers, chills, malaise may not be present early in the disease but indicate an immune response to the infection.
- Past medical history of diabetes mellitus, vascular disease, immunodeficiency, heart failure, cirrhosis, or prior surgery may predispose to infection.
- Physical exam may reveal erythema, swelling, tenderness, warmth, fluctuance, visible drainage, and eschar.
- Open wounds may be present with exposed subcutaneous fat, muscle, fascia, or bone.
- Pain out of proportion to physical exam findings or crepitus are concerning physical exam findings for necrotizing fasciitis.

IMAGING

- Despite its inability to well characterize fluid collections, standard multiple view radiographs are the first initial test to identify any bony injury or radiopaque foreign bodies as well as gas from anaerobic bacteria. Subtle soft tissue changes may also be demonstrated but are harder to appreciate by the untrained examiner.
- Ultrasonography may show cobble stoning of the subcutaneous tissues, which is indicative of edema. Discrete, hypoechoic fluid collections may also be identified. For patients with isolated abscesses, please see the chapter on drainage of abscesses of foot and ankle.
- Cross-sectional imaging with CT or MRI may better evaluate the extremity to determine the extent of infection.[1]

DIFFERENTIAL DIAGNOSIS

- Cellulitis
- Abscess
- Necrotizing fasciitis
- Plantar fasciitis
- Gout
- Skin cancer
- Venous stasis ulcer or dermatitis
- Impetigo
- Erysipelas

NONOPERATIVE MANAGEMENT

- Simple infections such as folliculitis or impetigo may improve with topical antibiotics alone.
- Cellulitis and more superficial infections require oral or intravenous antibiotics.
- Infected open wounds without burden of necrotic tissue may be treated with local wound care and antibiotics with careful monitoring for clinical worsening in poor surgical candidates.

SURGICAL MANAGEMENT

- The goal of surgery is to identify and debride all nonviable tissue, and a planned second look operation may be considered in severe infections where debridement is limited by critical structures.

Preoperative Planning

- In patients who are hemodynamically unstable or with suspected necrotizing infection, empiric antibiotic therapy should be ordered while drawing blood cultures and should not be delayed for wound cultures.
- In patients who are otherwise stable, consider deferring antibiotics until wound cultures have been obtained.
- If hardware is present, consider need for removal with orthopedic surgery consultation, as well as need for bony debridement.
- Ensure medical comorbidities are addressed. Patients with infected wounds due to vascular ulcers may require preoperative revascularization. Diabetics should have tight glycemic control.
- Ensure appropriate laboratory investigations are obtained including complete blood count, basic metabolic panel, C-reactive protein, sedimentation rate, and blood cultures.
- Antibiotic selection should cover gram-positive organisms with MRSA coverage, and due to prevalence of gram-negative organisms in foot infections, gram-negative coverage should also be provided while awaiting culture results.

Positioning

- Supine position is usually sufficient for exposure.

TECHNIQUES

■ Debridement of Soft Tissue Infections

- Identify the affected area of the leg or foot and prep well beyond the border with healthy tissue (**TECH FIG 1A**).
- Identify necrotic or nonviable tissue and sharply debride without the use of cautery.
  - Avoiding cautery will allow using the presence of bleeding to guide when sufficient debridement has been performed.
- Necrotic tissue is picked up with forceps and trimmed with curved mayo scissors, Metzenbaum scissors for finer tissue, or scalpel.
- Tissue may be sent to pathology and microbiology for culture and Gram stain.
- Presence of tunneling or disruption of fascial planes should be examined to identify necrotizing fasciitis.

- Probe the wound for any areas of tunneling. Areas of tunneling with fascial disruption and/or presence of "dishwater-" appearing fluid raises concern for presence of necrotizing fasciitis.
- If tunneling found, most overlying tissue should be opened to explore extent of infection, debride overlying tissue that is nonviable.
- Irrigate the cavity with at least 3 L of saline, which is easily done with cysto tubing (**TECH FIG 1B**).
- Obtain hemostasis with electrocautery.
- Pack the open wound with surgical packing.
- Consider ultimate reconstructive goal, including healing by secondary intention with wound care, wound Vacuum-assisted closure (VAC), skin grafting, local flap, or free flap (**TECH FIG 1C**).

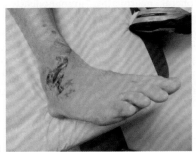 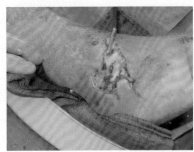 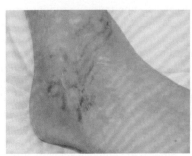

A   **B**   **C**

TECH FIG 1 • A. Infected lateral malleolar wound after trauma. **B.** Debridement with high-pressure water. **C.** Healed wound with split-thickness skin graft.

PEARLS AND PITFALLS

Preoperative workup	■ Failure to obtain blood cultures ■ Failure to identify patients needing revascularization before making larger wound ■ Delaying antibiotic therapy in severe infections ■ Nutritional optimization
Technique	■ Incomplete debridement resulting in need for additional surgery ■ Incompletely exploring extent of wound/tunneling ■ Use copious irrigation
Postoperative care	■ Placing wound VAC on infected wound ■ Neglecting medical comorbidities or nutritional status

POSTOPERATIVE CARE

- Continue broad spectrum antibiotics while awaiting culture speciation
- Continue local wound care with at least twice daily dressing changes until wound is confirmed to be clear of infection, afterward specialty dressings or wound VAC may be applied which may be changed less frequently.
- Silver sulfadiazine or other silver impregnated dressings controls both bacterial growth and facilitates wound healing.
- Continue to optimize medical comorbidities and smoking cessation.
- Allow for at least passive range of motion exercises if weight-bearing surface is affected.
- Elevation of the extremity and pressure off-loading.

COMPLICATIONS

- Persistent infection
- Missed diagnosis of necrotizing infection
- Injury to neurovascular structures
- Hematoma

REFERENCES

1. Anakwenze OA, Milby AH, Gans I, et al. Foot and ankle infections: diagnosis and management. *J Am Acad Orthop Surg.* 2012;20(11):684-693.
2. Stevens DL, Bryant AE. Necrotizing soft-tissue infections. *N Engl J Med.* 2017;377(23):2253-2265.

10
CHAPTER

Debridement of Infected Bone of the Foot and Ankle

Michael C. Holland and Scott L. Hansen

DEFINITION

- Osteomyelitis of the foot and ankle is defined by bacterial or less commonly fungal infection of bones of the lower third of the leg and foot.
- Spectrum of severity can range from chronic, indolent infections to acute, suppurative infections resulting in sepsis.
- Often resulting from existing soft tissue wound extending deep to underlying bone; however, seeding (eg, from bacteremia), direct inoculation (eg, trauma, puncture wounds), or healing of prior soft tissue defects can result in isolated osteomyelitis in the absence of soft tissue signs or symptoms.
- Frequently associated with hardware and prior fractures necessitating removal or replacement of hardware.
- The management of acute osteomyelitis is primarily medical, whereas the management of chronic osteomyelitis is mainly surgical in combination with antibiotic therapy.[1]

ANATOMY

- The ankle is formed by the distal aspect of the tibia (medial) and fibula (lateral) articulating with the talus of the foot.
- The foot is composed of 26 bones functionally homologous to bones of the hand and wrist.
- The hindfoot is composed of the talus, which is seated on the calcaneus.
- The midfoot articulates with the bones of the hindfoot and is composed of the cuboid navicular and three cuneiform bones (medial, intermediate, and lateral).
- The forefoot is composed of the 5 metatarsal bones and 14 phalanges.
- Two sesamoid bones underlying the first toe metatarsal phalangeal joint also are present in adults, with infrequently found accessory sesamoid bones at other joints.[2]

PATHOGENESIS

- Infection most often arises from soft tissue wounds, open fractures, complications from orthopedic reduction of closed fractures, hematogenous seeding from bacteremia or endocarditis, or inoculation from trauma

PATIENT HISTORY AND PHYSICAL FINDINGS

- History of diabetes mellitus, vascular insufficiency, venous hypertension, peripheral neuropathy, immunodeficiency, prior fracture, presence of hardware, prior surgery, and prior podiatric procedures are important to identify preoperatively in order to determine whether or not adjuvant therapy may be beneficial to precede operative intervention.
- Diminished sensation, paresthesias, and claudication are symptoms that may indicate the presence of these above comorbidities.
- Presence of open wounds with or without visible bone, erythema, fluctuance, and bony tenderness can indicate active infection.
- Decreased Semmes-Weinstein monofilament test, prior scars, palpable hardware, and venous ulceration are physical exam findings that may indicate higher-risk populations for developing osteomyelitis.

IMAGING

- Three-view plain radiographs of the foot and ankle are the first test to order, and will help give clear definition of bony anatomy, presence of hardware or radiopaque foreign bodies, and can detect subtle changes of osteomyelitis as early as 10 to 14 days but typically requires 3 weeks of active infection before changes will be found.[3]
  - Periosteal reaction (**FIG 1A**), lytic lesions, endosteal scalloping, loss of bone density, or trabecular architecture are findings indicative of osteomyelitis.[4]
- CT scan is useful for demonstrating extent of osteomyelitis and may detect radiologic changes earlier than plain radiographs; however, sensitivity is limited at around 67%[5] and may have findings obscured by hardware artifact. Utility may be found in ability to evaluate extent of disease and to create three-dimensional reformats for reconstructive planning.

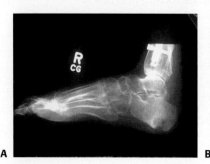

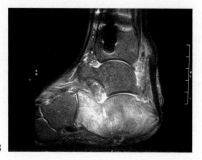

FIG 1 • A. Radiograph of the right foot demonstrating periosteal reaction of the calcaneus indicating osteomyelitis. **B.** Corresponding MRI of the right foot demonstrating the extent of calcaneus osteomyelitis.

- MRI is the most sensitive and specific modality for diagnosis of osteomyelitis, as early as 3 to 5 days (**FIG 1B**).[6,7]

DIFFERENTIAL DIAGNOSIS

- Gout
- Cellulitis
- Plantar fasciitis
- Sickle cell anemia
- Neoplasm (primary or metastasis)

NONOPERATIVE MANAGEMENT

- Acute osteomyelitis without abscess or necrotic component can frequently be treated with isolated intravenous antibiotic therapy for a duration of at least 6 weeks. However, if nonoperative management fails, operative management is indicated.

SURGICAL MANAGEMENT

- Surgical debridement should always be considered and is mandatory for osteomyelitis with any necrotic component and, in combination with antibiotic therapy, is the mainstay of treatment for chronic osteomyelitis.

Preoperative Planning

- Identify need for glucose control, preoperative revascularization, smoking cessation, nutrition optimization, initiation of antiretroviral therapy, address patients ultimate reconstructive goal (eg, flap vs amputation).

- Coordinate with orthopedic surgeon if hardware is in place in order to determine plan for replacement with antibiotic spacer or removal.
- Consider orthopedic surgery consult if large amount of debridement is expected with possible destabilization of ankle joint or foot requiring spanning ex-fix or other temporary stabilization.
- Obtain infectious disease consultation for antibiotic selection and duration.
- A second look procedure should be anticipated and discussed with patient.
- Laboratory studies including complete blood count, sedimentation rate, C-reactive protein, metabolic profile, and blood cultures should be obtained and trended throughout therapy.

Positioning

- Place patient in supine position.
- Prep affected extremity from toes to groin with Betadine.
- Apply either lower extremity drape or split sheet to create sterile field.

Approach

- Principles of therapy include wide debridement, stabilization of remaining bony architecture, culture-guided antimicrobial therapy, and reconstruction of resultant bony defects.[8]

■ Wide Debridement of Bone Infection

- If a wound is present with exposed bone (**TECH FIG 1A**), the wound edges are debrided sharply until healthy, bleeding tissue is reached (**TECH FIG 1B**).
- The underlying bone is inspected for viability.
- Any soft or necrotic bone must be removed with rongeur, curette, or osteotome, until healthy, viable bone is reached (**TECH FIG 1C,D**).
  - If hardware is present, it must also be removed at this time.
- Removed bone is sent to pathology and microbiology for culture and Gram stain.

- The resultant defect is examined for viability. Any remaining nonviable tissue must be removed to prevent reinfecting compromised bone.
- The wound is irrigated copiously with at least 3 L of saline.
- Any dead space must be obliterated with antibiotic beads, cement, or soft tissue to prevent fluid accumulation.
- Bony stabilization can be further provided with plating, screws, or external fixation.
- A sterile, temporary dressing may be applied if second look is anticipated.
- After final debridement, soft tissue coverage must be applied by primary closure, local flap, or free flap.

TECHNIQUES

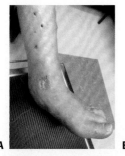
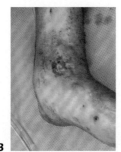
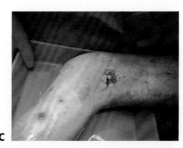
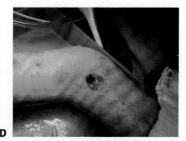

A   B   C   D

TECH FIG 1 • A. Medial malleolar chronic wound with underlying bone involvement. **B.** After wound care, there is no significant change. **C.** Wound after soft tissue debridement. **D.** Wound after debridement of infected bone.

PEARLS AND PITFALLS

Preoperative planning	▪ Lack of patient optimization resulting in poor wound healing. ▪ Lack of plan with orthopedic surgeon for need for removal of hardware, stabilization. ▪ Not considering patient preferences for early amputation and reconstructive goals. ▪ 6-week antibiotics. ▪ Premature, early weight bearing and subsequent fracture.
Technique	▪ Not performing wide enough debridement to reach healthy margins. ▪ Not taking intraoperative cultures for culture-guided therapy. ▪ Not taking a second look.
Postoperative	▪ Inadequate antibiotic duration, failure to follow culture-directed therapy.

POSTOPERATIVE CARE

▪ The patient is continued on antibiotics that may be narrowed when culture data return.

▪ Laboratory values are checked every few days to monitor for response to treatment.

▪ Postoperative radiographs are obtained to document degree of bony resection.

▪ Infectious disease consultation is considered if not already obtained.

▪ The patient is allowed to work with physical therapy but is kept nonweight bearing until final orthopedic reconstruction is completed or stability determined to be sufficient. If soft tissue reconstruction performed, positioning restrictions may vary depending on appearance of flaps.

OUTCOMES

▪ Patients frequently require multiple surgeries for adequate debridement to viable tissue.

▪ With adequate debridement, need for subsequent amputation has been reported to be around 18%, minor 11.7% and major 6.3%.[9]

▪ Long-term limb salvage (avoiding need for major amputation) with surgical management is around 82%.[9]

▪ Persistent infection can be as high as 36% after debridement, underscoring need for adequate debridement of all nonviable tissue.[10]

▪ Overall perioperative mortality has been reported to be 1.6%[11]

COMPLICATIONS

▪ Persistent infection
▪ Fracture

▪ Minor amputation
▪ Major amputation

REFERENCES

1. Parsons B, Strauss E. Surgical management of chronic osteomyelitis. *Am J Surg.* 2004;188(1A suppl):57-66.
2. Nwawka OK, Hayashi D, Diaz LE, et al. Sesamoids and accessory ossicles of the foot: anatomical variability and related pathology. *Insights Imaging.* 2013;4(5):581-593.
3. Pineda C, Espinosa R, Pena A. Radiographic imaging in osteomyelitis: the role of plain radiography, computed tomography, ultrasonography, magnetic resonance imaging, and scintigraphy. *Semin Plast Surg.* 2009;23(2):80-89.
4. Kothari NA, Pelchovitz DP, Meyer PJ. Imaging of musculoskeletal infections. *Radiol Clin North Am.* 2001;39:653-671.
5. Termaat MF, Raijmakers PG, Scholtein HJ, et al. The accuracy of diagnostic imaging for the assessment of chronic osteomyelitis: a systematic review and meta-analysis. *J Bone Joint Surg Am.* 2005;87:2464-2471.
6. Kocher MS, Lee B, Dolan M, et al. Pediatric orthopedic infections; early detection and treatment. *Pediatr Ann.* 2006;35:112-122.
7. Lee YJ, Sadigh S, Mankad K, et al. The imaging of osteomyelitis. *Quant Imaging Med Surg.* 2016;6(2):184-98.
8. Zarutsky E, Rush SM, Schuberth JM. The use of circular wire external fixation in the treatment of salvage ankle arthrodesis. *J Foot Ankle Surg.* 2005;44(1):22-31.
9. Aragón-Sánchez J. Treatment of diabetic foot osteomyelitis: a surgical critique. *Int J Low Extrem Wounds.* 2010;9(1):37-59.
10. Nehler MR, Whitehill TA, Bowers SP, et al. Intermediate-term outcome of primary digit amputations in patients with diabetes mellitus who have forefoot sepsis requiring hospitalization and presumed adequate circulatory status. *J Vasc Surg.* 1999;30:509-517.
11. Henke PK, Blackburn SA, Wainess RW, et al. Osteomyelitis of the foot and toe in adults is a surgical disease: conservative management worsens lower extremity salvage. *Ann Surg.* 2005;241:885-892.

Bony Reconstruction of Foot and Ankle (Bone Grafts)

11

CHAPTER

Kenneth Hunt and Loretta Chou

INTRODUCTION

- Recent decades have witnessed a dramatic increase in available bone graft harvest techniques, bone graft substitutes, and orthobiologic technologies. Despite the extensive availability and marketing of bone graft substitutes, and their purported advantages, autogenous bone graft remains the standard for augmenting healing during arthrodesis and nonunion surgery.
- Autograft bone is the only naturally occurring material purported to possess osteoconductive, osteoinductive, and osteogenic properties. Still, the use of bone grafts in orthopedic surgery has given rise to a multibillion dollar industry but has by no means eradicated nonunions in foot and ankle surgery.[1,2] This chapter will discuss current bone grafting techniques and technologies for foot and ankle procedures in the context of the most common conditions and patient risk factors requiring augmentation for effective healing.

DEFINITION

- Bone grafts in the foot and ankle are most commonly utilized for three indications: (a) increase the union rate for arthrodesis in revisions or joints with a known propensity for nonunion, (b) increase union rate for nonunited fractures, and (c) replace or add bone structure due to chronic or acute bone loss. The focus of this chapter is bone grafting techniques to illustrate these three indications. We include some specific, common foot pathology that requires bone grafting, but an inclusive review of foot and ankle pathologies and disease processes is outside of the scope of this chapter.
- By far, the most common use of bone graft in the foot and ankle is to aid in healing for joint arthrodesis. The degeneration of joints requiring fusion can occur as a result of a number of disease processes, including post-traumatic arthritis, degenerative joint disease (DJD), posterior tibial tendon insufficiency, trauma, congenital deformity, inflammatory or crystalline arthropathy, Charcot neuropathy, diabetes, avascular necrosis, tumor, and many other causes.
- Bone graft is generally incorporated to aid in healing when the risk of nonunion is unacceptably high. This is the case in patients who might have a suboptimal biologic healing response, including those with a history of smoking, diabetes, neuropathy, obesity, or a history of nonunion.[3-5]
- The procedures in the foot and ankle that most commonly involve bone graft application include ankle, subtalar (ST), tibiotalocalcaneal (TTC), triple, tibiocalcaneal (TC),

talonavicular (TN), calcaneocuboid (CC), naviculocuneiform (NC), and tarsometatarsal (TMT) arthrodesis, and most nonunion repairs. Due to the paucity and inconsistency of literature on the topic, the decision to use bone graft, and which type or material to use (ie, cancellous vs structural, harvest site, autograft vs allograft, bone graft substitutes, etc.), is dependent upon a host of patient factors and surgeon experience.

- Generally speaking, cancellous autograft generally has a higher surface area and greater content of growth factors and remains the standard for its ability to induce more new bone formation than cortical (ie, structural) autograft or allografts.[6] Structural autograft is often required when significant bone loss or deformity is present, as a means of restoring length, height, and/or alignment. The fast-growing arsenal of "orthobiologics" as substitutes for autograft are purported to rival autograft in terms of timing and rate of healing, without the morbidity of autograft harvest.

ANATOMY

- The foot and ankle is composed of 28 bones. There are multiple joints, muscles, tendons, and ligaments. The foot can be divided into the medial and lateral columns. The medial column includes the talus, navicular, cuneiforms, and medial three metatarsals. The lateral column is made up of the calcaneus, cuboid, and lateral two metatarsals. Any injury, deformity, or defect can result in length alterations or stiffness in one or more columns of the foot. This can lead to pain, imbalance, and problems with weight bearing on a foot that is not plantigrade, unstable, or painful.
- The ankle joint allows for most of the extension and flexion. The subtalar joint provides inversion and eversion, whereas the transverse tarsal joint (talonavicular and calcaneal cuboid) gives adduction and abduction.
- The foot and ankle is responsible for gait. The heel is the first point of contact in the normal gait cycle. As the foot rolls forward, the foot changes from a flexible valgus position to a rigid varus position for push off.
- The anatomy of the iliac crest, for the purposes of graft harvest discussed herein, is fairly easy to identify and superficial. The graft harvests described below are generally harvested from 2 to 4 cm above the anterior superior iliac spine (ASIS). The crest at this location can usually be palpated. Keeping the incision and dissection at least 2 cm proximal to the ASIS to avoid injury to the lateral femoral cutaneous nerve.

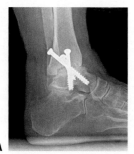 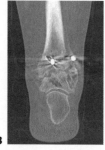

FIG 1 • A. Plain lateral radiograph. **B.** Coronal and sagittal CT scan images depicting a nonunion of ankle arthrodesis.

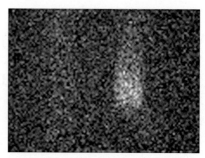

FIG 2 • Tagged WBC study demonstrating increased uptake in the left ankle compared to the right.

PATHOGENESIS

- The foot and ankle are the most peripheral structures in the body and are dependent during most physical activities. As a result, the foot and ankle are at higher risk of peripheral neuropathy, peripheral vascular disease, and other contributors to delayed or nonhealing of fusions or fracture fixation.
- The weight-bearing role of the foot and the complexity of biomechanics for normal foot and ankle function place many regions of the foot and ankle at higher risk for abnormal loading, further contributing to delayed- or nonunion of fractures, arthrodesis, or osteotomies.
- Patient risk factors known to contribute to nonhealing of bone include smoking, diabetes, age and osteoporosis, peripheral vascular disease, neuropathy, noncompliance, infection, and soft tissue injury.[4]

NATURAL HISTORY

- The disorders of the foot and ankle are broad and significant and include trauma, arthritis, congenital, acquired, sports injuries, and degenerative conditions. With severe deformities or trauma, structural loss or nonhealing of fractures or fusions frequently lead to worsening of the disorder and pain and function, over time. Reconstructive operations may be required to repair such problems. In cases where there is need to add structural bone, or add biology, bone grafting procedures are commonly considered.

PATIENT HISTORY AND PHYSICAL FINDINGS

- A thorough history is essential preoperatively. Patients are asked about injuries, chronicity, comorbidities, previous operations, and nonoperative treatment. Also, the patient's occupation and social situation are important considerations.
- Medical history should be considered when determining risk factors and the best bone graft to use. Social history is also important because patients may have particular traditions and beliefs governing whether autograft or allograft materials are acceptable. The beliefs should, and generally can, be respected during development of a treatment plan.
- The physical examination takes place with the patient undressed from the knees to the toes. Gait is evaluated, as well as the skin, noting edema, scars, erythema, masses, and bony deformities. The neurovascular status is carefully examined. Evaluating potential graft sites is also important.

- The foot and ankle examination can help guide surgical approach and counseling. Incisions should be made where soft tissue disruption, particularly of the well-vascularized periosteum, can be minimized. Old incisions should be incorporated whenever possible, especially when the procedure was recent.

IMAGING

- Most nonunions and malunions of fractures, fusions, and osteotomies can be diagnosed on plain radiographs (**FIG 1A**).
- For joints that are difficult to see on plain radiographs, or for complicated procedures with a large fixation construct, a CT scan is the best study to diagnose nonunion (**FIG 1B**).
- MRI scan plays little role in diagnosing nonunion but can be helpful to evaluate soft tissue structures, which may contribute to symptoms, and is a sensitive study for osteomyelitis.
- Nuclear medicine studies can aid in diagnosis of infection and osteomyelitis, which is a common contributor to nonhealing of bone (**FIG 2**).

DIFFERENTIAL DIAGNOSIS

- Hypertrophic nonunion
- Oligotrophic nonunion
- Septic (infected) nonunion
- Malunion
- Avascular necrosis of bone
- Failure of fixation

NONOPERATIVE MANAGEMENT

- Nonoperative treatment for many foot and ankle disorders include activity modification, ambulatory aid, such as a cane or crutch. Physical therapy, brace, or orthotic device may be helpful. Oral medications can help reduce pain, although one must be aware of risks (eg, NSAIDs can contributed to delayed healing, narcotic analgesics carry risk of dependency).
- Severe deformities may be difficult to accommodate or fit into a brace, and surgical options should be considered.
- In general, if patients have persistent pain, dysfunction, problems working or participating in activities of daily living, or if there are risks to other structures or to the patient by continuing nonoperative management, surgery should be considered.

SURGICAL MANAGEMENT

- The decision to augment a fusion, osteotomy, or fracture with graft is dependent on many factors, including surgeon preference and experience. Grafts should, in general, be added to increase both the likelihood and the timing of bone union in cases where nonunion or delayed union is unacceptably high. Examples include revision cases and patients with risk factors outlined above.
- The authors prefer autograft iliac crest bone graft for most indications where there is high risk of nonunion. When structural grafts are necessary to span a cortical gap in bone, structural autograft from the iliac crest is generally sufficient for most procedures in the foot. Ankle and hindfoot bone loss often requires larger allografts, such as femoral head or fibular grafts.
- Orthobiologics can be used in lieu of, or in addition to, other graft materials, or to add a large dose of specific growth factors to the fusion site. Examples of such orthobiologic therapies include platelet-rich plasma (PRP), bone marrow aspirate concentrate (BMAC), bone morphogenetic proteins (BMP), and platelet-derived growth factor (PDGF). The enormous recent growth of the number of available biologic products carries with it a high cost and a paucity of data on safety, effectiveness, and clinical outcomes for many products, particularly compared to the iliac crest bone graft standard. It is the responsibility of the surgeon to judiciously utilize these products with a thorough knowledge of their mechanism(s) of action, approved indications, side effect profiles, and cost.
- The ultimate goal of any fusion, osteotomy, or fracture repair operation is bone healing, pain relief, and return to optimal function while avoiding complications, prolonged hospitalization, and revision operations. When a graft is selected, the surgeon must balance necessity, cost, comorbid factors, and risk and have a keen understanding of the selected graft(s) and technique.

Preoperative Planning

- Plain weight-bearing radiographs of the foot and/or ankle are necessary for complete evaluation (**FIG 3A**).
- Other imaging studies may be helpful. MRI may show extent of infection or the presence of avascular necrosis. CT scans confirm nonunion and show bone quality and structural bone loss, bony defects and deformities (**FIG 3B,C**).
- A complete evaluation of the skin and adjacent structures must be performed, using radiographs when prudent. This should include the surgical site in the foot or ankle and any potential graft harvest site.

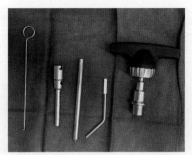

FIG 4 • Photograph illustrating components of a coring reamer setup for harvesting of autograft cancellous bone graft. These include a coring reamer (7 mm diameter pictured here), a tipped trochar, and a T handle. Alternatively, power tools can be utilized with caution.

- A thorough discussion of risks and the postoperative course (which can be prolonged) should be had with the patient because compliance is vital to success.
- Ensure that appropriate equipment is available prior to starting the case. A good coring reamer is helpful for cancellous graft harvest (**FIG 4**). Osteotomes and retractors can help to expose and harvest cortical grafts. Allografts and biologics should be requested if these might be required.
- Plan for size and volume. It is important to estimate the amount of graft that will need to be harvested for a given procedure.

Positioning

- Most cases are performed with the patient in a supine position. This also facilitates graft harvest for most sites.
- The patient is typically positioned toward the edge of the bed to facilitate access to the foot and ankle.
- Generally, the autograft is harvested on the ipsilateral extremity. The graft site undergoes sterile preparation and draping along with the surgical extremity (**FIG 5A**).
- With distal lower extremity autografts, we advised that the patient have protected weight bearing in a cast or brace for the primary procedure, which also allows for healing of the harvest site.

Approach

- In the primary surgery setting, the decision to use bone graft is complex and based on the criteria outlined above. Once this decision is made, preoperative planning using available imaging should be undertaken. The surgical approach should ensure avoidance of injury to neurovascular structures and minimizing soft tissue disruption.

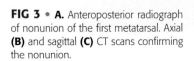
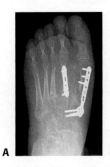
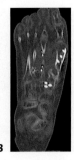
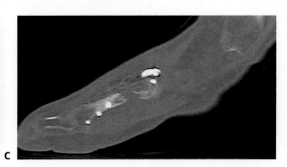

FIG 3 • **A.** Anteroposterior radiograph of nonunion of the first metatarsal. Axial **(B)** and sagittal **(C)** CT scans confirming the nonunion.

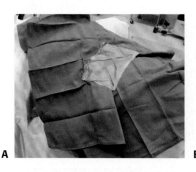

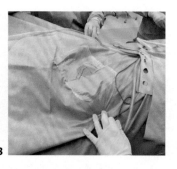

FIG 5 • A,B. Prep and draping of iliac crest harvest site.

- For nonunion surgery, once a symptomatic nonunion is diagnosed and appropriate conservative measures have been taken toward healing and restoration of function, the use of bone graft is considered for revision surgical options.
- The approach for graft harvest is based on access to sufficient graft volume for the indication while avoiding

large bone defects, bleeding, and injury to surrounding structures. We will specifically discuss and illustrate the four most common graft harvest sites for foot and ankle indications: the anterior iliac crest (structural and/or cancellous), the proximal tibia, and the calcaneal tuberosity.

■ Technique 1: Iliac Crest Autograft Harvest (Tricortical Structural)

- This technique is described in another chapter.
- Briefly, the ipsilateral hip is positioned with a well-padded bump. The area is draped after sterile surgical prep. An iodine barrier may be placed (**FIG 5B**).
- The incision site may be injected with lidocaine plus epinephrine to decrease bleeding.
- The anatomic landmarks are palpated, and a longitudinal incision is made along the iliac crest, starting 2 cm above the ASIS. The soft tissue is bluntly dissected until the periosteum is exposed.
- The periosteum is incised in line with the incision and the crest. Once bone is identified, subperiosteal dissection is performed to expose the crest. Great care must be taken to avoid penetration of the medial structures, especially if the inner table is required as part of the graft harvest.

- The size of the graft must be determined at this point, based on the defect size (**TECH FIG 1A,B**).
- Structural cortical or tricortical graft is removed with a saw or osteotomes (**TECH FIG 1C**).
- The graft is shaped to fit the defect (**TECH FIG 1D–F**). Additional cancellous graft can be harvested from the crest if needed to fill gaps.
- Appropriate fixation is applied to stabilize the graft (**TECH FIG 1G,H**).
- Following harvest, the iliac crest area can be packed with Gelfoam and thrombin to aid in hemostasis.
- Allograft cancellous chips can be used to pack the harvest site. This can provide hemostasis as well as filling of the defect.
- Periosteum is closed after hemostasis is achieved followed by layered closure of the overlying soft tissue and skin (**TECH FIG 1I**)

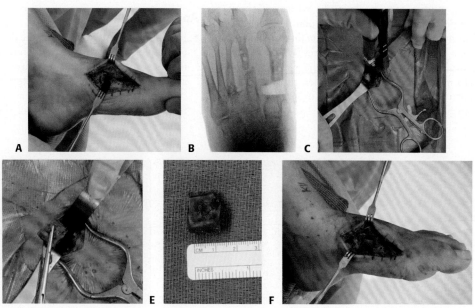

TECH FIG 1 • A. Clinical photograph of bone defect requiring structural graft. **B.** Intraoperative fluoroscopic image showing the defect. **C.** Photograph of sagittal saw used for iliac crest structural harvest. **D–F.** Harvesting of iliac crest bone segment measuring 1.3 cm, appropriate to fill defect.

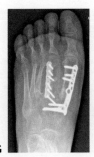 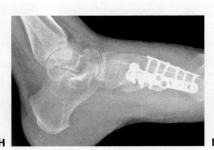 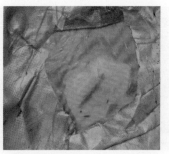

TECH FIG 1 (Continued) • **G.** Anteroposterior. **H.** Lateral radiographs showing fixation of structural graft. **I.** Closure of iliac crest harvest site with absorbable subcuticular stitch.

Technique 2: Iliac Crest Autograft Harvest (Cancellous)

- This technique is for cases where cancellous autograft is indicated. The iliac crest cancellous bone contains the highest concentration of growth factors of the sites described in this chapter. Because it is a non–weight-bearing bone, this also mitigates risk of fracture postoperatively.
- As above, the ipsilateral hip is positioned with a well-padded bump. The area is draped after sterile surgical prep. An iodine barrier may be placed.
- The incision site may be injected with lidocaine plus epinephrine to decrease bleeding.
- The landmarks are palpated, and a small longitudinal incision is made along the iliac crest (usually about 1 cm in length), starting 2 cm above the ASIS. The soft tissue is bluntly dissected until the periosteum is exposed.
- The periosteum is incised in line with the incision and the crest. Once bone is identified, a trochar is used to create a defect in cortical bone (**TECH FIG 2A**).
- Next, a coring reamer is used to penetrate cortical bone penetrating up to 2 cm deep into the crest (**TECH FIG 2B–D**).
- Up to three passes (central, distal, proximal) can be made through one bone window. If additional graft is required, a second bone window should be created proximal to the end of the most proximal reaming pass.
- The periosteum is closed after hemostasis is achieved followed by layered closure of overlying soft tissue and skin.

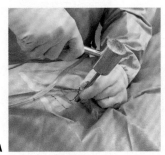 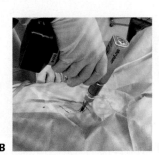 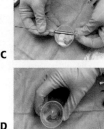

TECH FIG 2 • **A.** Trochar and mallet used to create starting point in iliac crest for cancellous harvest. **B–D.** Coring reamer used to harvest iliac crest cancellous bone.

Technique 3: Proximal Tibia Autograft Harvest

- As with iliac crest autograft, it is ideal to obtain proximal tibia autograft from the ipsilateral tibia.
- The patient is placed in the supine position. A thigh tourniquet is used to create a bloodless field.
- A longitudinal incision is made medial to the tibia tubercle, about 1 cm (**TECH FIG 3A**).
- The periosteum is elevated, and the tibia metaphysis is identified. Small drill holes are made in a circular pattern.
- An osteotome is used to connect the drill holes, beveling the cortical window. The window is saved (**TECH FIG 3B**).
- Curettes or gouges are used to remove cancellous bone (**TECH FIG 3C,D**).
- The window is replaced and the wound closed in layers.

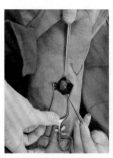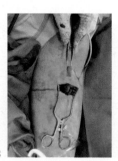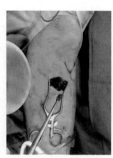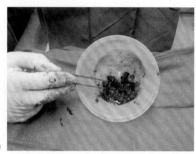

TECH FIG 3 • A. Incision for proximal tibia cancellous graft harvest. Marked V indicates tibial tubercle, **(B)** cortical window allowing access to cancellous bone of proximal tibia. **C.** Photograph illustrating curettage of cancellous bone from the proximal tibia, and **(D)** sample of typical harvest yield from proximal tibia.

■ Technique 4: Calcaneal Autograft Harvest

- Calcaneal bone graft is generally obtained from the ipsilateral calcaneus.
- In order to mitigate the risk of donor site fracture, this graft harvest is best selected in the setting of a procedure that will require a period of nonweight bearing.
- The patient is placed in the supine position. A calf or thigh tourniquet is used.
- Landmarks are identified first, including the tip of the calcaneal tuberosity, the peroneal tendons, and the distal fibula.
- A 2-cm oblique incision is made parallel and inferior to the peroneal tendons through the skin only, with blunt dissection down to bone and protection of the branches of the sural nerve (**TECH FIG 4A**).

- Elevation of the periosteum of the lateral calcaneus is performed to expose the cortical bone.
- A small diameter (7–8 mm) coring reamer is used to harvest cancellous bone from of the posterior tuberosity of the calcaneus (**TECH FIG 4B**). Multiple passes can be made through the same window, depending on volume need.
- The graft is collected in a small cup or receptacle such that appropriate volume can be assessed before discontinuing graft harvest (**TECH FIG 4C**).
- If required, additional bone can be curetted from the area, but use caution not to penetrate the far cortices.
- The skin is closed with 4-0 monofilament absorbable subcutaneous sutures, skin tape, and a period of nonweight bearing determined by the primary procedure.

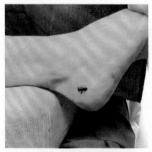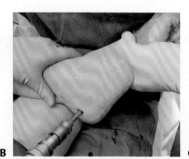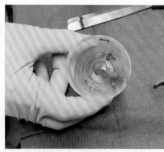

TECH FIG 4 • A. Incision for calcaneal graft harvest. **B.** Coring reamer for calcaneal graft harvest. **C.** Resulting yield of calcaneal graft harvest.

■ Technique 5: Bone Marrow Aspirate Concentrate

In cases where structural graft is not necessary, but there is a desire to supplement biology with autograft marrow rich in stem cells, autograft bone marrow can be a valuable adjunct. This is usually harvested from the ipsilateral iliac crest, because this is the location with the greatest concentration of growth factors.[7]

- Bone marrow aspirate can be administered in three ways:
  - As an isolated graft injection
  - Combined with demineralized bone matrix (DBM)
  - Bone marrow aspirate concentration (BMAC) of growth factors

- Harvesting of bone marrow from the iliac crest:
  - The iliac crest undergoes sterile prep at the same time as the ipsilateral foot.
  - A separate sterile drape is used after prep, using sterile towels, followed by sterile iodoform drape. After the final sterile drape is placed, a small hole is cut in the drape and a second iodoform drape is used to seal the crest site (see **FIG 5**).
  - Bone marrow should be harvested just prior to its administration to optimize the viability of cells. A small incision is made with a no. 15 blade. It is essentially a puncture, just the width of the blade, providing room for the Jamshidi needle.

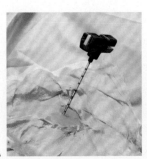 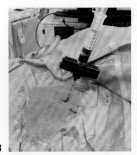 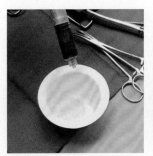 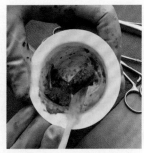

TECH FIG 5 • A. Jamshidi needle placed in iliac crest through percutaneous incision. **B.** Syringe attaches to Jamshidi needle and 2 cc of iliac crest withdrawn. **C.** Bone marrow aspirate can be combined with DBM to create a cellular putty to fill small defects.

- A Jamshidi needle is advanced to the iliac crest. Direct palpation assures that the needle is centered in the crest and directed centrally, between the inner and outer tables (**TECH FIG 5A**). It is important to ensure that the inner table is not penetrated during harvest.
- Advance the needle about 1 to 2 cm into the crest and aspirate 2 cc. Then, redirect and advance the needle about 2 cm and withdraw an additional 2 cc. This can be repeated until sufficient volume has been harvested (**TECH FIG 5B**). The highest concentration of cells is in the first 2 cc at each location.[8]

- The BMA can be combined with DBM to create a cellular putty (**TECH FIG 5C**). This can be administered where small defects are present in joints and fractures with oligotrophic nonunions. This can be injected percutaneously in some cases to avoid disruption of blood supply.[9]
- Alternatively, larger volumes of bone marrow can be harvested and concentrated using a commercially available system and injected into the fracture or fusion site.[10]

▪ Technique 6: Concentrated Synthetic Growth Factors

There are many synthetic growth factors available to help augment healing of nonunions and at-risk procedures in the foot and ankle. Although a more thorough discussion is beyond the scope of this chapter, this is an important consideration for bone graft options. More detailed descriptions can be found elsewhere in the literature.[11–13]

- Examples of available bone graft substitutes along with a brief description include the following:
  - Bone morphogenetic protein (BMP-2)
  - Platelet-derived growth factor (PDGF)
  - Demineralized bone matrix (DBM)
  - Hydroxyapatite
- Limitations to utilization of these substances can include cost, FDA approval status (often limited for foot and ankle indications), and availability.

PEARLS AND PITFALLS

Hemostasis	▪ Hemostasis must be obtained at the graft site prior to closure of skin in order to avoid bleeding, hematoma, and wound complications.
Controlling hemostasis	▪ Lidocaine with epinephrine helps to control bleeding from the subcutaneous tissue. ▪ Gelfoam and thrombin helps reduce postoperative bleeding.
Volume yield	▪ The iliac crest bone graft harvest yields the greatest amount of cancellous graft. ▪ Autograft from the proximal tibia may yield sufficient cancellous graft for many foot and ankle procedures.
Technique	▪ Beveling the cortical window will prevent the window from falling into the tibia.
Wound closure	▪ Closure with an absorbable monofilament subcuticular stitch and skin tape can provide a more cosmetic and less painful scar.
Plan ahead	▪ Ensure that appropriate equipment for harvest and/or graft material is available for the procedure. ▪ Estimate the volume and quality of graft required such that appropriate harvest sites and techniques can be utilized.

POSTOPERATIVE CARE

■ Generally, the autograft is harvested from the ipsilateral limb, to facilitate protected weight bearing and frequently with a splint or cast. Crutches or knee scooter devices are used in many of the procedures. The harvest site may heal in 6 to 12 weeks. Sutures may be removed at 2 weeks. Range of motion exercises may then begin at that time.

OUTCOMES

■ There are a considerable number of reports in the literature addressing bone grafting techniques and their impact on fusion rates following reconstructive surgeries. Contributing factors include the breadth of procedures and diagnoses, the impact (or poor reporting) of patient factors, and inconsistent indications for bone grafting. Although most available data come from level IV and V data, some meaningful conclusions can be drawn.

■ Lareau et al.[14] reported a systematic review of the literature on bone grafting for the foot and ankle. While underscoring the need for more level I and II evidence to better guide our use of bone graft adjuvants during foot and ankle surgery, their pooled data demonstrated a trend toward favoring the use of cancellous autograft, structural autograft, or cancellous allograft over using no graft material during fusion surgery.[14] They suggest that using no graft leads to nonunion rates of only about 10% (ie, a greater than 90% union rate), whereas the addition of cancellous autograft, structural autograft, or cancellous allograft reduced the nonunion rate by half.

COMPLICATIONS

■ Complications from autograft from the iliac crest include infection, nerve injury, painful scar, nonunion, and pain. Harvest from the proximal and distal tibia or calcaneus may result in infection, numbness, and rarely fracture through the graft site. Superficial infections may be treated with local wound care and oral antibiotics. Rarely, the infection is deep, requiring surgical debridement and intravenous antibiotics.

REFERENCES

1. Mann RA, Prieskorn D, Sobel M. Mid-tarsal and tarsometatarsal arthrodesis for primary degenerative osteoarthrosis or osteoarthrosis after trauma. *J Bone Joint Surg Am.* 1996;78(9):1376-1385.
2. Thevendran G, Younger A, Pinney S. Current concepts review: risk factors for nonunions in foot and ankle arthrodeses. *Foot Ankle Int.* 2012;33(11):1031-1040.
3. O'Connor KM, et al. Clinical and operative factors related to successful revision arthrodesis in the foot and ankle. *Foot Ankle Int.* 2016;37(8):809-815.
4. Thevendran G, et al. Nonunion risk assessment in foot and ankle surgery: proposing a predictive risk assessment model. *Foot Ankle Int.* 2015;36(8):901-907.
5. Bettin CC, et al. Cigarette smoking increases complication rate in forefoot surgery. *Foot Ankle Int.* 2015;36(5):488-493.
6. Friedlaender GE. Bone grafts. The basic science rationale for clinical applications. *J Bone Joint Surg Am.* 1987;69(5):786-790.
7. Hyer CF, et al. Quantitative assessment of the yield of osteoblastic connective tissue progenitors in bone marrow aspirate from the iliac crest, tibia, and calcaneus. *J Bone Joint Surg Am.* 2013; 95(14):1312-1316.
8. Muschler GF, Boehm C, Easley K. Aspiration to obtain osteoblast progenitor cells from human bone marrow: the influence of aspiration volume. *J Bone Joint Surg Am.* 1997;79(11):1699-1709.
9. Hunt KJ, Anderson RB. Treatment of Jones fracture nonunions and refractures in the elite athlete: outcomes of intramedullary screw fixation with bone grafting. *Am J Sports Med.* 2011;39(9):1948-1954.
10. Murawski CD, Kennedy JG. Percutaneous internal fixation of proximal fifth metatarsal jones fractures (Zones II and III) with Charlotte Carolina screw and bone marrow aspirate concentrate: an outcome study in athletes. *Am J Sports Med.* 2011;39(6):1295-1301.
11. Arner JW, Santrock RD. historical review of common bone graft materials in foot and ankle surgery. *Foot Ankle Spec.* 2014;7(2): 143-151.
12. DiGiovanni CW, Lin S, Pinzur M. Recombinant human PDGF-BB in foot and ankle fusion. *Expert Rev Med Devices.* 2012;9(2):111-122.
13. Rearick T, Charlton TP, Thordarson D. Effectiveness and complications associated with recombinant human bone morphogenetic protein-2 augmentation of foot and ankle fusions and fracture nonunions. *Foot Ankle Int.* 2014;35(8):783-788.
14. Lareau CR, et al. Does autogenous bone graft work? A logistic regression analysis of data from 159 papers in the foot and ankle literature. *Foot Ankle Surg.* 2015;21(3):150-159.

Reconstruction of the Forefoot

Rachel Hein and Scott T. Hollenbeck

DEFINITION

- The primary goal in forefoot reconstruction is to preserve function of the lower extremity. Given the unique bony and skin arrangements in the foot as well as the high functional demand for this area, an understanding of multiple reconstructive approaches is necessary.

ANATOMY

- The forefoot contains the distal third of the foot from the base of the metatarsals to the distal phalanges of the toes on both the plantar and dorsal surfaces of the foot.
- The plantar surface of the foot has highly specialized glabrous skin with a thick epidermis. Beneath the skin and subcutaneous tissue is the plantar aponeurosis, which is a thick fibrous band adherent to the skin. This resists shearing forces as it attaches to the skin via the retinaculum cutis ligaments distal to the metatarsals. In contrast, the dorsal skin of the forefoot is extremely thin and relatively mobile.
- The bones of the forefoot are somewhat analogous to the hand with the first toe containing only a distal and proximal phalanx. The second through the fifth toes have a middle phalanx. There are five metatarsal bones, which span from the midfoot bones (cuneiforms and cuboid) to the proximal phalanx of each digit.
- There are four separate plantar fascia compartments and one dorsal fascial compartment that are divided by intermuscular septa. These separate the intrinsic muscles of the foot.
  - The medial and lateral compartments are the most relevant for reconstruction as the muscles are most superficial and amenable to flap use. Of note, the medial compartment contains the abductor hallucis (AH) and flexor hallucis brevis (FHB) whereas the lateral compartment contains the abductor digiti minimi (ADM) (**FIG 1**).
- There are extrinsic and intrinsic muscles of the foot.
  - The extrinsic muscles originate in the leg and insert onto the bones of the foot.
  - The peroneus tendons insert onto the 5th metatarsal and allow for foot eversion.
  - The extensor digitorum longus (EDL) tendons insert onto an extensor mechanism of each of the lateral four digits.
  - The extensor hallucis longus (EHL) tendon has its own muscular unit and inserts onto the first phalanx.

- In addition to the digit extending muscles, the foot may be brought into extension by the tibialis anterior (TA), which inserts onto the medial cuneiform/first metatarsal junction.
- Preservation of at least one of these three systems is needed to prevent a functional footdrop. The digital flexors have a similar arrangement to the extensors, with the flexor digitorum longus (FDL) inserting onto each of the lateral four digits and the flexor hallucis longus (FHL) tendon inserting onto the first toe.
- Plantar flexion is primarily driven by the Achilles mechanism of the heel, but digit flexors do have some importance as it pertains to the toe push off phase of the gait cycle.
  - The intrinsic muscles are contained in the compartments of the foot and primarily act on the toes.
- The flexor digitorum brevis (FDB) occupies the central aspect of the superficial muscles of the plantar surface of the foot. There are two additional deep layers of muscles in the plantar foot that are not commonly used in reconstructive surgery.
- Secondary action of intrinsic muscles includes maintaining posture and foot concavity.
- The dorsal aspect of the foot is primarily made up of the extrinsic tendons, deeper intrinsic digit extensors, and still deeper interosseous muscles.
- The main vascular supply to the foot comes from the posterior tibial artery. The artery splits into the medial and lateral plantar arteries beneath the flexor retinaculum. These two arteries join at the base of the metatarsals to form the deep plantar arch.
  - The lateral plantar artery is the dominant artery supplying the fourth and fifth toes through metatarsal and then proper digital arteries.
  - The medial artery supplies the first through third toes in a similar fashion. The dorsalis pedis artery supplies the dorsum of the foot and also gives terminal branches completing the plantar arch. For reconstructive purposes, the plantar intrinsic muscles of the foot are typically supplied via the medial and lateral plantar arteries (**FIG 2**).
- Cutaneous sensation to the forefoot is supplied via terminal branches of the sciatic nerve. The plantar surface of the forefoot sensation is mainly derived from the medial plantar nerve (tibial origin) and the lateral plantar nerves (tibial origin).

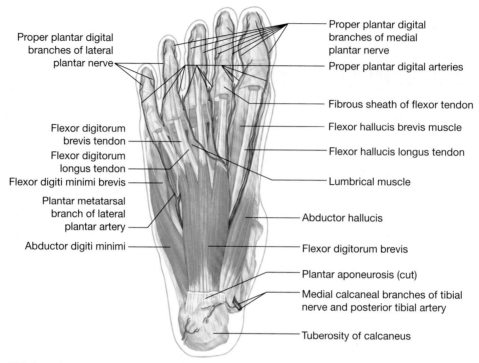

Proper plantar digital branches of lateral plantar nerve

Proper plantar digital branches of medial plantar nerve

Proper plantar digital arteries

Fibrous sheath of flexor tendon

Flexor digitorum brevis tendon

Flexor digitorum longus tendon

Flexor digiti minimi brevis

Plantar metatarsal branch of lateral plantar artery

Abductor digiti minimi

Flexor hallucis brevis muscle

Flexor hallucis longus tendon

Lumbrical muscle

Abductor hallucis

Flexor digitorum brevis

Plantar aponeurosis (cut)

Medial calcaneal branches of tibial nerve and posterior tibial artery

Tuberosity of calcaneus

FIG 1 • Sole of foot.

- The dorsal forefoot sensation is mainly derived from the superficial peroneal nerves (common peroneal origin) and the unique first web space distribution of the deep peroneal nerve (common peroneal, sciatic, L5 origin).
- Motor innervation of the intrinsic foot muscles is mainly through the medial and lateral plantar nerves[1] (see **FIG 2**).

PATHOGENESIS

- Traumatic foot injuries are typically associated with high-energy events. This may lead to extensive and complex wounds involving lacerations, contusions, skin degloving, open fractures, and severe crush injuries.

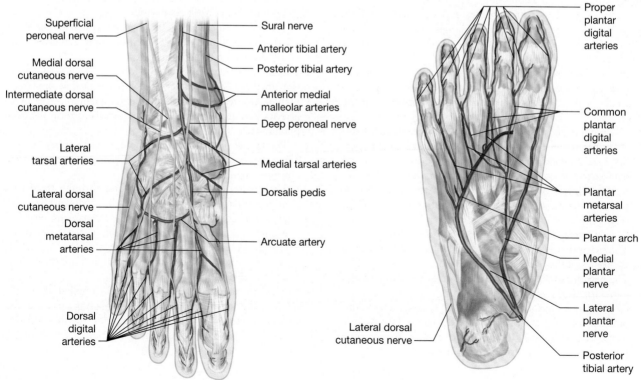

Superficial peroneal nerve

Medial dorsal cutaneous nerve

Intermediate dorsal cutaneous nerve

Lateral tarsal arteries

Lateral dorsal cutaneous nerve

Dorsal metatarsal arteries

Dorsal digital arteries

Sural nerve

Anterior tibial artery

Posterior tibial artery

Anterior medial malleolar arteries

Deep peroneal nerve

Medial tarsal arteries

Dorsalis pedis

Arcuate artery

Proper plantar digital arteries

Common plantar digital arteries

Plantar metatarsal arteries

Plantar arch

Medial plantar nerve

Lateral plantar nerve

Posterior tibial artery

Lateral dorsal cutaneous nerve

A

B

FIG 2 • **A,B.** Anatomy of the foot, vessels, and nerves.

- Cancerous lesions may require extensive surgical resection and reconstruction within the foot. Many of these are amenable to isolated digit or ray amputation but some may require large skin resections on weight-bearing areas of the foot.
- Postsurgical complications following foot and ankle surgery may also present with complex problems involving necrotic skin, exposed tendons, colonized hardware and bony nonunion.
- Chronic vascular disease including venous stasis and peripheral vascular disease can be a cause of tissue loss within the forefoot. This should mainly be addressed by controlling the inciting factor. Amputation and debridement are often needed in these cases prior to any consideration of reconstruction.
- Diabetes is a major contributor to forefoot wounds and ulcers. Many of these patients have diabetic neuropathy and develop pressure-related ulcers over the metatarsal heads. Prior to consideration of reconstruction, the patient's status should be optimized and nonsurgical options should be considered. This may include weight-bearing restrictions and/or use of shoe inserts to deflect pressure away from the affected area.[2]

NATURAL HISTORY

- The lower extremity is commonly involved in motor vehicle injuries, and this is the most common scenario requiring forefoot reconstruction. These are often complex injuries and may involve multiple levels of the lower extremity and multiple systems within the patient. Standard principles of trauma care must be followed. Once the patient has been stabilized, foot reconstruction may involve a multidisciplinary limb salvage team including plastic and orthopedic surgeons.
- A unique trauma scenario involving the forefoot is that related to lawn mower injuries and amputations. These are often isolated foot injuries but may be severe in nature.
- Replantation of amputated digits is not typically performed in the lower extremity.

PATIENT HISTORY AND PHYSICAL FINDINGS

- Gait cycle and biomechanics
  - Reconstructive surgeons managing wounds of the foot should be familiar with the gait cycle as it pertains to functional outcomes. Classically, there are three cycles of the stance phase of ambulation including heel strike, midstance, and propulsion. This is followed by the noncontact swing phase.
  - For the purpose of forefoot injuries, it is important to note that high pressures occur during propulsion and include the final contact point at the first toe. Higher pressures and abnormal gait may lead to skin breakdown and development of wounds over the forefoot.[3]
- Evaluation of forefoot wounds
  - Initial evaluation of a patient with an acute traumatic injury to the foot includes assessment of the mechanism, energy, and contamination associated with the event. This often occurs during the initial washout and debridement of the wound. The associated soft tissue injury and underlying bony injury should be appreciated as well as the integrity of the vascular and neurologic systems within the foot.

- Understanding a patient's underlying comorbidities as well as preinjury functional status and work demands is also important.
- Doppler examination is useful to determine arterial perfusion as well as planning for operative intervention. However, severe edema may prevent accurate Doppler assessment, and additional angiographic studies may be required. Any presumed acute arterial injury warrants a vascular surgery consultation and subsequent evaluation for compartment syndrome.[4]
- Neurologic evaluation of the injured foot may be limited due to associated neuropraxia and tissue edema. Declaration of a nonsalvageable foot based on neurological injury should be deferred during the acute injury phase.
- For chronic wounds, duration of wound and measurements should be taken including length, width, and depth. Involvement of skin, dermis, fascia, muscle, tendon, and bone should be noted as well as any concurrent cellulitis. Photographs should be taken, and previous therapies should be noted. Gait analysis is also important in these patients as disease processes can affect weight bearing over the forefoot. Vascular and neurological status is also important to take into account.

IMAGING

- The physical exam will dictate the imaging studies needed when evaluating foot wounds. In the trauma setting, plain films are typically obtained first to rule out fractures. In some circumstances, a CT scan or MRI is obtained for better bony and ligamentous imaging. Angiography is typically reserved when evaluating more proximal injuries, but may be useful on certain occasions.
- Chronic infectious wounds such as diabetic ulcers and postoperative wound breakdown require plain films to rule out pathologic fractures and gas in the subcutaneous tissues along with MRI to rule out osteomyelitis. Bone biopsies are the standard, but MRI may help delineate operative management in these cases. Ankle-brachial indices and duplex arteriogram should be obtained to assess arterial insufficiency and need for possible vascular intervention.

DIFFERENTIAL DIAGNOSIS

- Traumatic
- Postsurgical
- Infectious
- Diabetic
- Acute arterial
- Venous ulceration
- Connective tissue disorder

NONOPERATIVE MANAGEMENT

- Traditionally, dressing changes are helpful for managing small superficial wounds through healing by secondary intent. Negative pressure wound therapy (NPWT) may also be used to achieve secondary healing or to prepare a complex wound bed for a skin graft or flap.
- Newer wound dressings have also aided in the treatment of open forefoot injuries including semipermeable dressings, hydrocolloids, and hydrogels. These new dressings can aid in chemical debridement as well as hydration of the wound.

Additionally, synthetic products and xenograft products exist and may have some utility in managing these wounds. More data are needed to prove the clinical efficacy of these treatments.

- Hyperbaric oxygen (HBO) treatment may be used as an adjunct to traditional wound healing methods but remains somewhat unproven in its efficacy for foot wounds. HBO works by promoting angiogenesis and ultimately increasing the amount of vascularity in the wound bed, thereby promoting wound healing. It may be indicated in crush injuries, refractory osteomyelitis, and gas gangrene.

SURGICAL MANAGEMENT

Preoperative Planning

- Debridement remains one of the most important preoperative principles in lower extremity salvage. For an acute wound, it is important to perform serial debridement if necessary until all nonviable tissue has been removed. Chronic wounds should be serially debrided until negative cultures are obtained. Comorbidities should be managed for optimization.
- Once a decision has been made to proceed with reconstruction, the timing of intervention should be determined. Typically, this will be based on the underlying source of the wound.
  - In acute trauma settings, debridement and bony fixation should be complete. An understanding of vascular and nerve injury should be established. At this point, the extent of the reconstruction will be known and a proper approach may be determined.
  - The ideal window to operate on traumatic injuries is within the first week, if not sooner. Bacterial contamination and traumatic edema make reconstruction more difficult and warrant delay.

Positioning

- A modification of standard supine positioning is required for most procedures. For plantar defects, it is often best to place the patient in a lateral decubitus or possibly prone position. Of course the positioning will be influenced by the planned reconstruction. A thigh or calf tourniquet is often used during these procedures to optimize visualization. Bipolar cautery should be available when procedures involve deep structures near the neurovascular bundles.

Approach

- Reconstructive options for forefoot wounds include secondary closure, skin graft or skin substitute, local or random patterned flap, pedicled flap, or free flap with microvascular anastomosis.
- Function and aesthetics must be taken into account. For example, a split-thickness skin graft to a wound bed is not likely to be a durable option for a plantar defect. Likewise, a large bulky flap placed on the dorsal forefoot is likely to make shoe fitting difficult. The specific approach for each reconstructive option is listed below.
  - *Delayed primary closure* is often difficult to perform secondary to refractory edema and minimal skin laxity of the foot.

- *Tissue expansion* is often not an option for the same reasons listed above.
- *Skin substitutes* have become popular in recent years and are used as dermal replacements in patients who would otherwise require flap reconstruction. A secondary skin graft is often needed. These products are directly applied to the wound bed after debridement.
- *Local random patterned flaps* are an option in patients with small foot wounds who may not be good free flap candidates. These flaps are inherently difficult to move in the foot.
- *Pedicled flaps* are useful in the forefoot due to rapid harvest and inset; however, for many of these flaps to reach the forefoot they must be based on unreliable distal perfusion. Another approach is to slide the flap with a component of plantar tissues in a V to Y pattern. These flaps can include both muscle and fasciocutaneous elements.
  - The reverse abductor digit minimi (ADM) flap is harvested along the lateral aspect of the plantar surface near the 5th metatarsal. The distally based flap and reverse based flap are useful for plantar forefoot wounds.
  - The reverse AH flap may be used for plantar defects of the forefoot. This muscle originates from the medial border of the calcaneus and inserts on the base of the proximal phalanx of the great toe.
  - The reverse FDB flap and the FDB based V-Y advancement flap are used in distal plantar surface wounds of the arch. For the reverse flap to be used, the dorsalis pedis and anterior tibialis must be intact as the medial plantar artery perforator is divided.
  - The toe fillet flap is a form of pedicled flap and is used after a toe amputation to cover a plantar- or volar-based wound associated with the effected digit.
  - The reverse dorsalis pedis fasciocutaneous flap can be designed up to 10 cm in size and is based on the dorsalis pedis artery. The pedicle of a standard dorsalis pedis flap is based on the dorsalis pedis artery; however, its reverse is based on the deep plantar arch and thus completeness of the arch must be assessed.
  - Reverse medial plantar artery flap: This flap contains the skin of the instep or non–weight bearing area of the plantar surface from the head of the first metatarsal to the navicular bone proximally.[5-7]
- *Free flaps* entail harvesting tissue from a different site along with its blood supply and transferring it to the recipient site. This requires a microvascular anastomosis. Both fasciocutaneous and muscle flaps work well on the forefoot and depend on goals of reconstruction.
  - Important aspects of the approach for free flap reconstruction include choosing a donor flap that will easily cover the defect. If the flap is too small, the closure will be tight.
  - Vessel size needs to be considered to match the flap with the foot recipient vessels. Also, the vascular anastomosis needs to be performed outside of the zone of injury which may even be at or above the ankle. Finally, the flap must be of sufficient bulk to obliterate any underlying dead space.

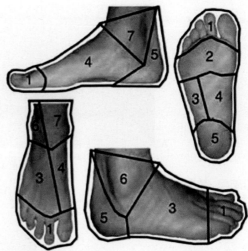

Subunit	Demands Tissue Needs	Optimal Flaps
1	Low functional, Moderate aesthetic: small, thia and pliable.	Radial forearm > lateral arm
2	High functional, Low aesthetic: durable and minimal bulk.	(*): Radial forearm > lateral arm > gracilis with STSG > ALT
3/4	Low functional, High aesthetic: smooth, thin and pliable	Radial forearm > ALT > scapular > latissimus dorsi
5	High functional Low aesthetic: durable and moderate bulk.	(*): ALT > gracilis with STSG > latissimus dorsi > scapular > lateral arm > radial forearm
6/7	Moderate functional, Moderate aesthetic: may vary from smooth, thin and pliable to Large and bulky.	Gracitia with STSG, latissimus dorsi, ALT, rectus abdominis, lateral arm, radial forearm, scapular

STSG: Split thickness skin graft
ALT: Anterolateral thigh
*: Nerve coaptation may be considered.

FIG 3 • Four separate views of foot and ankle demonstrating different aesthetic and functionally different subunits. There are four different relevant subunits of the forefoot. (Reprinted from Hollenbeck S, et al. Longitudinal outcomes and application of the subunit principle to 165 foot and ankle free tissue transfers. *Plast Reconstr Surg.* 2010;125(3):924-934, with permission.)[8]

- Free flap choice: Considerations on choice of free flap include size of wound, defect composition, pedicle size and length, and state of wound. Location of wound also precludes itself to choice of flap. The foot may be broken into seven subunits, which have been established for functional and aesthetic reconstructive goals. With respect to the forefoot, there are four relevant subunits (**FIG 3**). Each has its own aesthetic and functional concerns with regards to reconstruction.

■ Secondary Healing Using Regenerative Matrix

- Skin substitutes have become more popular in the recent years and are used in patients who may otherwise require flap reconstruction.
- Contraindications include exposed hardware; relative contraindications include exposed tendon or bone.
- Begin by obtaining adequate debridement. All nonviable tissue should be removed. Healthy bleeding tissue or bone should be visualized. If covering a chronic wound, ensure that negative cultures have been obtained (**TECH FIG 1A**).
- Apply the wound matrix to the exposed area generously. Similar principles to application of a skin graft applies and includes ensuring adequate contact of matrix to wound bed.
- After application, the matrix is fixated per surgeon preference including absorbable sutures such as chromic or staples that may be removed postoperatively. A hydrated dressing should be applied. This includes a negative pressure wound dressing or semipermeable colloid dressing. This remains in place for 1 to 4 weeks (**TECH FIG 1B**).
- Depending on the type of matrix applied, a bilayer may require removal around 4 weeks with the final result being total skin closure or a granulation bed that requires skin grafting (**TECH FIG 1C**)

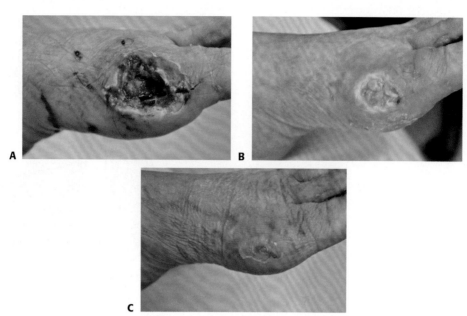

TECH FIG 1 • A. The left foot with a full-thickness defect down to bone following elective orthopedic surgery. Adequate debridement is obtained to healthy bleeding tissue. **B.** After 4 weeks of application of regenerative matrix (porcine bladder elements), an appropriate dressing should be applied that obliterates the dead space and keeps the wound hydrated to encourage granulation. **C.** Six weeks postoperatively. Full closure with minimal eschar remains. Regenerative matrix may be sufficient for small wounds that would otherwise require flap coverage.

■ Reverse Fasciocutaneous Flap (Reverse First Dorsal Metatarsal Artery [1st DMTA] Flap)

- Begin by obtaining adequate debridement. All nonviable tissue should be removed. Healthy bleeding tissue or bone should be visualized. If covering a chronic wound, ensure that negative cultures have been obtained (**TECH FIG 2A**).
- A Doppler should be used to identify the first dorsal metatarsal artery on the dorsum of the foot. The flap is then designed around this using the measurements needed to fill the defect. The proximal extension of the flap is designed so that once rotated it will fit into the defect (**TECH FIG 2B**).
- Dissection begins around the marked flap, first beginning over the dorsal skin and continuing through the fascia exposing the underlying tendons. Care is taken to preserve the paratenon associated with the tendons (**TECH FIG 2C**).
- The flap is then rotated around the axis of the 1st DMTA, which is located typically underneath the first interosseous muscle and adjacent to the metatarsal bone. The flap can be kept as a peninsula or as an island (**TECH FIG 2D**).
- It is important to ensure that the inset is relatively tension free. The flap donor defect is covered with a split-thickness skin graft (**TECH FIG 2E**).[9]

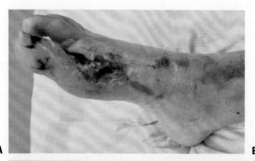

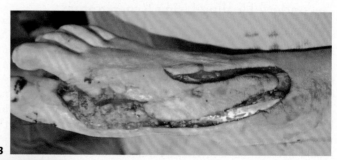

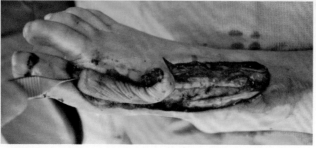

TECH FIG 2 • A. Chronic dorsal great toe wound, debrided back to healthy tissue. Negative cultures obtained. **B.** First dorsal metatarsal artery flap, marked and dissected to level tendon, keeping paratenon intact. Flap is undermined taking care to ensure the perforator is not inadvertently divided. **C.** Proximal end of flap is rotated 180 degrees to fill the defect. One must ensure a relatively tension-free closure.

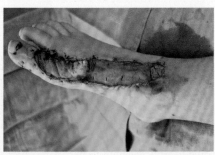
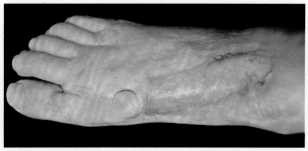

TECH FIG 2 (Continued) • **D.** A split-thickness skin graft is harvested to fill the donor site. There is typically some venous congestion of the distal portion of the rotated flap; however, in our experience this has done well with time. **E.** Six weeks postoperatively with a completely healed wound and donor site.

■ Free Gracilis for Osteomyelitis

- The gracilis free flap may be used over the plantar surface of the forefoot in weight-bearing areas. It is a Mathes and Nahai II flap with its main blood supply from the medial circumflex artery off of the profunda femoral artery. The muscle itself is 30 cm long, 5 cm wide and 2 cm thick.
- The gracilis muscle is an excellent option for chronic defects of a weight-bearing area in association with osteomyelitis (**TECH FIG 3A**). Debridement should include all nonviable tissues and affected areas. Negative cultures should be obtained.
- For this type of defect (**TECH FIG 3B**), local types of closure are not an option. A free tissue transfer (gracilis) has been chosen.

- The dorsalis pedis artery is dissected proximally out of the zone of injury and is isolated. Attention is now turned to the donor site.
- For harvest, the patient is placed in supine and frog-leg position. A line is drawn from the medial pubic tubercle to the medial femoral condyle.
- The gracilis should include the proximal portion along with the length needed to obliterate the defect.
- Transfer and inset takes place (**TECH FIG 3C**) via the dorsalis pedis artery. Primary closure of the donor site is obtained, and a split-thickness skin graft is used to cover the newly inset flap. This provides stable coverage and good shoe fitting (**TECH FIG 3D**).[10]

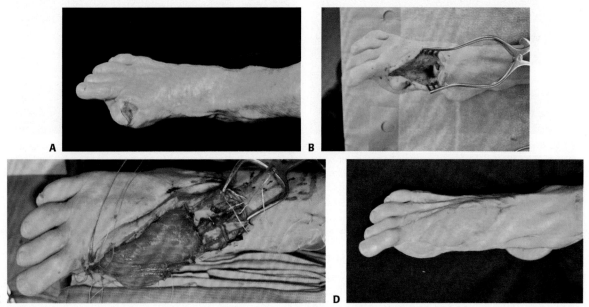

TECH FIG 3 • **A.** This patient suffered from chronic osteomyelitis of the first metatarsal head as a postoperative complication and eventually underwent ray amputation of the first toe as pictured. **B.** Debridement of entire affected segment and remaining metatarsal head and shaft. This has left the patient with a large defect that is not amenable to local types of closure. **C.** After inset of free gracilis. It is important that the tissue transfer obliterates dead space of the wound. Closure should be relatively tension free. **D.** Two months postoperatively. The patient has completely healed the wound and has an overall aesthetically pleasing result.

TECHNIQUES

■ Free Flap for Distal Skin Defect

- The radial forearm free flap is the flap of choice for most forefoot reconstruction defects. This flap meets both the aesthetic and functional needs including being both thin and pliable. It varies in size and can be harvested from the wrist to the antecubital crease. This flap is primarily a fasciocutaneous flap but may be harvested also as a myocutaneous or osteocutaneous. Its blood supply is the radial artery.
- In this example, free tissue transfer may be used in chronically infected wounds or in wounds with exposed hardware. This patient did not have a sizeable tissue defect and thus radial forearm flap was a great match due to pliability, coverage, and aesthetic result (**TECH FIG 4A**).
- First, obtain adequate debridement; in this patient debridement was conservative due to acute osteotomies with nonunion and exposed hardware.

- For harvest, the nondominant arm is typically utilized. An Allen's test is performed preoperatively to ensure that the palmar arch is intact.
- Doppler is utilized to identify the radial artery. A flap matching the size of the defect is marked with the radial most aspect over the radial artery.
- Dissection proceeds distally through skin, elevating fascia with the flap. Ensure to leave paratenon intact. The radial artery is dissected out proximally and ligated according to pedicle length need.
- The flap is then inset over the defect and anastomosed to the dorsalis pedis artery (**TECH FIG 4B**). Antibiotics are utilized due to exposed and presumed infected nature of the hardware. This will be kept for up to 6 weeks. Long-term coverage of the dorsal foot with a radial artery flap provides excellent contour (**TECH FIG 4C**).
- Donor site may be closed primarily depending on defect size and if tourniquet was used (**TECH FIG 4D**). If defect is large, split-thickness skin graft may be utilized.[11]

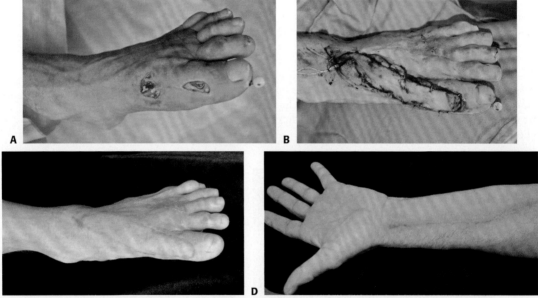

TECH FIG 4 • A. This patient has exposed hardware after orthopedic procedure presumed to be infected. This was unable to be removed due to nonunion. The patient was taken to the operating room for proper debridement. **B.** Radial forearm free flap after anastomosis and inset. Good size and thickness match is noted. **C.** Defect 2 months postoperatively. The forefoot is well healed with no signs of exposed hardware or chronic infection. The patient remained on a course of IV antibiotics for 6 weeks. **D.** Donor site. The patient's donor site was amenable to primary closure due to the small size of the defect. The patient has completely healed donor site with good perfusion of the hand and no chronic paresthesias.

■ Free Flap For Mangled Foot—Latissimus

- Latissimus is one of the largest muscles in the body and is used for covering large defects. The muscle may be harvested up to 35 cm in size and may be used as a muscle or myocutaneous flap. This is a Mathes and Nahai type V flap with the main blood supply coming from the thoracodorsal artery and vein.
- In this example, the patient suffered from a severe mangled foot after a crush injury. Acute debridement is performed in several stages along with external fixation.

It is important to determine the viability of the surrounding tissue prior to reconstruction (**TECH FIG 5A**).
- The free latissimus is chosen for reconstruction. The patient is placed in a lateral decubitus position for both harvest and inset.
- The harvest site is prepared; in this case, the anterior tibial vessels are used and dissected out proximally out of the zone of injury.
- The latissimus is now harvested as a muscle flap in its usual fashion. The donor site may be closed primarily over a suction drain.

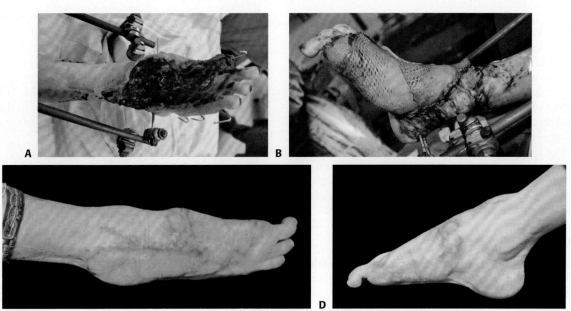

TECH FIG 5 • A. The right lower extremity after a severe crush and degloving injury. The patient undergoes external fixation along with adequate debridement performed in several days. **B.** After inset and skin grafting of latissimus flap over mangled foot. External fixator still in place. **C.** Two months postoperatively with acceptable contour. Wound well healed. **D.** Six months postoperatively, fully healed and with great aesthetic result that will fit in shoe or prosthesis.

■ The muscular flap is inset over the defect and anastomosed to the anterior tibial vessels, taking care to obliterate the dead space (**TECH FIG 5B**). A split-thickness skin graft is used to cover the muscular flap. A tension-free closure should be obtained.

■ A muscle flap with a split-thickness skin graft may provide excellent durable long-term coverage of the dorsal and plantar foot allowing for ambulation (**TECH FIG 5C,D**).[12]

PEARLS AND PITFALLS

Function	■ Amputation may be a reasonable option for wounds involving the forefoot. However, there will be some degree of functional loss associated with disruption of the propulsion phase of the gait cycle.
Tendon coverage	■ Reconstruction of the forefoot may involve wounds that are associated with flexors or extenders of the ankle. Preservation of these insertion points may impact leg function significantly.
Local flaps	■ Local flaps may be limited in the foot as there is minimal skin laxity for advancing and rotating these flaps. Ideally, incisions should not be placed on the weight-bearing areas of the foot.
Flap options	■ Free flap choices can be guided by consideration of the defect location and functional demand of the area in combination with aesthetic considerations and shoe fitting requirements. Microvascular anastomosis should be performed out of the zone of injury. Secondary thinning may be required especially for bulky fasciocutaneous flaps.
Outcomes	■ Free flap failure in the foot and ankle may be as high as 10% and is often related to a tight skin closure or poor distal extremity perfusion. Success is measured in stable skin coverage, bony healing, painless ambulation, and shoe fitting.

POSTOPERATIVE CARE

■ At the time of reconstruction, patients are typically placed in a posterior slab splint to minimize movement. A hole may be cut as a window to view the surgical site. This splint is typically kept until the patient begins transfers at which a formal splint will be applied.

■ Leg elevation is an important aspect of foot reconstruction, especially in the setting of trauma. A typical protocol for free flaps is strict bed rest and leg elevation until postoperative

day 4. At this point, the patient may begin working with physical therapy for dangling the lower extremity during transfers for 5 minutes 3 times daily. Weight-bearing status is dictated by orthopedic restrictions. Activity and dependent positioning should progress over the next several weeks. At this point, a compression garment may be applied to help with edema. During this course, it is important to utilize a prophylactic anticoagulant dose to prevent venous thromboembolism.

- CAM boots are typically used to offload pressure from the forefoot as the patient begins weight bearing. Sutures are typically kept in place for 3 to 4 weeks, but should be removed prior to ambulation to prevent callus formation or postoperative ulceration.
- Range of motion exercises are typically initiated in the noninvolved joints immediately postoperatively to prevent stiffness. Exercises in involved joints of reconstruction are begun somewhere between 5 days and 2 weeks.
- Postoperative follow-up should be frequent and consistent. This should involve a multidisciplinary team including plastic surgery, orthopedics, vascular surgery, podiatry, physical therapy, and wound care as needed. Many centers have limb salvage programs that incorporate these aspects of care for their patients.

OUTCOMES

- The majority of patients undergoing flap reconstruction with local or free flap transfer have a successful recovery. Free flap viability rates have been quoted to be 90% to 93% in lower extremity reconstruction. In those with primary flap failure, treatment consists of debridement and wound care with consideration for further reconstruction. Patients that experience flap failure are at increased risk for amputation.
- Some patients will have long-term wound healing issues, with ulceration around the site of flap inset. This may occur anywhere from months to years after surgery and typically occurs on the weight-bearing surfaces of the foot at the flap interface.
- Secondary procedures are common in forefoot reconstruction and are most commonly associated with debulking procedures, especially when free tissue transfer is performed. Instability or nonunion is infrequently seen in the forefoot.
- Amputation may be indicated in the primary setting or after reconstruction failure. Functional loss of an amputation needs to be weighed against morbidity of limb salvage. For the forefoot, options include isolated digit amputation, ray amputation, or transmetatarsal amputation. For those with vascular disease or open fractures, a higher level of amputation may be required.[8,12]

COMPLICATIONS

- Given the high risk nature of the patient population, complications can occur. Acute complications may be related to poor perfusion within the flap. This may occur when distally based flaps are used or when free flaps become compromised from pressure. Infections related to fractures and hardware placement are not uncommon in foot reconstruction. These are treated with flap elevation and further debridement.
- Long-term complications include flap ulceration or callus, typically around the flap–native skin interface. In these circumstances, excision of the ulcer with flap advancement is usually sufficient.

REFERENCES

1. Themes U. Comprehensive lower extremity anatomy. February 21, 2016. Retrieved September 18, 2017, from https://plasticsurgerykey.com/comprehensive-lower-extremity-anatomy/
2. Wrobel JS, Mayfield JA, Reiber GE. Geographic variation of lower-extremity major amputation in individuals with and without diabetes in the Medicare population. *Diabetes Care.* 2001;24(5):860-864.
3. Alexander IJ, Chao EY, Johnson KA. The assessment of dynamic foot-to-ground contact forces and plantar pressure distribution: a review of the evolution of current techniques and clinical applications. *Foot & Ankle.* 1990;11(3):152-167. doi:10.1177/107110079001100306
4. Lassen NA, Tonnesen KH, Holstein P. Distal blood pressure. *Scand J Clin Lab Invest.* 1976;36:705.
5. Attinger CE, Ducic I, Cooper P, et al. The role of intrinsic muscle flaps of the foot for bone coverage in foot and ankle defects in diabetic and non diabetic patients. *Plast Reconstr Surg.* 2002;110:1047-1054.
6. Man D, Acland RD. The microarterial anatomy of the dorsalis pedis flap and its clinical applications. *Plast Reconstr Surg.* 1980; 65(4):419-423.
7. Emmett A. The filleted toe flap. *Br J Plast Surg.* 1976;29(1):19-21. doi:10.1016/0007-1226(76)90083-7
8. Hollenbeck ST, Woo S, Komatsu I, et al. Longitudinal outcomes and application of the subunit principle to 165 foot and ankle free tissue transfers. *Plast Reconstr Surg.* 2010;125(3):924-934. doi:10.1097/prs.0b013e3181cc9630
9. Hallock GG. The first dorsal metatarsal artery perforator propeller flap. *Ann Plast Surg.* 2016;76(6):684-687. doi:10.1097/sap.0000000000000264
10. Eom JS, Sun SH, Hong JP. Use of the upper medial thigh perforator flap (gracilis perforator flap) for lower extremity reconstruction. *Plast Reconstr Surg.* 2011;127(2):731-737. doi:10.1097/prs.0b013e3181fed789
11. Chicarilli ZN, Price GJ. Complete plantar foot coverage with the free neurosensory radial forearm flap. *Plast Reconstr Surg.* 1986;78: 94-101.
12. Zhu Y, Wang Y, He X, et al. Foot and ankle reconstruction: An experience on the use of 14 different flaps in 226 cases. *Microsurgery.* 2013;33(8):600-604. doi:10.1002/micr.22177

CHAPTER 13

The Medial Plantar Flap

Arash Momeni and Subhro K. Sen

DEFINITION

- The medial plantar flap is suitable for reconstruction of heel and lateral plantar defects.[1,2]
- The medial plantar flap is harvested from the non–weight-bearing instep area of the foot.
- In the majority of cases, the donor site must be skin grafted. Narrow flaps up to 2 cm in width may be closed primarily.
- Volar hand and finger, as well as contralateral foot defects, may be reconstructed with the free medial plantar flap, as it is an excellent source of glabrous skin.[3,4]

ANATOMY

- The medial plantar flap is centered on an axis extending from the medial aspect of the first metatarsal head distally to the medial horizontal calcaneal eminence (talar shelf) proximally (**FIG 1**).
- Perfusion to the flap is via perforators from the medial plantar artery and venae comitantes that course between the abductor hallucis and flexor digitorum brevis muscles (**FIG 2**).
- Subcutaneous veins can be incorporated into the flap to augment venous drainage.
- The medial plantar flap may be raised as a sensate flap by including branches of the medial plantar nerve.
- It is critical to avoid including the weight-bearing regions of the foot (plantar forefoot, lateral plantar area, and heel) when harvesting this flap (**FIG 3**).

PATIENT HISTORY AND PHYSICAL FINDINGS

- Preoperative evaluation of patients with plantar foot wounds includes a detailed history, focused physical examination, as well as assessment of the functional limitations associated with the foot defect.

- History
  - A thorough history of pre-existing medical conditions as well as their severity must be obtained. Important conditions to identify and address preoperatively include peripheral vasculopathy, diabetes mellitus, and smoking.
    - Peripheral vasculopathy must be corrected prior to any attempt at reconstructing an existing ischemia-related soft tissue defect.
    - Diabetes mellitus management needs to be optimized to increase the likelihood of an uneventful recovery.
    - Preoperative smoking cessation is mandatory to decrease the risk of delayed wound healing.
  - A focused history of the foot wound with particular emphasis on etiology, duration, changes in size, previous wound-related complications (eg, infections), and previous attempts at treatment is critically important.
- Physical examination
  - The foot wound is inspected and its location and dimensions documented.
  - The foot is inspected for pre-existing scars that may preclude harvest of the medial plantar flap.

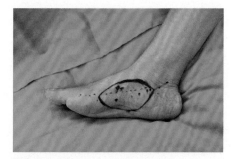

FIG 1 • Design of medial plantar flap.

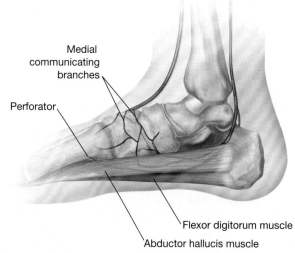

FIG 2 • Perfusion to the medial plantar flap is via perforators from the medial plantar artery and venae comitantes that course between the abductor hallucis and flexor digitorum brevis muscles.

Medial communicating branches

Perforator

Flexor digitorum muscle

Abductor hallucis muscle

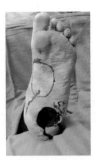

FIG 3 • Note that the medial plantar flap is designed in a manner to not include the weight-bearing regions of the foot.

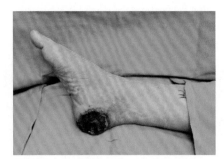

FIG 4 • Heel defect.

■ A thorough neurovascular exam of the lower extremity is performed.
  • Pulses, that is, dorsalis pedis and posterior tibial artery, are palpated.
    • Doppler examination is used to confirm the presence of the medial plantar artery and identify its course.
    • Absence of perfusion to the foot via the dorsalis pedis artery represents a possible contraindication to utilizing the medial plantar flap, depending on arterial inflow via the peroneal artery.
  • Sensory examination using Semmes-Weinstein monofilaments is performed in the distribution of the tibial as well as deep and superficial peroneal nerves.
■ The foot is evaluated for any acquired or congenital deformities, as these could influence the weight-bearing areas of the foot, thus, affecting flap design.

IMAGING

■ Preoperative imaging is not routinely required prior to harvest of the medial plantar flap.
  ■ Traditional or CT angiography can be obtained to confirm the presence of suitable pedicle vessels for patients with peripheral vasculopathy in whom there is concern for involvement of the pedicle vessels or patients with traumatic defects with the possibility of involvement of the medial plantar artery/posterior tibial artery.
■ Handheld pencil Doppler examination is typically sufficient to localize the medial plantar artery as well as intermuscular perforators emanating between the abductor hallucis medially and the flexor digitorum brevis muscle laterally.

SURGICAL MANAGEMENT

■ Patients with defects of glabrous skin containing areas are generally considered for reconstruction with the pedicled medial plantar flap based on the principle of "replacing like with like."
  ■ Typical indications include heel and lateral plantar midfoot defects (**FIGS 4** and **5**).
  ■ It may be transferred as a free flap for reconstruction of the contralateral foot as well as volar hand and finger defects.
■ It is critical to examine the foot and identify weight-bearing areas so not to include these regions in the flap. The weight-bearing areas include the plantar forefoot over the metatarsophalangeal heads, lateral plantar foot, and the heel.

Preoperative Planning

■ Preoperative radiographs of the affected extremity are obtained to assess the bone underlying the defect. It is critical to establish whether osteomyelitis is present. If osteomyelitis is present, it should be adequately treated with debridement and antibiotics prior to reconstructing any existing soft tissue defect.
  ■ Preoperative magnetic resonance imaging (MRI) may be indicated to preoperatively delineate the extent of osseous and soft tissue involvement.[5]
■ Handheld pencil Doppler examination is performed to outline the course of the medial plantar artery.
■ The medial plantar flap is centered on an axis extending from the base of the first metatarsal distally to the sustentaculum tali. The sustentaculum corresponds to the medical eminence of the calcaneus.
  ■ It is critical to avoid incorporating weight-bearing skin areas of the foot into the flap.
  ■ The flap can be designed with its proximal skin bridge intact or as an island flap depending on the needs of the defect.[6]

Positioning

■ The patient is typically placed in the supine position with the leg externally rotated and knee flexed ("frog leg"). Prone positioning is likewise possible depending on defect location and surgeon preference.
■ A well-padded tourniquet is placed on the thigh to provide for a bloodless operative field, which substantially facilitates identification of key structures during flap dissection.

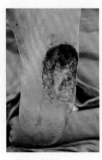

FIG 5 • Lateral plantar midfoot defect.

■ Medial Plantar Flap Harvest

- Landmarks: first metatarsal head, medial calcaneal eminence, midline of the plantar surface of the foot, navicular bone.
- The flap is designed within the boundaries of these landmarks, with particular attention paid not to include any weight-bearing areas of the foot (see **FIGS 1** and **3**).
- The foot wound is debrided until healthy-appearing tissue is encountered.
- The lower extremity is elevated, exsanguinated with an Esmarch bandage, and the tourniquet inflated to 100 mm Hg above the systolic blood pressure value.
- Skin incision is made along the borders of the flap, extending through the plantar aponeurosis.
  - Although the authors prefer to include the plantar aponeurosis, inclusion of this structure is not mandatory.
- Distally, the abductor hallucis and flexor digitorum brevis muscles are identified.
- Perforators between these muscles are identified, the abductor hallucis muscle is retracted medially, and the perforators are traced to their origin (**TECH FIG 1**).
  - The medial plantar artery is visualized, along with the accompanying medial plantar nerve and venae comitantes.

- The medial plantar artery is distally ligated and divided, followed by a distal-to-proximal flap dissection.
  - It is important to maintain all superficial attachments between the medial plantar artery and the overlying skin to ensure flap vascularity.
- In order to avoid sensory loss of the distal medial plantar foot and toes, the medial plantar nerve is not routinely transected.
  - Instead, a nerve-splitting internal neurolysis technique is employed, in which the nerve fibers entering flap are split from the medial plantar nerve, thus preserving distal sensory innervation as well as providing for a sensate flap.
- Dissection is continued proximally until a sufficient arc of rotation is obtained to allow transposition/rotation into the defect.
  - Occasionally, it may be necessary to divide the lateral plantar artery, the abductor hallucis muscle, and the flexor retinaculum to increase the arc of rotation in pedicled flap transfer or to increase pedicle length in cases of microvascular transfer.
  - Release of the tarsal tunnel may be necessary. It may be necessary to follow the medial plantar artery to its origin from the posterior tibial artery. The posterior tibial vessels can also be used for microsurgical anastomosis in the case of free tissue transfer.

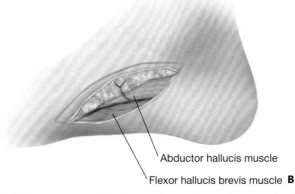
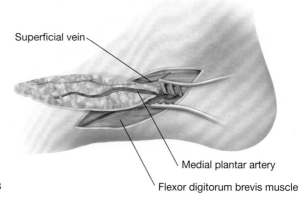

A Abductor hallucis muscle
Flexor hallucis brevis muscle **B**

Superficial vein
Medial plantar artery
Flexor digitorum brevis muscle

TECH FIG 1 • A. During flap harvest, the perforators between the abductor hallucis and flexor digitorum brevis muscles are identified. **B.** The abductor hallucis muscle is retracted medially, and the perforators are traced to their origin.

■ Donor Site Closure

- The donor site of narrow medial plantar flaps up to 2 cm in width may be closed primarily.
- The majority of donor sites require skin grafting for closure.

- The exposed abductor hallucis and flexor digitorum brevis muscles are reapproximated to provide for a well-vascularized wound bed, amenable to receipt of a split-thickness skin graft (**TECH FIG 2**).
- A negative pressure wound dressing can be applied over the skin graft as a bolster.

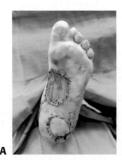
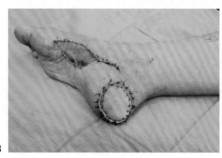

TECH FIG 2 • **A.** Split-thickness skin graft to donor site. **B.** Split-thickness skin graft to donor site.

PEARLS AND PITFALLS

Indications	▪ Heel and lateral plantar defects (pedicled flap transfer). ▪ Any defect requiring reconstruction with glabrous skin (microvascular-free tissue transfer).
Contraindications	▪ Previous surgical intervention or injury that violate the area of medial plantar flap harvest. ▪ Peripheral vascular disease with occlusion or stenosis of pedicle vessels of significant microvascular disease. ▪ Occlusion of dorsalis pedis artery.
Imaging	▪ Handheld pencil Doppler examination outlining the course of the medial plantar artery typically sufficient. ▪ Routine use of preoperative imaging is not indicated. ▪ In cases of peripheral vascular disease or traumatic defects with the pedicle vessels at risk, traditional or CT angiography is useful.
Flap dissection	▪ Avoid incorporating weight-bearing skin areas into the flap. ▪ Distal-to-proximal flap dissection. ▪ Preserve the medial plantar nerve, ie, employ a nerve-splitting approach. ▪ May increase pedicle length/arc of rotation by dividing the lateral plantar artery, abductor hallucis muscle, and flexor retinaculum, and dissect the pedicle to the posterior tibial artery.
Donor site closure	▪ Up to 2 cm width can be closed primarily. ▪ Typically donor site closure requires the use of a skin graft.

POSTOPERATIVE CARE

▪ The patient is instructed to keep the donor leg elevated for 2 weeks.

▪ The bolster dressing on the donor site skin graft is typically removed on postoperative day 5, and routine skin graft care is initiated.

▪ In cases of soft tissue reconstruction only without any underlying fractures, patients are allowed to ambulate once the flap suture lines and donor site skin graft have healed and are stable. In cases on underlying fractures, weight-bearing status will be determined by orthopedic surgery.

▪ Meticulous foot care, particularly in patients with diabetes mellitus, is paramount.

▪ Referrals should be made to an experienced podiatrist for evaluation and possible alterations of foot wear to decrease the likelihood of wound recurrence.

OUTCOMES

▪ **FIGS 6** to **8** demonstrate representative cases of long-term postoperative outcomes following plantar reconstruction using the medial plantar flap (**FIGS 6** to **8**).

▪ Siddiqi et al. presented their experience in 18 patients who underwent reconstruction of the weight-bearing heel with the medial plantar artery flap.[2]

  ▪ Indications for reconstruction included trauma, pressure sores, and unstable plantar scars.

  ▪ No flap loss was reported. Merely one case of partial skin graft loss that healed by secondary intention was observed.

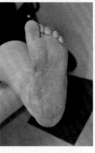

FIG 6 • Long-term outcome after heel reconstruction with the medial plantar flap.

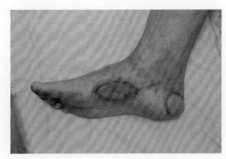

FIG 7 • Long-term outcome after heel reconstruction with the medial plantar flap.

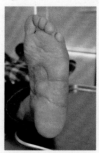

FIG 8 • Long-term outcome after reconstruction of a lateral plantar midfoot defect with the medial plantar flap.

- Patients were able to wear normal footwear.
- No functional donor site morbidity was reported.
- Schwarz and Negrini reported on 51 medial plantar artery flaps that were performed in 48 patients.[7]
  - Indications included defects of the posterior heel (*N* = 25), lateral border of the foot (*N* = 12), anterior heel (*N* = 10), and an over the Achilles tendon (*N* = 4).
  - Complications were encountered in 25.5% of the procedures (13/51), with the most common complications being delayed wound healing (*N* = 6) and infection (*N* = 3).
  - One flap loss was reported in addition to 9 ulcer recurrences in 7 ft.

COMPLICATIONS

- Postoperative complications requiring surgical intervention are uncommon.
- Complications, however, can include the following:
  - Infection
  - Wound dehiscence
  - Delayed wound healing
  - Skin graft loss
  - Flap loss

- Injury to the medial plantar nerve with consecutive altered sensation of the medial forefoot and toes
- Gait disturbance
- Pain
- Unstable scar

REFERENCES

1. Shanahan RE, Gingrass RP. Medial plantar sensory flap for coverage of heel defects. *Plast Reconstr Surg.* 1979;64:295-298.
2. Siddiqi MA, Hafeez K, Cheema TA, Rashid HU. The medial plantar artery flap: a series of cases over 14 years. *J Foot Ankle Surg.* 2012;51:790-794.
3. Koshima I, Urushibara K, Inagawa K, et al. Free medial plantar perforator flaps for the resurfacing of finger and foot defects. *Plast Reconstr Surg.* 2001;107:1753-1758.
4. Huang QS, Wu X, Zheng HY, et al. Medial plantar flap to repair defects of palm volar skin. *Eur J Trauma Emerg Surg.* 2015;41:293-297.
5. Pineda C, Espinosa R, Pena A. Radiographic imaging in osteomyelitis: the role of plain radiography, computed tomography, ultrasonography, magnetic resonance imaging, and scintigraphy. *Semin Plast Surg.* 2009;23:80-89.
6. Harrison DH, Morgan BD. The instep island flap to resurface plantar defects. *Br J Plast Surg.* 1981;34:315-318.
7. Schwarz RJ, Negrini JF. Medial plantar artery island flap for heel reconstruction. *Ann Plast Surg.* 2006;57:658-661.

14 CHAPTER

Reconstruction of Heel and Plantar Defects: Free Flap

Goo-Hyun Mun and Kyong-Je Woo

DEFINITION

- Heel and plantar soft tissues perform a special role of weight bearing while walking or standing. The heel sustains up to 115% of body weight during slow walking and up to 260% of body weight during running.[1]
- Heel and plantar defects may result from several causes such as trauma, diabetes, infection, peripheral vascular disease, frostbite injuries, and tumor resections.
- The goal of reconstruction is aimed at not only providing stable wound healing but also achieving functional restoration of the salvaged limb and maintaining acceptable appearance.

ANATOMY

- The weight-bearing plantar skin is a highly specialized part of the foot that is able to withstand and absorb the forces exerted during gait or running cycles. The epidermis and dermis are much thicker in plantar skin ("glabrous skin") than in other parts of the body.
- Subcutaneous fat in combination with the vertical fibrous connective tissue provides a cushioning effect to weight bearing.
- The three arteries at the ankle level and their terminating branches in the foot that can be used as recipient vessels for free flaps include the anterior tibial-dorsalis pedis artery, posterior tibial-medial and lateral plantar artery, and peroneal-lateral calcaneal artery.
  - Anterior tibial-dorsalis pedis artery: the dorsalis pedis artery passes under the extensor retinaculum at the midpoint between the medial and lateral malleoli. It usually runs across and beneath the extensor hallucis longus (**FIG 1A**). It passes to the proximal end of the first intermetatarsal space, where it turns into the sole between the heads of the first dorsal interosseous to complete the plantar arch and provides the first plantar metatarsal artery

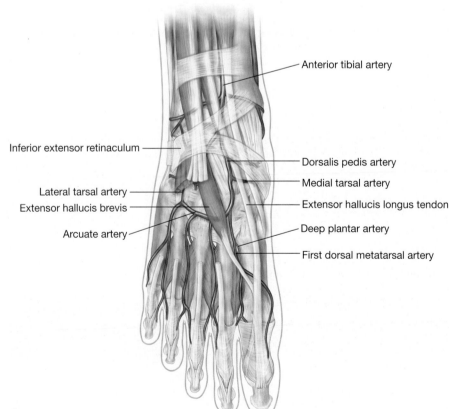

Anterior tibial artery

Inferior extensor retinaculum —

Lateral tarsal artery —

Extensor hallucis brevis —

Arcuate artery —

— Dorsalis pedis artery

— Medial tarsal artery

— Extensor hallucis longus tendon

— Deep plantar artery

— First dorsal metatarsal artery

A

FIG 1 • A,B. Anterior tibial-dorsalis pedis artery.

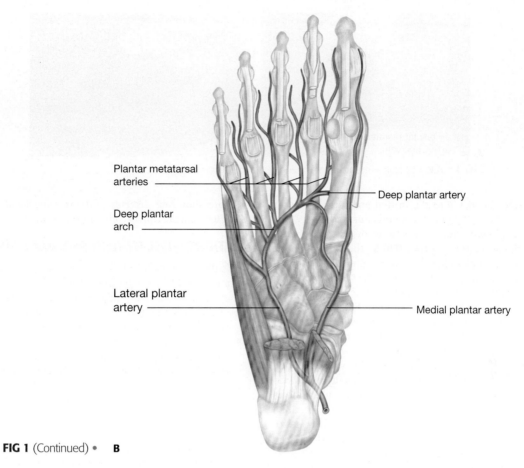

Plantar metatarsal arteries

Deep plantar artery

Deep plantar arch

Lateral plantar artery

Medial plantar artery

FIG 1 (Continued) • **B**

(**FIG 1B**). In heel and plantar reconstruction with a free flap, the dorsalis pedis artery can be reached for the recipient vessel by using a remote incision and subcutaneous tunneling (**FIG 2**). The first plantar metatarsal artery can be used in the plantar forefoot reconstruction (**FIG 3**).

■ Posterior tibial-medial and lateral plantar artery: posterior tibial artery runs midway between the medial malleolus and the medial calcaneal tubercle under the laciniate ligament. It is located between the flexor digitorum longus and flexor hallucis longus tendons (**FIG 4**). The posterior

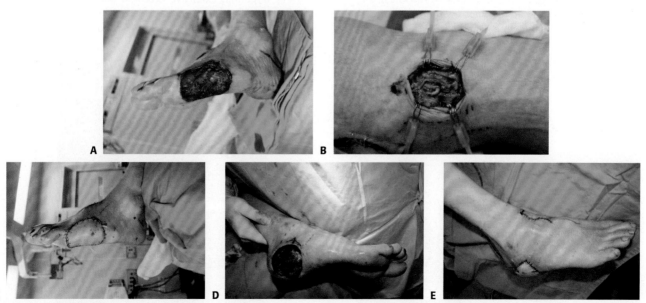

FIG 2 • **A.** The dorsalis pedis artery was used as a recipient artery for defect on lateral forefoot. A remote incision and subcutaneous tunneling was performed to reach the recipient vessels. **B.** Microvascular anastomosis. **C.** Immediate postoperative photo. **D.** Another case with defect on the lateral heel. Dorsalis pedis vessels were used as recipient vessel through a remote incision and subcutaneous tunneling. **E.** Immediate postoperative photo.

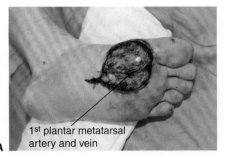
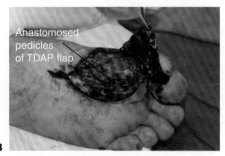

FIG 3 • A,B. First plantar metatarsal artery and vein for the recipient vessel.

tibial artery divides into the medial and lateral plantar arteries under the origin of the abductor hallucis. While the medial plantar artery runs between the abductor hallucis and flexor digitorum brevis (**FIG 5**), the lateral plantar artery, being usually larger, travels from medial to lateral position under the proximal third of the flexor digitorum brevis and then continues distally between flexor digitorum brevis and abductor digiti minimi (**FIG 6**).

■ Peroneal-lateral calcaneal artery: peroneal artery terminates into lateral calcaneal artery around the lateral malleolus (**FIG 7**). The lateral calcaneal artery was introduced as a pedicle for local flap, but a recent anatomical study suggests that it could be used as a recipient blood vessels for free flap.[2,3] The lateral calcaneal artery originates either from peroneal artery (80.3%), posterior tibial artery (13.1%), or a common branch from both the peroneal and posterior tibial arteries (6.6%) and runs between lateral malleolus and Achilles tendon.[3,4]

■ The principal superficial veins are termed long (great) and short (small) saphenous veins (**FIG 8**). The long (great) saphenous vein passes anterior to the medial malleolus, whereas the short (small) saphenous vein ascends from the lateral side of the foot. It ascends posterior to the lateral malleolus, passing along the lateral border of the Achilles tendon. A deep venous system runs near the corresponding arteries and develops communication with the great and small saphenous veins. Both deep veins of the

corresponding arteries and the superficial veins can be selected as recipient veins in the foot.

PATIENT HISTORY AND PHYSICAL FINDINGS

■ A thorough medical history and examinations for sensation and presence of diabetes, peripheral vascular disease, and existence of osteomyelitis need to be obtained. Deformities of the foot and a postoperative rehabilitation plan should also be considered in the selection of reconstruction methods.

■ Vascular anatomy and patency must be evaluated. In this regard, noninvasive Doppler ultrasound exam is a simple and useful evaluation method. Recently, computed tomography (CT) or magnetic resonance (MR) angiography methods are also recommended for vascular imaging.

IMAGING

■ The authors routinely perform preoperative CT angiographic examination of the lower extremities, except when contraindicated.

■ Bone assessment includes plain radiography and bone scan or MR imaging for the diagnosis of osteomyelitis.

SURGICAL MANAGEMENT

■ For large and extensive heel and plantar defects, the free flap transfer procedure is preferred because it can provide a large amount of tissue with various tissue components

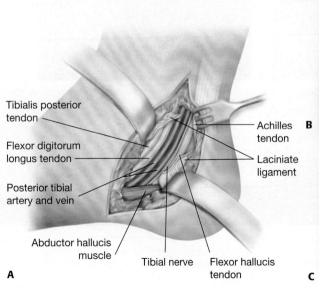
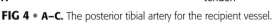
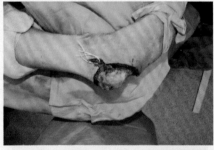
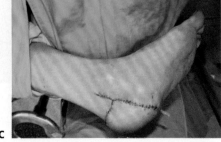

FIG 4 • A–C. The posterior tibial artery for the recipient vessel.

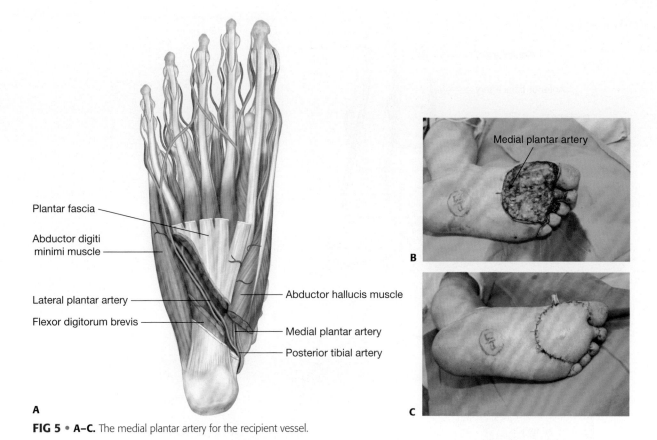

Plantar fascia

Abductor digiti minimi muscle

Lateral plantar artery

Flexor digitorum brevis

Abductor hallucis muscle

Medial plantar artery

Posterior tibial artery

Medial plantar artery

A

B

C

FIG 5 • A–C. The medial plantar artery for the recipient vessel.

for obliterating deep and/or extensive wounds. The early and definitive reconstruction of compound defects leads to a dramatic improvement in the rate of lower extremity salvage and restoration of the weight-bearing function and normal gait pattern.

■ The final choice of most suitable flap depends on the surgeon's preference and the patient's needs. A form of durable, permanent, pain-free, and functionally and aesthetically

satisfying coverage should be achieved in the heel and plantar reconstruction.

■ Free muscle flap versus fasciocutaneous flap: free muscle flap (rectus abdominis, latissimus dorsi, or gracilis) has been used commonly for extensive foot defects. A muscle flap has advantages, including the large amount of tissue availability, and ability to obliterate dead space especially in defects with irregular contours, where there is greater ease

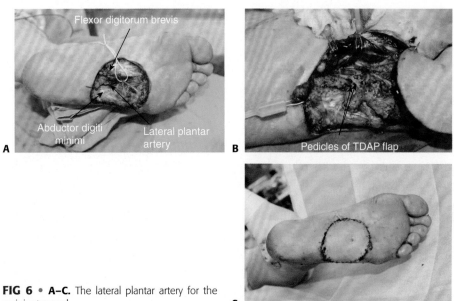

Flexor digitorum brevis

Abductor digiti minimi

Lateral plantar artery

A

Pedicles of TDAP flap

B

C

FIG 6 • A–C. The lateral plantar artery for the recipient vessel.

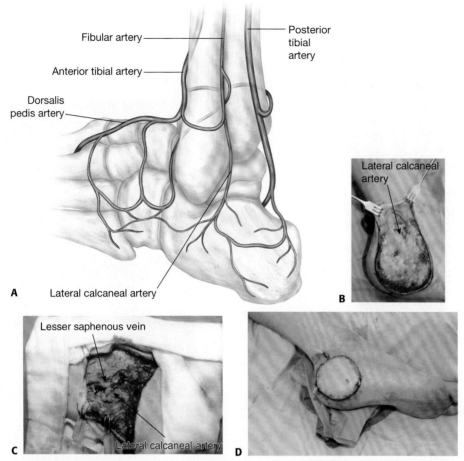

FIG 7 • A–D. The lateral calcaneal artery for the recipient vessel.

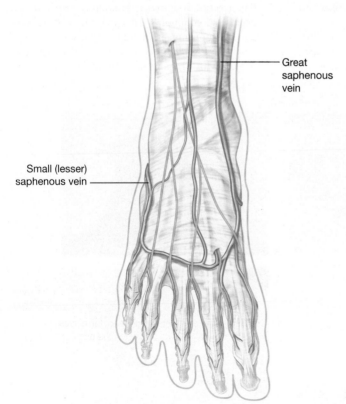

FIG 8 • A superficial venous system of the foot.

to form three-dimensional (3D) shapes.[5] In contrast, recent clinical studies have demonstrated that fasciocutaneous flaps (anterolateral thigh, thoracodorsal artery perforator [TDAP] flap) provide a sufficient amount of bulk, large, and pliable skin flap, with acceptable donor site morbidities.[6,7] The donor site morbidities caused by harvesting the muscle flap and additional donor site for skin graft can be avoided by using the fasciocutaneous flap.

- The authors prefer the TDAP flap for many foot defects because it provides thick skin from the back that has negligible incidence of atherosclerosis of the vascular pedicle, which is relatively long. Furthermore, the TDAP can be tailored to include different tissue types such as muscle (latissimus dorsi) and/or bone (scapula) depending upon the requirements for reconstruction. The anterolateral thigh flap is also useful when supine position of the patient is favorable.
- Muscle-chimeric perforator flap is useful to obliterate dead space when it is necessary (see **FIG 12B,C**).
- Innervated (sensate) flap: although it seems reasonable to assume that plantar reconstruction requires a sensate flap to avoid recurrent ulceration, there is no evidence suggesting that innervated flaps on weight-bearing portion of the foot is superior in terms of rates of ulceration. A noninnervated fasciocutaneous flap showed progressive improvement in sensitive thresholds, achieving good protective sensitivity, similar to that of an innervated flap.[9]
- The status of an underlying skeletal anatomy is a critical factor in the durability of the soft tissue reconstruction. Abnormally high pressure points on the plantar surface lead to the recurrent breakdown after reconstruction, and the abnormalities should, therefore, be corrected.
- In the heel and plantar reconstructions, restoration of 3D configuration of the heel and plantar foot is essential to wear a normal shoe and to regain normal gait pattern. The primary defatting and wedge resection of the flap facilitates making 3D configuration.

Preoperative Planning

- The patient had a large malignant melanoma on the left heel. Wide excision of the tumor and reconstruction of the heel were planned (**FIG 9**).
- CT angiographic evaluation showed all major vessels of the foot had normal anatomy with no atherosclerosis or vascular occlusion. The presence of a sizable lateral calcaneal

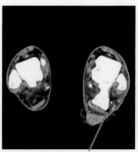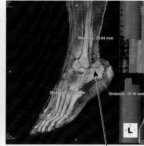

A Lateral calcaneal artery   **B** Lateral calcaneal artery

FIG 10 • **A,B.** CT angiographic image of lateral calcaneal artery.

artery on the patient's left foot was also confirmed, and the course could be followed by 3D reconstruction of the CT images (**FIG 10**).

- A TDAP flap, instead of an anterolateral thigh flap, was planned to be used for several reasons in the described case. Lateral position was better than supine position for both tumor resection and inset of the flap. In addition, it might have been necessary to perform a skin graft for the anterolateral thigh flap donor site if the flap was more than 10 cm wide.

Positioning

- The procedure can be performed in the lateral decubitus position, with the affected leg placed on the upper side. An ipsilateral TDAP flap can be harvested following tumor resection, without changing the position, at the same time as dissecting the lateral calcaneal artery as the recipient artery.
- When the posterior tibial artery is planned to be the recipient vessel, a TDAP flap is harvested from the contralateral side in a position of lateral decubitus with the recipient foot placed on lower side (**FIG 11**).

Approach

- When a recipient vessel can be found in the defect, it is approached directly. Otherwise, an extended incision starting from the defect or a separate incision with subcutaneous tunneling is used as an approach to preparing the recipient vessels.

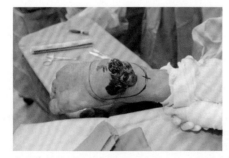

FIG 9 • A clinical case with malignant melanoma on the left heel.

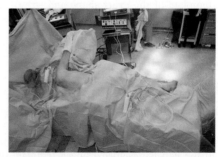

FIG 11 • Lateral decubitus position for harvesting TDAP flap on the contralateral side of the defect when the posterior tibial artery is used as recipient vessel.

Note: Each step of techniques is included in the video clip.

■ Wound Preparation

- It is critical that there is complete debridement or excision of pathologic, necrotic, or infected tissue under tourniquet control (**TECH FIG 1**).

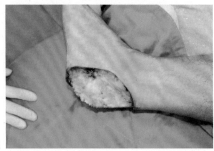 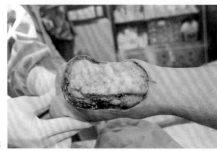

A   **B**

TECH FIG 1 • A,B. Defect of the heel after tumor resection.

■ Recipient Vessel Preparation

- Patency and location of the lateral calcaneal artery for use as the recipient artery are checked using handheld pencil Doppler.
- Small saphenous vein is preserved and dissected for use as the recipient vein.
- The lateral calcaneal artery runs superficially between lateral malleolus and the Achilles tendon. The vessel traverses anterior to the calcaneal tendon and posterior to the small saphenous vein (**TECH FIG 2**). Opening the extensor retinaculum and deep fascia exposes the lateral calcaneal artery with its associated venae comitantes.

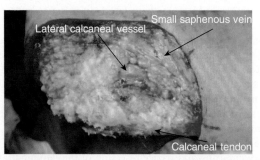

TECH FIG 2 • Dissection of lateral calcaneal vessels.

■ Assessment of the Defect

- After deflating the tourniquet, meticulous hemostasis is performed, which is followed by irrigation with saline.
- A template of the exact shape and size of the defect is made by using a transparent plastic or paper to be used when designing the flap.

- Wedge-shaped excision of the skin flap is necessary in case of the total heel resurfacing. The area for planned wedge excision is incorporated when estimating the flap dimensions.

■ Flap Harvest

- Outline of the relevant muscle and landmarks are marked on the skin.
- Perforators are located using handheld pencil Doppler, and the flap is designed using a template of the defect. The perforator can be located eccentrically, considering the area of wedge excision (**TECH FIG 3A**).
- A limited incision is made, and a suprafascial dissection is performed until the targeted perforator is identified.

- Once the perforator is evaluated and deemed suitable, then the whole skin paddle is elevated and meticulous intramuscular dissection of pedicle with bipolar forceps is commenced.
- Motor nerve branches to the muscle are preserved, and the pedicle is divided when sufficient length is obtained (**TECH FIG 3B**).
- A closed suction drain is placed, and the donor site is primarily closed in layers (**TECH FIG 3C**).

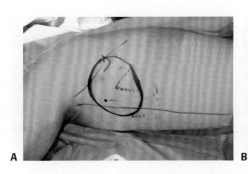
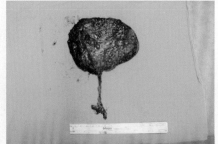
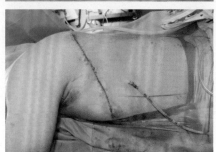

TECH FIG 3 • A–C. Flap design and elevation.

Microanastomosis with Temporary Inset

- Temporary inset of flap can be performed using a skin stapler.
- It is critically important to avoid twisting of the pedicle. If excessively long, the vascular pedicle under the flap is positioned in lazy-S shape to avoid kinking.
- The pedicle artery is anastomosed to the lateral calcaneal artery, and the vein is anastomosed to the short (small) saphenous vein (**TECH FIG 4**).
- Vascular clamps are removed after completion of the anastomosis. Warm saline is applied onto the vessels and flap, and inflow and outflow of the flap are checked after waiting for several minutes.

- A thorough microscopic evaluation is conducted to find any bleeding points along the vascular pedicle.

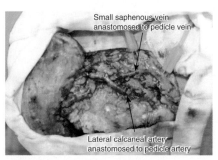

Small saphenous vein anastomosed to pedicle vein

Lateral calcaneal artery anastomosed to pedicle artery

TECH FIG 4 • Microanastomosis.

Final Inset

- Defatting of the flap is performed before the final inset. The deep fat and part of the superficial fat may be carefully removed with scissors according to the required thickness of tissue. Thinning can be done with or without loupe, but microscope magnification is not usually necessary. This procedure is important to obtain an optimal contour of the reconstructed foot. The authors prefer primary (immediate) defatting to secondary (delayed) defatting because it provides well-contoured reconstruction in one stage, reduces tension of closure, and is a safe procedure. Alternatively, secondary defatting is a viable option, which can avoid potential risk of circulatory problem associated with primary thinning.
- In contrast to the conventional fasciocutaneous flap that includes deep fat and fascia, a perforator flap with a thin subcutaneous layer composed of the superficial fat lobules surrounded by dense fibers allows the skin to anchor tightly to the surface and to glide less.[6,7] Generally, perforator flap is thinned accordingly to match the contour of adjacent plantar tissue.
- Redraping of the flap for the final inset is attempted only after the defatting procedure is completed because this may change the pliability and extensibility of the flap. Dimensional excess should be corrected at this stage by careful trimming to obtain durable weight-bearing surface against anticipated shear forces (**TECH FIG 5**).
- The wound is closed over a drain placed under the flap to prevent fluid collections.
- Fluffed gauze is gently applied to the flap, but the part of flap including the location of captured perforator is left exposed for postoperative monitoring using the hand-held pencil Doppler.

T
E
C
H
N
I
Q
U
E
S

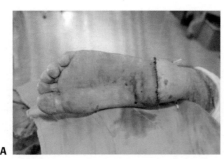
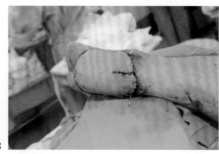

TECH FIG 5 • A,B. Inset of the flap after defatting and wedge-shaped excision.

PEARLS AND PITFALLS

Reconstruction goal	■ The weight-bearing plantar skin is highly specialized to withstand and absorb forces exerted during gait or running cycles. ■ The reconstructive goal is not only to provide stable wound healing but also to achieve functional restoration of the salvaged limb with an acceptable appearance.
Flap selection	■ Free muscle flaps (rectus abdominis, latissimus dorsi, and gracilis) have been commonly selected for the extensive foot defects. ■ Cutaneous perforator flaps now provide favorable functional and aesthetic outcomes in heel and plantar reconstruction.
Selection of recipient vessel	■ The three named arteries at the ankle level and their terminating branches can be candidates for recipient vessels; anterior tibial-dorsalis pedis artery, posterior tibial-medial and lateral plantar artery, and peroneal-lateral calcaneal artery. ■ CT angiography is a valuable tool to evaluate the arterial and venous flows and the presence of atherosclerosis.
Assessment of the defect	■ Before designing the flap, the size and shape of the defect are measured exactly by making a template. ■ Required vascular pedicle length and flap thickness are also assessed.
Flap inset	■ Defatting of the flap at the time of insetting is important to obtain a desirable contour of the reconstructed foot. Alternatively, secondary defatting is an option. ■ Excessive skin dimension is carefully corrected to have the flap closely tailored to the defect.

POSTOPERATIVE CARE

■ The leg is elevated to help with edema for a better venous return while the patient is lying in bed.

■ Care should be taken to avoid any compression along the course of the superficial vein of the leg when it is used as an outflow vessel.

■ There is no consensus regarding the use of medications for thromboprophylaxis such as aspirin, heparin, and dextran. The authors do not routinely use any of these medications but low molecular weight heparin is given for chemoprophylaxis of the venous thromboembolism while patient is immobilized in bed.

■ For postoperative monitoring, the flap can be checked every 1 to 3 hours for the first 48 hours, followed by every 4 to 6 hours for the next 48 hours after the surgery. Monitoring is done by physical examination and handheld pencil Doppler examination.

■ Diet is usually allowed 24 hours after surgery in the authors' practice.

■ Although the duration of immobilization time varies based on the orthopedic and bony status, in general, progressive weight bearing and ambulation are achieved once the flap maturation is assured. At 2 weeks, compressive garment is applied to prevent edema of the flap and foot. Bearing weight on the site of flap is usually allowed in 4 weeks after the surgery.

■ Abnormal weight-bearing patterns and gait abnormalities correlate with the development of chronic ulcers. An early orthotic use and physical therapy in rehabilitation unit may prevent ulceration and wound breakdown.

■ Patient education on meticulous foot care with frequent inspections to recognize any area of wound breakdown is essential for a successful and durable result.

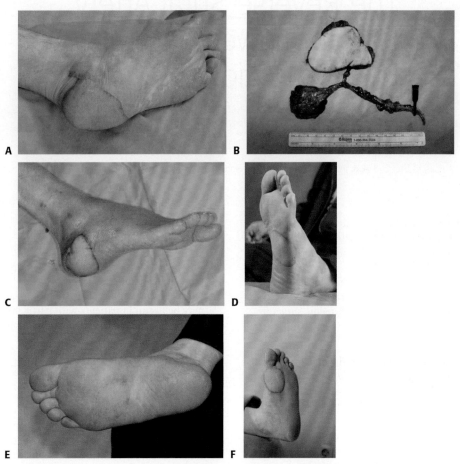

FIG 12 • A. Total heel reconstruction using TDAP flap. Posterior tibial vessels were the recipient vessels. **B,C.** Reconstruction for small heel defect with muscle-chimeric TDAP flap. Anterior tibial vessels are the recipient vessel. **D.** Reconstruction of the plantar midfoot with TDAP flap, using lateral plantar vessels as a recipient vessel. **E.** Reconstruction of lateral forefoot with TDAP flap, using posterior tibial vessels as a recipient vessel through subcutaneous tunneling. **F.** Reconstruction of medial forefoot with TDAP flap, using the first plantar metatarsal vessels as a recipient vessel.

OUTCOMES

- Microvascular free flap for foot reconstruction is, at present, a safe and reliable procedure, with high success rate.[10] Recently, the plantar reconstruction using the perforator flaps showed a success rate of between 97.5% and 98.5%, with acceptable functional and aesthetic outcomes.[5,6]
- Microvascular free flap is a reliable reconstructive option for a variety of size defects on various locations of the heel and plantar foot (**FIG 12A**). Multiple tissue components such as cutaneous and chimeric muscle (**FIG 12B,C**) can be used according to tissue requirements.

COMPLICATIONS

- Vascular complications such as venous and arterial thrombosis.
- Hematoma: early diagnosis of a hematoma under the flap is critical for its evacuation to prevent the obstruction of anastomotic site from the expanding hematoma.
- Infection.
- Ulcerations: ulceration is one of the most common complications of free flap reconstruction of the heel. Although flap-specific factors may contribute to its development, it is possible that flap extrinsic factors such as the recipient bed, bony prominence, Contouring of the flap, and footwear may be more important.

REFERENCES

1. Folman Y, Wosk J, Voloshin A, Liberty S. Cyclic impacts on heel strike: a possible biomechanical factor in the etiology of degenerative disease of the human locomotor system. *Arch Orthop Trauma Surg.* 1986;104:363-365.
2. Chang H, Kwon SS, Minn KW. Lateral calcaneal artery as a recipient pedicle for microsurgical foot reconstruction. *J Plast Reconstr Aesthet Surg.* 2010;63:1860-1864.
3. Woo KJ, Park JW, Mun GH. The lateral calcaneal artery as an alternative recipient vessel option for heel and lateral foot reconstruction. *Microsurgery.* 2018;38:164-171.
4. Burusapat C, Tanthanatip P, Kuhaphensaeng P, et al. Lateral calcaneal artery flaps in atherosclerosis: cadaveric study, vascular assessment and clinical applications. *Plast Reconstr Surg Glob Open.* 2015;3:e517.
5. May JW Jr, Halls MJ, Simon SR. Free microvascular muscle flaps with skin graft reconstruction of extensive defects of the foot: a clinical and gait analysis study. *Plast Reconstr Surg.* 1985;75:627-641.
6. Hong JP, Kim EK. Sole reconstruction using anterolateral thigh perforator free flaps. *Plast Reconstr Surg.* 2007;119:186-193.
7. Jeon BJ, Lee KT, Lim SY, et al. Plantar reconstruction with free thoracodorsal artery perforator flaps. *J Plast Reconstr Aesthet Surg.* 2013;66:406-413.
8. Lee KT, Park SJ, Mun GH. Reconstruction outcomes of oncologic foot defect using well-contoured free perforator flaps. *Ann Surg Oncol.* 2017;24:2404-2412.
9. Santanelli F, Tenna S, Pace A, Scuderi N. Free flap reconstruction of the sole of the foot with or without sensory nerve coaptation. *Plast Reconstr Surg.* 2002;109:2314-2322.
10. Zhu YL, Wang Y, He XQ, et al. Foot and ankle reconstruction: an experience on the use of 14 different flaps in 226 cases. *Microsurgery.* 2013;33:600-604.

15 CHAPTER

The Reverse Sural Artery Flap for Lower Extremity Reconstruction

Ashkaun Shaterian and Amber R. Leis

DEFINITION

- The reverse sural artery flap was first described by Donski and Fogdestam[1] and later by Masquelet et al.[2] and represents a fasciocutaneous flap used in lower extremity reconstruction.
- As a one-stage or two-stage operation that does not require microsurgical techniques, the reverse sural flap is an option available to most reconstructive and orthopedic surgeons.

ANATOMY

- The blood supply for the skin paddle of the distal two-thirds of the leg depends on the sural arteries along its most proximal course and the peroneal artery perforators more distally.
- The reverse sural artery flap receives retrograde arterial flow through septocutaneous perforators that originate from the peroneal artery and directly anastomose with the superficial sural artery.
- There are typically two to five perforators located 5 to 7 cm proximal to the lateral malleolus.[3]
- The venous drainage for this flap is composed of a venous network of the superficial sural vein, the lesser saphenous vein, and the associated veins of the peroneal artery.

PATIENT HISTORY AND PHYSICAL FINDINGS

- Assessment of the defect begins with evaluation for missing tissues, exposed vital structures, and presence of underlying orthopedic hardware.
  - If healthy subcutaneous or granulation tissue presides, the wound may be amenable to skin grafting.
  - If exposure of tendon, artery, vessel, or bone are present, more definitive coverage with fasciocutaneous or muscle flaps is often necessary.
  - The size of the defect will also influence the reconstructive choice.
- The reverse sural artery flap can be used to cover defects of the posterior aspect of heel and Achilles tendon, anterior and lateral ankle, dorsum of the foot, lateral aspect of the hindfoot, and the anterior crest of lower third of the leg.
- Physical exam to evaluate the vascular status of the extremity, and to evaluate for peripheral artery disease or venous insufficiency, is necessary as they may influence flap survival.
- Patient comorbidities of diabetes mellitus, lower extremity venous insufficiency, and peripheral artery disease have been associated with flap necrosis and represent relative contraindications.
- The presence of an occluded anterior or posterior tibial artery does not represent an absolute contraindication to

this flap; however, most consider occlusion of the peroneal artery to preclude its use.[4-6]

IMAGING

- Rarely are radiographs necessary except in the evaluation of bone abnormalities.
- Preoperative angiograms are not routinely obtained but may be useful in patients with pertinent exam findings or in traumatic wounds of the lower extremity.

SURGICAL MANAGEMENT

Preoperative Planning

- The reverse sural artery flap is a fasciocutaneous flap that can be designed with either a complete skin bridge overlying the pedicle or as an island skin flap with an adipofascial pedicle.
- Preoperatively, the peroneal perforators and lesser saphenous vein are identified with Doppler ultrasonography.
- The lesser saphenous vein is used to determine the oblique axis of the pedicle and the flap.
- The flap is designed on the posterior aspect of the calf between the two heads of gastrocnemius at the junction of upper and middle third of the leg (**FIG 1**).
- The dimensions of the flap are determined by the arc of rotation and the size of the defect; however, a reliable flap should not exceed a ratio of length to width of pedicle of 4:1.
- The flap dimensions can reach 15 cm in length and 12 cm in width, but when the flap is less than 3 to 4 cm wide, the donor site defect can be closed primarily.
- The pivot point of the pedicle is dependent on the main perforator and is located 5 cm or three fingerbreadths proximal to the tip of the lateral malleolus and posterior to the fibula.
- The flap may also be designed based on more distal perforators, but the dissection becomes more risky, the width of pedicle decreases, and reliability of the flap declines.

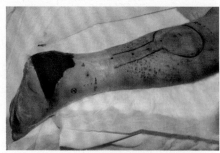

FIG 1 • Flap markings for a reverse sural artery flap with a fasciocutaneous pedicle.

Positioning

- To provide the best exposure, the patient is placed in a prone or lateral position depending on the location of the defect.
- In the lateral position, flexion and adduction of hip and flexion of knee allow for easier access.
- The surgeon is positioned on the same side as the flap and the assistant on the contralateral side.

- All bony prominences should be well padded and the upper extremities and neck placed in positions of safety.

Approach

- The flap is approached from the posterior lower leg after identifying the vascular pedicle and completing the appropriate markings.

■ Reverse Sural Artery Flap

- A well-padded lower extremity tourniquet is applied.
- The skin incision begins along the location of the pedicle and continues around the proximal edge of the flap (**TECH FIG 1A**).
- The subcutaneous tissue is dissected along the pedicle and most proximally to identify and expose the sural nerve, superficial sural artery, sural vein, and lesser saphenous vein.
- At the proximal margin of the flap, the nerve and the vessels are ligated and divided.
- The flap including the skin and subcutaneous tissues containing the neurovascular structures are elevated off the surface of the gastrocnemius muscle in a subfascial plane to the level of the chosen pivot point (**TECH FIG 1B,C**).
- These tissue layers are elevated as a single fasciocutaneous unit and continue distally to isolate the pedicle.

- The pedicle should be at least 2 to 3 cm in width after its dissection from the surrounding tissues.
- The pedicle is dissected free at the pivot point, mobilized, and the flap repositioned to cover the recipient site. It is important that the arc of rotation does not kink or place undue tension on the pedicle.
- Transposition of the flap through either a wide subcutaneous tunnel or an excised skin bridge allows for flap inset.
- The donor site is closed primarily or covered with a split-thickness skin graft.
- At the completion of the case, dressings are applied. The skin graft (if needed) is covered with nonadherent dressings and antibiotic ointment. Nonadherent gauze is used to cover suture lines.
- A well-padded posterior plaster splint with a window for flap monitoring is applied to cover and protect the surgical site.

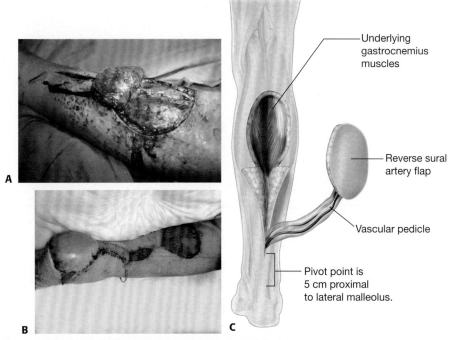

Underlying gastrocnemius muscles

Reverse sural artery flap

Vascular pedicle

Pivot point is 5 cm proximal to lateral malleolus.

TECH FIG 1 • **A.** Flap dissection with the fasciocutaneous pedicle incised. **B.** Flap after inset (as a second stage following a delay procedure) with split-thickness skin grafting to the donor site. **C.** Reverse sural artery flap after flap dissection and elevation.

TECHNIQUES

■ Delayed Reverse Sural Artery Flap

- The delayed reverse sural artery flap aims to improve longitudinal blood flow along the axial pedicle and decrease flap necrosis and is especially useful in patients with vascular comorbidities.
- The described techniques have included raising the flap in the typical subfascial plane but without incising the proximal portion of the skin island flap.

- The skin is closed and 1 to 2 weeks later completely elevated and transposed.
- Others have described complete elevation of the flap at the first stage following flap transfer at the second stage.
- These staged techniques establish improved flap circulation prior to the trauma of flap transfer.

■ Supercharged Reverse Sural Artery Flap

- The supercharged reverse sural artery flap aims to improve venous drainage and bypass venous valves that prevent retrograde venous outflow.

- Described techniques include anastomosing the proximal segment of the less saphenous vein to a vein located at the recipient site or exteriorizing the proximal segment to allow for intermittent drainage upon signs of vascular congestion.[4]

PEARLS AND PITFALLS

Imaging	■ Consider imaging to evaluate the patency of the peroneal artery in traumatic wounds of the lower extremity.
Technique	■ A longer pedicle will allow for tension-free twisting; excessive pedicle rotation at the pivot point can result in a kinked pedicle and flap failure.
	■ It is preferable to incise the skin bridge between the pivot point and recipient site to prevent retractile tissue from compressing the pedicle.
	■ The pivot point of the flap can be revised at a later operation (ie, delayed flaps).
	■ The use of a skin pedicle (vs adipofascial) improves venous return but limits rotation of the flap.
	■ A pedicle width of at least 4 cm has been recently shown to improve venous drainage and flap viability.[3]
	■ The reverse sural flap is often at risk for venous congestion where impaired venous drainage is thought to be a major contributor to flap failure. Widening the pedicle, performing a delayed flap, or supercharging the flap may overcome this problem.

POSTOPERATIVE CARE

- In the immediate postoperative period, direct pressure on the flap must be avoided and strict elevation of the lower extremity is instructed.
- The splint and dressings are removed at 5 to 7 days to allow for complete evaluation of the flap and assessment of skin graft viability.
- Prolonged use of a splint beyond the first week is discouraged but may be continued based on the underlying orthopedic status of the bone.
- Nonadherent dressings are reapplied and maintained for 2 to 3 weeks.
- The patient is maintained nonweight bearing for 1 to 2 weeks and restricted weight bearing for 4 to 6 weeks until flap viability and healing is established.

OUTCOMES

- The reverse sural artery flap has a low complication profile with 82% of flaps healing without any flap-related complications on meta-analysis.[4]
- Morbidity associated with selection of this flap includes loss of sensation over the donor site and lateral foot, presence

of a donor site scar, and excess foot bulk that may preclude proper footwear.

COMPLICATIONS

- Rate of specific complications range in the literature and include partial or complete flap necrosis, venous congestion, infection, hematoma, delayed healing, wound dehiscence, and skin graft loss.
- Patients with vascular comorbidities (ie, diabetes, venous insufficiency, peripheral artery disease), for example, have a five- to sixfold increase in complication rate relative to their healthier counterparts.[7]
- Age over 40 has also been shown to correlate with flap failure.[4,7]

REFERENCES

1. Donski PK, Fogdestam I. Distally based fasciocutaneous flap from the sural region. A preliminary report. *Scand J Plast Reconstr Surg.* 1983;17(3):191-196.
2. Masquelet AC, Romana MC, Wolf G. Skin island flaps supplied by the vascular axis of the sensitive superficial nerves: anatomic study and clinical experience in the leg. *Plast Reconstr Surg.* 1992;89(6): 1115-1121.

3. Sugg KB, et al. The reverse superficial sural artery flap revisited for complex lower extremity and foot reconstruction. *Plast Reconstr Surg Glob Open.* 2015;3(9):e519.

4. Follmar KE, Baccarani A, Baumeister SP, et al. The distally based sural flap. *Plast Reconstr Surg.* 2007;119(6):138e-148e.

5. Hsieh CH, et al. Distally based sural island flap for the reconstruction of a large soft tissue defect in an open tibial fracture with occluded anterior and posterior tibial arteries—a case report. *Br J Plast Surg.* 2005;58(1):112-115.

6. Jolly GP, Zgonis T. Soft tissue reconstruction of the foot with a reverse flow sural artery neurofasciocutaneous flap. *Ostomy Wound Manage.* 2004;50(6):44-49.

7. Baumeister SP, et al. A realistic complication analysis of 70 sural artery flaps in a multimorbid patient group. *Plast Reconstr Surg.* 2003;112(1):129-140.

16
CHAPTER

Ankle Reconstruction With Free Flap

Sean S. Li, Ahmed Suliman, and Deepak M. Gupta

DEFINITION

- The ankle has limited soft tissue for protection of vital structures, and trauma or tumor extirpation often leads to exposed tendons, bone, vessels, or nerves.
- There are few reliable local flaps that can be used for coverage in this area.
- Impaired blood flow is also typical of the distal lower extremity especially in high-risk patients with comorbidities such as smoking, diabetes, peripheral arterial disease, and venous insufficiency, which may result in ulceration, infection, and necrosis of the soft tissues ultimately requiring free flap coverage.
- Due to the complexity of the ankle, reconstruction ideally should be approached in a multidisciplinary fashion consisting primarily of collaboration between plastic and orthopedic surgeons but also with consideration of consultation of infectious disease and vascular surgery.

ANATOMY

- The ankle is a hinge joint with articulations between the tibia, fibula, and talus.
- Defects in the ankle commonly expose bone or orthopedic hardware, usually at the tibia or the medial and lateral malleoli.
- Five nerves supply the foot and ankle—saphenous, sural, deep peroneal, superficial peroneal, and tibial nerves.
- Knowledge of the ankle's vascular anatomy is essential for limb salvage. The distal lower extremity's arterial supply is primarily supplied by three vessels: posterior tibial (PT), anterior tibial (AT), and peroneal.
- The AT artery branches from the popliteal artery, and its course across the ankle is shown (**FIG 1**, left).
- The PT and peroneal arteries originate from the tibioperoneal trunk, and their courses across the ankle are shown (**FIG 1**, right).

PATHOGENESIS

- Defects of the ankle requiring free flap reconstruction originate from trauma (**FIG 2**), tumor extirpation, and peripheral vascular disease.

PATIENT HISTORY AND PHYSICAL FINDINGS

- Evaluation of the patient begins with history and physical focusing on the following:
  - Eliciting the etiology of the wound and presence of comorbidities including smoking, diabetes, obesity, and peripheral vascular disease

- Assessing the overall function of the patient and considering the potential outcomes for the patient and bearing in mind the patient's rehabilitative potential, motivation, and compliance. Location, size, depth, character of the wound, and exposed structures
- Neurological, vascular, and skeletal evaluation of the lower extremities utilizing physical exam, imaging, and Doppler

IMAGING

- Plain films of the defect should be obtained to evaluate for fractures and bony defects with further computed tomography imaging to be considered depending on complexity of the injury.
- If physical or Doppler exam reveals inconclusive vascular status or if peripheral vascular disease is suspected, preoperative arteriography may be obtained.
- Computed tomographic angiography (CTA) (**FIG 3**) can obtain vascular information valuable for flap planning and assessing the recipient site without risk of complications associated with arterial puncture of the groin.
- Selective preoperative CTA may be considered in patients who have lost peripheral pulses, had a neurological deficit secondary to the injury, or of a compound fracture that has undergone reduction and external or internal fixation.[2]

NON OPERATIVE MANAGEMENT

- Defects in the ankle that typically require free flap reconstruction have exposed hardware, tendon devoid of paratenon, vessels, nerves, open joint(s), or bone denuded of periosteum.
- These defects if managed nonoperatively will not heal and can potentially lead to further tissue loss, osteomyelitis, loss of function, or amputation.

SURGICAL MANAGEMENT

- The goal of reconstruction is to achieve a healed wound to allow function.
  - In the ankle, the aims are to allow the patient to wear normal footwear, avoid bulky flaps, and return to weight bearing and ankle motion.
  - Selection of flaps is based on morbidity of the donor site and accessibility of local tissue.
  - Regardless of the flap selection, the principles for reconstruction include adequate debridement, restoring skeletal support, and anastomosing of the flap vessels outside of the zone of injury.[3]

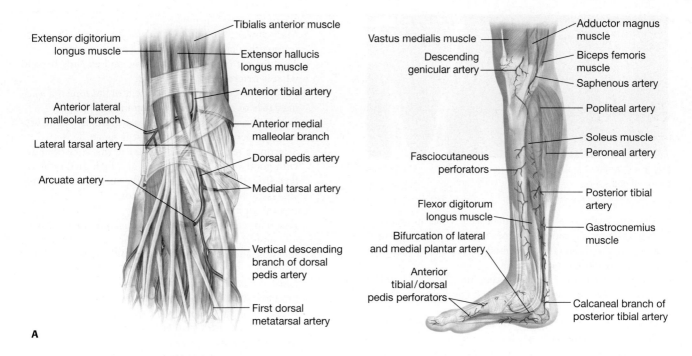

A

Extensor digitorium longus muscle

Tibialis anterior muscle

Extensor hallucis longus muscle

Anterior tibial artery

Anterior lateral malleolar branch

Lateral tarsal artery

Anterior medial malleolar branch

Arcuate artery

Dorsal pedis artery

Medial tarsal artery

Vertical descending branch of dorsal pedis artery

First dorsal metatarsal artery

Vastus medialis muscle

Adductor magnus muscle

Descending genicular artery

Biceps femoris muscle

Saphenous artery

Popliteal artery

Fasciocutaneous perforators

Soleus muscle

Peroneal artery

Flexor digitorum longus muscle

Posterior tibial artery

Bifurcation of lateral and medial plantar artery

Gastrocnemius muscle

Anterior tibial/dorsal pedis perforators

Calcaneal branch of posterior tibial artery

B

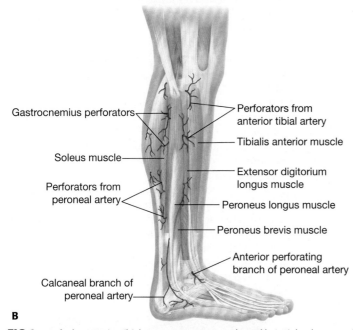

Gastrocnemius perforators

Perforators from anterior tibial artery

Tibialis anterior muscle

Soleus muscle

Extensor digitorium longus muscle

Perforators from peroneal artery

Peroneus longus muscle

Peroneus brevis muscle

Anterior perforating branch of peroneal artery

Calcaneal branch of peroneal artery

FIG 1 • *Left*: the anterior tibial artery course across the ankle.[1] *Right*: the posterior tibial artery and peroneal artery course across the ankle.[1]

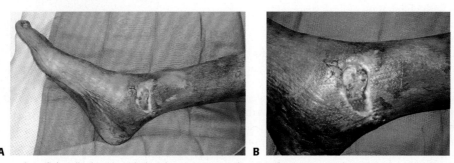

A   **B**

FIG 2 • **A.** Exposed bone of medial malleolus, denuded of the periosteum, chronic inflammation, and scarring of surrounding soft tissues. **B.** Necrotic bone within medial malleolus wound.

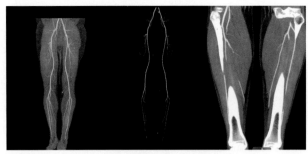

FIG 3 • CTA shows normal angiogram of bilateral thighs and three vessel runoff of the legs.

- After the evaluation of the patient as a whole in regard to their systemic conditions, socioeconomic factors, extent of injury, and rehabilitative potential, a decision for amputation versus salvage can be made.
  - The decision for free flap reconstruction goes hand-in-hand with the patient's orthopedic injuries and potential for functional recovery.
- Scores such as the Mangled Extremity Severity Score (MESS), Predictive Salvage Index, and the Limb Salvage Index can be used to assist in the decision-making for amputation versus salvage.[4]
  - Absolute indications for amputation include complete disruption of the posterior tibial nerve in adults and crush injuries with warm ischemia time greater than 6 hours.
  - Relative indications of amputation include serious associated polytrauma, severe ipsilateral foot trauma, and prolonged anticipated course to soft tissue coverage and tibial reconstruction.

Preoperative Planning

- If reconstruction is indicated, the following must be considered:
  - Bony stability is first established by utilizing external or internal fixation devices.
    - External devices are usually preferred if there is significant bone loss or bone devascularization.
  - In contaminated wounds, multiple stages of debridement may be required until an adequate wound bed without devitalized or infected tissues is achieved.
    - Vacuum-assisted closure decreases need for dressing changes and can promote healing.[5]
    - Osteomyelitis can follow severe open fractures with massive contamination or devascularized tissue; management includes resection of dead or infected bone, flap coverage with obliteration of dead space, and antibiotic treatment.[6]
  - Timing of reconstruction
    - If the general condition of the patient and the status of the wound are adequate, definitive coverage should not be delayed.
    - Ideally, the wound should be covered in the first week after injury in the acute phase as further delay causes the wound to enter into the subacute and chronic phases when there is a higher rate of infectious complications and flap failure.[7,8]

- Zone of injury[9]
  - Many lower extremity wounds result from high-energy trauma that creates a significant "zone of injury."
  - This zone is highly thrombogenic and extends beyond what is macroscopically evident.
  - Failure to recognize the true extent of the zone is a leading cause of microsurgical anastomotic failure.
  - Within this zone, there is increased friability of the vessels and increased perivascular scar tissue.
  - Selecting a recipient vessel outside of this zone of injury with good vessel wall pliability and high-quality blood flow from the transected end of the vessel is essential for successful microsurgical anastomosis.
- Coverage after tumor extirpation
  - Free flap reconstruction must withstand radiation therapy and/or chemotherapy with the goal of preserving function and achieving an acceptable appearance and function.
  - Close cooperation with oncologists and knowledge of prognosis/risk of recurrence/survival, tumor characteristics, behavior, and adjuvant treatment is necessary to plan for the correct type of reconstructive procedure.
- Exposed hardware
  - Traditionally management involved irrigation and debridement, antibiotics, and removal of hardware.
  - However, if the hardware is clinically stable, exposure is less than 2 weeks, the infection is controlled, and the hardware is utilized for bony consolidation, then the likelihood of salvage with soft tissue coverage is increased.[10]
- Reconstruction in patients with a two- or one-vessel extremity
  - Consider vascular bypass surgery.
  - End-to-side anastomosis during free flap reconstruction can preserve the existing main arteries.
  - A flow-through free flap can be utilized where an anastomosis is made both proximally and distally to vessels in the leg (**FIG 4**).
  - Some have reported that an anastomosis can technically also be made to a distal stump of a recipient vessel to rely on arterial backflow[11]; however, this should be a last resort and consideration should be made for possible low flow state.
- Muscle versus fasciocutaneous free flaps
  - Controversy exists over selecting the type of flap for lower extremity defects.

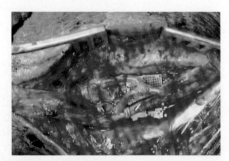

FIG 4 • The flap has been anastomosed end-to-end to the posterior tibial artery. After flowing through, another end-to-end anastomosis allows circulation to the foot through the posterior tibial artery via the rectus femoris branch.

- Reconstruction of wounds with muscle flaps has been shown experimentally to have increased blood flow and antibiotic delivery, increased oxygen tension, increased phagocytic activity, and decreased bacterial counts when compared to fasciocutaneous flaps.[12]
- Arguably muscle flaps are technically less challenging, can fill larger defects, and can be harvested with decreased operative time compared with fasciocutaneous flaps (eg, vastus lateralis flap versus anterolateral thigh flap).[13]
- Donor site morbidity of muscle flaps can be greater than fasciocutaneous flaps depending on the muscle selected.
- Selection of a flap depends on the defect, condition of the wound, goals of reconstruction, and surgeon and patient preference.

Positioning

- Patient positioning in free flap surgery is an important issue that needs to be considered preoperatively. Most cases can be done in supine, supine frog leg, or lateral decubitus position.
- The goal is to avoid unnecessary repositioning of the patient intraoperatively in order to save anesthetic and operative time.
- The location of the defect or choice of recipient vessels may determine the positioning of the patient and to some extent, the flap choice.
- For example, anterior defects favor the use of the anterolateral thigh flap, gracilis flap, rectus abdominis flap, etc.
- Posterior tibial recipient vessels (medial leg approach) may favor either supine or lateral decubitus position and the concordant flap choices.

Approach

- The approach to flap harvest depends on the flap selection and considering the positioning of the patient as noted above.

- The approach to the ankle wound depends on the location of the defect and selection of recipient vessels.
- The posterior tibial artery is the most commonly used recipient vessel.
  - It is easily accessible by a medial approach and is found between the deep posterior and superficial posterior compartments. In other terms, it is deep to the soleus muscle.
  - The most favorable positioning for the patient is either lateral or with frog leg positioning.
  - It is the preferred vessel for defects of the posterior or medial ankle.
  - It may also be used for lateral defects, and there are several options for pedicle routing, such as under the Achilles tendon.
- The anterior tibial artery is the second most commonly used recipient vessel.
  - It is easily accessible in the anterior compartment.
  - The most favorable positioning of the patient is supine.
  - Some may favor the anterior tibial vessels for defects of the anterior and lateral ankle.
- The peroneal artery is usually the last choice for recipient vessel because of difficulty of accessibility, which may require removal of fibular bone.
- The two major superficial veins of the lower extremity are the great and small saphenous veins, which run superficial to the fascia cruris.
  - The great saphenous vein is accompanied by the saphenous nerve and is located anterior to the medial malleolus.
  - The small saphenous vein arises from the lateral side of the foot, posterior to the lateral malleolus, and passes along the border of the Achilles tendon.
  - Any superficial vein with adequate caliber can be used as a recipient vein in addition to the venae comitantes of the major arteries.
  - Anastomosis of two recipient veins for each artery is optional. If undertaken, it is preferable to anastomose to separate drainage systems (eg, one deep vein and one superficial vein).

■ Vastus Lateralis

- Take into account all of the preoperative factors as noted in the preoperative planning section.
- Assess the defect.
- Approach your recipient vessel as mentioned in the various approaches above, and dissect back to healthy vessel outside of the zone of injury (**TECH FIG 1A**). Use of tourniquet may be considered.
- Elevate the flap as previously described.[13]
  - With the patient positioned supine, a line is drawn between the anterior superior iliac spine and the superolateral corner of the patella on the donor thigh.
  - An incision is then made along the middle third of the line. Carry the incision through the muscle fascia until the interval between the rectus femoris and the vastus lateralis is identified. Extend the incision as needed as you go along. Take care to identify any branches of the lateral cutaneous femoral nerve so as not to injure them.
  - Separate the rectus femoris and vastus lateralis and identify and preserve the pedicle (the descending

branch of the lateral circumflex femoral artery), which is generally visible along the medial border of the vastus lateralis.
- Perform a lateral subfascial dissection superficial to the muscle until the width of muscle flap needed has been visualized. Continue this dissection proximal and distal along the superficial surface of the muscle until the dimensions of muscle flap needed have been achieved.
- Identify the motor nerve branches, which typically enter the midportion of the muscle; only sacrifice branches directly involved in the transferred portion of muscle.
- Dissect the pedicle from distal to proximal. Continue the dissection until adequate pedicle length and vessel caliber has been obtained. One may encounter vascular branches to the vastus intermedius or rectus femoris, which can typically be sacrificed. Nerve branches should be spared.
- Divide the muscle along the required dimensions. Ligate and divide the pedicle when the recipient area is ready.

TECHNIQUES

- Perform your anastomosis (**TECH FIG 1B**) and inset the flap (**TECH FIG 1C**). Consider use of penrose drains around the microvascular anastomoses. Some additional de-epithelialization or resection of leg skin may be required to accommodate flap and/or pedicle lie.

- Harvest split-thickness skin graft for the flap. Meshing of the skin graft may be considered (**TECH FIG 1D**).
- The donor site can usually be closed primarily over closed suction drains.

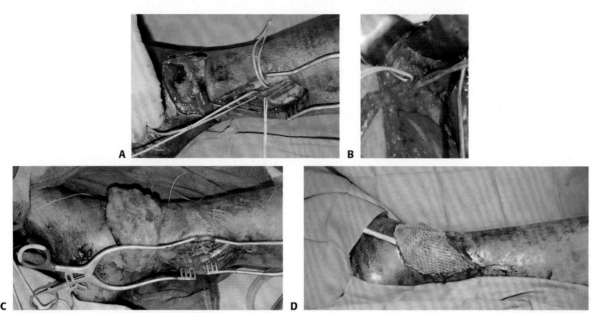

TECH FIG 1 • A. The posterior tibial artery and two venae comitantes have been dissected proximal to the zone of injury. **B.** The descending branch of the lateral circumflex femoral artery has been dissected (*blue loop*) to its origin along with the rectus femoris branch (*red loop*). **C.** The flap has been anastomosed in flow through configuration outside the zone of injury. The inset is partially completed with Vicryl sutures. Intervening leg skin was subsequently de-epithelialized to accommodate flap and pedicle lie. **D.** The flap has been inset and covered with a meshed split-thickness skin graft.

■ Anterolateral Thigh (ALT)

- Take into account all of the preoperative factors as noted in the preoperative planning section.
- Assess the defect.
- Approach your recipient vessel as mentioned in the various approaches above, and dissect back to healthy vessel outside of the zone of injury. Use of tourniquet may be considered.
- Elevate the flap as previously described.[14]
   - With the patient positioned supine, a line is drawn between the anterior superior iliac spine and the superolateral corner of the patella on the donor thigh.
   - Draw a 3-cm circle centered at the midpoint of this line. Map the cutaneous perforators with a portable, handheld pencil Doppler probe. The majority of perforators will be found in the inferolateral quadrant of this circle.
   - The flap is centered over the location of these vessels, and its long axis should be parallel to that of the thigh. The maximum width of the flap is judged with a pinch test.
   - Incise the medial border of the proposed flap and continue dissection deep and through the muscle fascia until you have identified fibers of rectus femoris.
   - Continue the subfascial dissection from medial to lateral. Take care to identify the interval between vastus lateralis and rectus femoris and not cross it. At this point, the dissection should be slowed so that one can identify and preserve any septocutaneous or

musculocutaneous perforators corresponding to the cutaneous Doppler signals.
   - Once the dominant perforator(s) have been identified, these are carefully dissected distal to proximal, to either free them from the vastus lateralis muscle or include them with a cuff of muscle.
   - Incise the skin paddle along its lateral aspect. Perform a subfascial dissection to the dissected perforators.
   - Depending on the vascular configuration, vastus lateralis muscle can also be dissected on a separate branch if a chimeric flap is needed.
   - Dissect the pedicle from distal to proximal. Continue the dissection until adequate pedicle length and vessel caliber has been obtained. One may encounter vascular branches to the vastus intermedius or rectus femoris, which can typically be sacrificed. Nerve branches should be spared.
   - Ligate and divide the pedicle when the recipient area is ready.
- Perform your anastomosis and inset the flap.
- The anterolateral thigh (ALT) donor site can usually be undermined and closed primarily over closed suction drains. The maximum width of the flap is judged with a pinch test. Donor sites that cannot be primarily closed may be skin grafted. Others have reported closing large donor sites using adjacent tissue transfer techniques.

▪ Gracilis

- Take into account all of the preoperative factors as noted in the preoperative planning section.
- Assess the defect.
- Approach your recipient vessel as mentioned in the various approaches above and dissect back to healthy vessel outside of the zone of injury. Use of tourniquet may be considered.
- Elevate the flap as previously described.[15]
  - With patient supine, position the lower limb in external hip rotation, and knee and hip in flexion as needed. Palpate the adductor longus tendon in the medial thigh.
  - The gracilis is posterior to the adductor longus. An incision is marked two to three finger breadths posterior to the adductor longus tendon. Keep in mind that the neurovascular pedicle enters the muscle approximately 10 cm below its bony origin.
  - An optional distal incision at the knee can be made to transect the distal tendon if the entire length of the flap is needed.
  - Carry the proximal incision down through the fat and muscular fascia to the muscle. Take care to identify the greater saphenous vein during this step and protect it by retracting if necessary.
  - Dissect superficial to the gracilis muscle to expose its surface.
  - Identify the interval between gracilis and adductor longus. Enter the interval carefully to identify the pedicle—the medial circumflex femoral artery and veins.
  - Dissect the pedicle from distal to proximal. Continue the dissection until adequate pedicle length and vessel caliber has been obtained. One may encounter vascular branches to the adductor longus, which can be sacrificed. Nerve branches should be spared.
  - Divide the muscle along the required dimensions. Ligate and divide the pedicle when the recipient area is ready.
- Perform your anastomosis and inset the flap.
- Harvest split-thickness skin graft for the flap.
- The donor site can usually be closed primarily over closed suction drains.

▪ Rectus Abdominis

- Take into account all of the preoperative factors as noted in the preoperative planning section.
- Assess the defect.
- Approach your recipient vessel as mentioned in the various approaches above, and dissect back to healthy vessel outside of the zone of injury.
- Elevate the flap as previously described.[16]
  - With the patient supine, the muscle can be exposed through a midline vertical, paramedian vertical, or lower transverse incision with the total length of the incision depending on the amount of muscle harvested.
  - Dissect down to the level of the rectus sheath, ligating perforators as they are found.
  - Divide the rectus sheath longitudinally and elevate the fascia medially and laterally taking care to tease off the inscriptions without damaging the muscle fibers.
  - Identify the deep inferior epigastric artery and its accompanying veins at the lateral edge of the inferior muscle within the fatty tissue. Dissect the pedicle from distal to proximal. Continue the dissection until adequate pedicle length and vessel caliber has been obtained.
  - Divide the muscle along the required dimensions. Ligate and divide the pedicle when the recipient area is ready.
- Perform your anastomosis, and inset the flap.
- Harvest split-thickness skin graft for the flap.
- Close the fascia with nonabsorbable suture. Close the donor site wound primarily. Use drains as needed.

▪ Latissimus Dorsi

- Take into account all of the preoperative factors as noted in the preoperative planning section.
- Assess the defect.
- Approach your recipient vessel as mentioned in the various approaches above, and dissect back to healthy vessel outside of the zone of injury.
- Elevate the flap as previously described.[17]
  - The flap harvest is usually done in lateral decubitus position with appropriate padding. The ipsilateral arm may also be prepped into the operative field depending on surgeon preference. The current authors prefer to use a padded and draped Mayo stand to position the arm.
  - The latissimus is marked by finding the surrounding landmarks—scapular tip superiorly, iliac crest inferiorly, spinous processes medially.
  - Choice of skin incision also depends on surgeon preference and size of flap needed. Incisions made include transverse (to hide within a bra line), oblique (extending from posterior axillary fold over the middle of the muscle belly), or vertical (uncommon).
  - Expose the latissimus by dissecting the skin and subcutaneous tissues off the muscle all the way to all its edges. Dissect the submuscular plane taking care not to elevate the serratus muscle or fat pad. It is easiest to being this dissection anteriorly or superiorly.

- Release the insertions near the midline of the back and then inferiorly. Proceed with the submuscular dissection from distal to proximal toward the axilla. The pedicle can be visualized along the deep surface of the muscle as one approaches the axilla.
- Identify the branch to the serratus muscle. Ligate it if necessary. The circumflex scapular branch may also be ligated if additional pedicle length or larger caliber is needed.

- Trim the muscle along the required dimensions. Ligate and divide the pedicle (including the thoracodorsal nerve) when the recipient area is ready.
- Reposition the patient if necessary.
- Perform your anastomosis and inset the flap.
- Harvest split-thickness skin graft for the flap.
- Close the donor site over suction drains.

PEARLS AND PITFALLS

Amputation vs limb salvage	Consider limb salvage on a case-to-case basis. If a long, protracted course for limb salvage is anticipated, consider the benefit of early mobilization and physical therapy after amputation.
Zone of injury	Microsurgical anastomosis outside the zone of injury is critical to success.
Timing of reconstruction	If possible, reconstruction within 7 days in the acute period leads to higher incidence of flap survival.
Sequence of salvage	Bony stability, thorough debridement to achieve favorable wound bed, flap reconstruction.
Flap selection	Select a flap with sufficient pedicle length to anastomose outside the zone of injury, does not require intraoperative repositioning, and has acceptable donor site morbidity.

POSTOPERATIVE CARE

- Immobilization of the extremity and bed rest is recommended for 5 to 14 days postoperatively.
- Dangling of the leg is then initiated, with increasing frequency and length continuously while the flap is carefully watched for swelling, congestion, or increasing pain.
- Compression stockings or wraps are applied after 4 weeks and continued for approximately 6 months.

OUTCOMES

- The goal is a healed wound, return to activity, and acceptable contour (**FIG 5**).
- Functional outcomes largely depend on the extent of the patient's injuries.

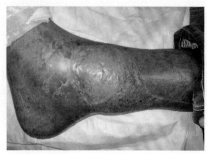

FIG 5 • The goal is a healed wound, return to activity, and acceptable contour.

- Prognosis for bony union and adequate neurovascular recovery must be considered.
- Patient compliance is important for best long-term results.
- Patients at high risk for amputation can be advised that reconstruction typically results in 2-year outcomes equivalent to those of amputation.[18]

COMPLICATIONS

- Osteomyelitis
- Chronic pain
- Nonunion
- Flap failure
- Contour abnormality
- Donor site morbidity
- Amputation

REFERENCES

1. Attinger CE, Evans KK, Bulan E, et al. Angiosomes of the foot and ankle and clinical implications for limb salvage: reconstruction, incisions, and revascularization. *Plast Reconstr Surg.* 2006;117:261s-293s.
2. Duymaz A, Karabekmez FE, Vrtiska TJ, et al. Free tissue transfer for lower extremity reconstruction: a study of the role of computed angiography in the planning of free tissue transfer in the posttraumatic setting. *Plast Reconstr Surg.* 2009;124:523-529.
3. Serafin D, Voci VE. Reconstruction of the lower extremity. Microsurgical composite tissue transplantation. *Clin Plast Surg.* 1983; 10:55-72.
4. Ong YS, Levin LS. Lower limb salvage in trauma. *Plast Reconstr Surg.* 2010;125:582-588.
5. Reddy V, Stevenson TR. MOC-PS(SM) CME article: lower extremity reconstruction. *Plast Reconstr Surg.* 2008;121:1-7.

6. Anthony JP, Mathes SJ. Update on chronic osteomyelitis. *Clin Plast Surg.* 1991;18:515-523.

7. Godina M. Early microsurgical reconstruction of complex trauma of the extremities. *Plast Reconstr Surg.* 1986;78:285-292.

8. Byrd HS, Cierny G III, Tebbetts JB. The management of open tibial fractures with associated soft-tissue loss: external pin fixation with early flap coverage. *Plast Reconstr Surg.* 1981;68:73-82.

9. Arnez ZM. Immediate reconstruction of the lower extremity—an update. *Clin Plast Surg.* 1991;18:449-457.

10. Viol A, Pradka SP, Baumeister SP, et al. Soft-tissue defects and exposed hardware: a review of indications for soft-tissue reconstruction and hardware preservation. *Plast Reconstr Surg.* 2009;123:1256-1263.

11. Park S, Han SH, Lee TJ. Algorithm for recipient vessel selection in free tissue transfer to the lower extremity. *Plast Reconstr Surg.* 1999; 103:1937-1948.

12. Calderon W, Chang N, Mathes SJ. Comparison of the effect of bacterial inoculation in musculocutaneous and fasciocutaneous flaps. *Plast Reconstr Surg.* 1986;77:785-794.

13. Kaminsky AJ, Li SS, Copeland-Halperin LR, Miraliakbari R. The vastus lateralis free flap for lower extremity gustilo grade III reconstruction. *Microsurgery.* 2017;37:212-217.

14. Wei FC, Jain V, Celik N, et al. Have we found an ideal soft-tissue flap? An experience with 672 anterolateral thigh flaps. *Plast Reconstr Surg.* 2002;109:2219-2226.

15. Franco MJ, Nicoson MC, Parikh RP, Tung TH. Lower extremity reconstruction with free gracilis flaps. *J Reconstr Microsurg.* 2017; 33:218-224.

16. Bunkis J, Walton RL, Mathes SJ. The rectus abdominis free flap for lower extremity reconstruction. *Ann Plast Surg.* 1983;11: 373-380.

17. May JW Jr, Lukash FN, Gallico GG III. Latissimus dorsi free muscle flap in lower-extremity reconstruction. *Plast Reconstr Surg.* 1981; 68:603-607.

18. Bosse MJ, MacKenzie EJ, Kellam JF, et al. An analysis of outcomes of reconstruction or amputation after leg-threatening injuries. *N Engl J Med.* 2002;347:1924-1931.

17 CHAPTER

Vascular Reconstruction of Lower Extremity, Foot, and Ankle

Michael D. Sgroi and Jason T. Lee

DEFINITIONS

- Peripheral arterial disease (PAD) affects 8 to 12 million people worldwide.
- Up to 40% of these patients suffer from poor quality of life due to impaired walking ability, nonhealing wounds, and need for amputation.
- Risk factors include male gender, age, hypertension, diabetes, hyperlipidemia, renovascular disease, and smoking.
- Sixty to ninety percent of patients with peripheral arterial disease also have coronary artery disease, and up to 25% have carotid artery stenosis.[1]
- The overall 5-year mortality rate among all patients with PAD is 15% to 30%, and the risk of nonfatal myocardial infarction or stroke is 20% at 5 years.[2]
- Patients with critical limb ischemia have an annual cardiovascular mortality of 25% and an annual amputation rate of 25%.[3]

ANATOMY

- Femoral artery usually lies one-third the distance from the pubic tubercle and two-thirds from the anterior superior iliac spine.
- Lateral dissection at the femoral artery should be minimized so not to disrupt the femoral nerve.
- Medial dissection at the femoral artery should be minimized so not to damage the femoral vein.
- Exposure of the common femoral artery should include the distal external iliac artery under the inguinal ligament.
- Care should be taken to identify all distal branches (superficial femoral artery (SFA) and profunda femoris).
- Anterior tibial artery runs in the anterior compartment of the leg.
- Anterior tibial artery is between the anterior tibialis and extensor digitorum longus muscles.
- Anterior tibial artery becomes the dorsalis pedis when it crosses the ankle joint.
- Dorsalis pedis can be palpated just lateral to extensor hallucis longus on the dorsum of the foot.
- Posterior tibial artery carries blood through the posterior compartment of the leg and plantar surface of the foot.
- Posterior tibial artery branches into the medial and lateral plantar arteries in the foot.
- Posterior tibial artery can be palpated midway between the medial malleolus and the Achilles tendon.

PATIENT HISTORY AND PHYSICAL FINDINGS

- Ischemic claudication (ie, arterial perfusion inadequate to meet the demands of the muscle) leads to cramping, aching pain.
- Claudication will usually occur one vascular level below the stenosis or occlusion.
- Ischemic rest pain (ie, chronic ischemic neuropathy that is positional) is often described as diffuse aching or burning while legs are up in recumbent position, which is improved after legs have been put in the dependent position.
- Vascular and neurogenic claudication must first be differentiated.
- Infrapopliteal disease is most often going to lead to ankle and foot disease.
- Patients with tibial disease are more likely to experience rest pain or have nonhealing wounds rather than claudication symptoms.
- Ulcers to the medial side of the ankle are more likely due to venous disease.
- Ulcers to the lateral food and ankle are more likely to be due to arterial disease.

IMAGING AND OTHER DIAGNOSTIC STUDIES

- An ankle-brachial index (ABI) may be obtained by dividing the systolic blood pressure of the lower leg/ankle by the systolic blood pressure of the upper arm (brachial artery) (**FIG 1**).
  - An ABI ≤ 0.9 is considered abnormal.
  - ABIs will most commonly be indeterminate because the tibial vessels become noncompressible and waveforms will be monophasic.
- Toe-brachial pressures (TBIs) will be more diagnostic in patients with tibial disease.
  - A TBI < 0.4 will indicate a wound is unlikely to heal without intervention.
- Arteriography should be performed to evaluate the tibial vessels prior to any distal lower extremity or foot reconstruction.
  - Patients with diabetes and end-stage renal disease most frequently are affected by small vessel disease, including tibial vessels and the microvascular circulation.

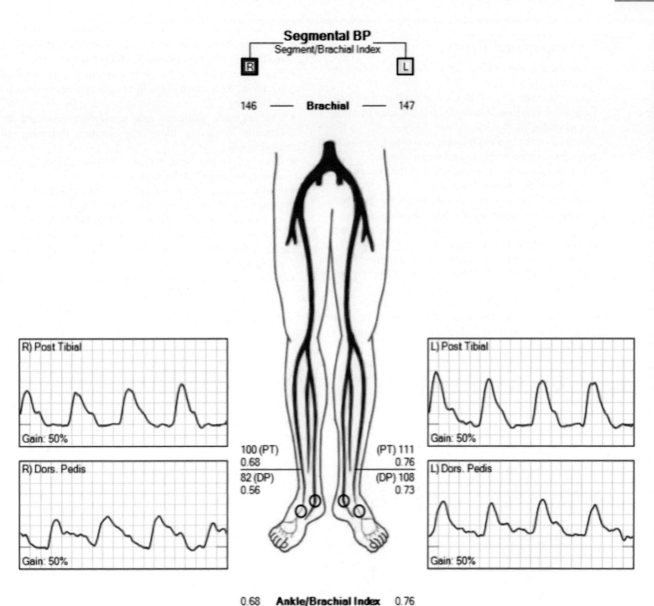

FIG 1 • Example of an abnormal ankle-brachial index study.

SURGICAL MANAGEMENT

- A patient must first have an appropriate inflow and outflow vessel identified for reconstruction.
- Autologous vein has superior rates of patency compared to prosthetic grafts.
- Vein mapping should be performed preoperatively, assuring at least a 3-mm conduit.
- Shorter bypass grafts have better patency.

- The most distal patent native vessel should be used as the proximal origin of the bypass graft.
  - For example, if the patient has a patent popliteal artery, this should be chosen over a femoral artery.
- Primary patency (the patency of a graft without any adjunctive therapies to keep it open), secondary patency (the patency rate once the graft has been completely abandoned and no further interventions are performed to keep it open), and limb salvage rates are 56.8%, 62.7%, and 78.2%, respectively, at 5 years for pedal revascularizations.

■ Femoropopliteal Bypass

- Identification of the femoral artery should be within the femoral triangle.
  - Femoral triangle consists of the inguinal ligament superiorly, sartorius muscle laterally, and the adductor magnus medially.
  - The floor of the femoral triangle consists of the iliacus, psoas major, pectineus, and adductor magnus.
  - The femoral artery is a continuation of the external iliac artery below the inguinal ligament.
  - Common femoral artery divides into the profunda femoral artery and the superficial femoral artery.
  - The profunda femoral gives branches to the thigh and collaterals to the lower extremity.
  - The superficial femoral artery is a continuation of the common femoral artery and progresses to the popliteal artery.
- Longitudinal incision is made over the pulse in the groin, which is usually located below the inguinal ligament approximately one-third lateral to the pubic tubercle (**TECH FIG 1A**).

- Dissection is taken down through the fascia lata, keeping medial to the sartorius muscle (**TECH FIG 1B**).
- The superior limit of the groin dissection is the inguinal ligament. Retraction of the ligament exposes the external iliac artery.
- The inguinal ligament can be further retracted by laterally dissecting along the ligament releasing all attachments.
- Once under the ligament, the inferior epigastric vein should be identified and ligated.
- Profunda femoral artery divides into the adductor fascia. Dissection along the anterior surface can be performed, identifying each of its branches (**TECH FIG 1C,D**).
- Care should be taken not to dissect into the deep lateral circumflex femoral vein, which lies across the proximal profunda.
- A lateral approach at the profunda can also be performed along the lateral surface of the sartorius.
  - The sartorius is then retracted medially while the rectus femoris and vastus medialis are retracted laterally.

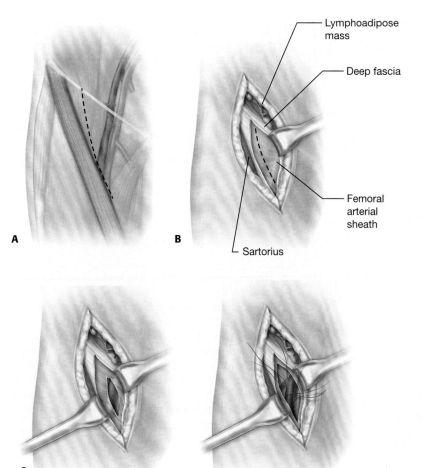

A. Longitudinal exposure of the common femoral artery. **B.** A longitudinal incision is medial to the sartorius muscle allowing exposure.

Lymphoadipose mass

Deep fascia

Femoral arterial sheath

Sartorius

TECH FIG 1 • A. Longitudinal exposure of the common femoral artery. **B.** A longitudinal incision is medial to the sartorius muscle allowing exposure. **C.** The femoral artery sits in the middle of the femoral sheath between the nerve and vein. **D.** Proper exposure includes vascular control of the common femoral, superficial femoral, and profunda femoral artery.

Above-Knee Popliteal Exposure

- Exposure of the above-knee popliteal artery starts with a longitudinal incision on the distal medial thigh in the intermuscular groove between the sartorius muscle and the vastus medialis (**TECH FIG 2**).
- Care should be taken not to damage the greater saphenous vein during this incision.

- Sartorius is then retracted posteriorly, while the adductor magnus is retracted anteriorly.
- Retraction of sartorius and adductor magnus gives exposure to the adductor canal.
- Dissection is then performed through the popliteal fat pad allowing exposure of the popliteal artery and vein.

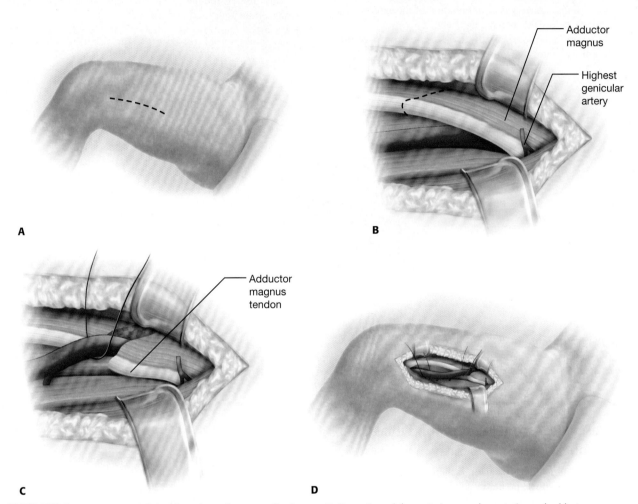

TECH FIG 2 • A. Exposure of the above-knee femoropopliteal artery. **B.** Retraction of the sartorius muscle posterior and adductor magnus anterior allows for exposure of adductor canal. **C.** The geniculate collaterals should be saved if possible. However, they can be ligated for higher exposure if necessary. **D.** Adductor magnus can also be cut if needed for more proximal control.

Below-Knee Popliteal Exposure

- A longitudinal incision should be made on the medial calf from the tibial condyle distally (**TECH FIG 3A**).
- Keeping the medial head of the gastrocnemius posterior (**TECH FIG 3B**), the soleus muscle arch will be identified. Superior to the soleus is the popliteal fat pad where the popliteal neurovascular bundle is located.
- The paired popliteal veins will be surrounding the artery and will need to be mobilized (**TECH FIG 3C**).

- The soleus muscle can be dissected away from the tibia if more distal control is needed.
- Autogenous vein grafts provide the best patency for use in arterial bypass for all infrainguinal reconstructions, regardless of the distal bypass target.
  - Reverse and in situ vein have equal effectiveness.[4]
  - If an above-knee bypass is performed, PTFE has equivalent 2- to 3-year patency rates to autogenous vein.[5]

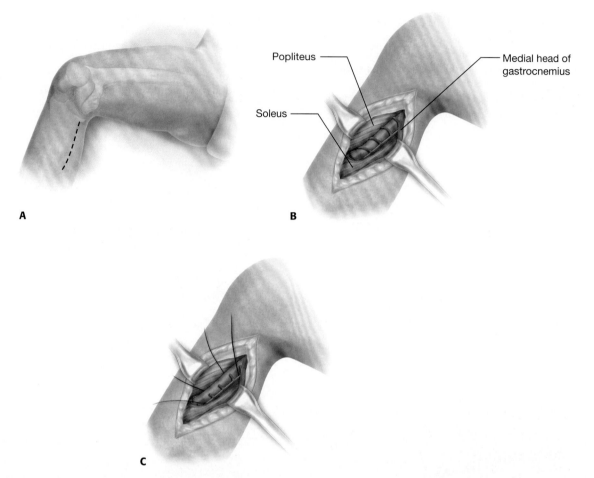

TECH FIG 3 • A. The below-knee popliteal artery is exposed from a medial incision starting at the tibial condyle and continuing distally. **B.** The medial head of the gastrocnemius muscle is then retracted posteriorly and popliteus muscle anteriorly. **C.** There are multiple crossing veins around the popliteal artery that will need to be controlled during popliteal artery exposure.

■ Vascular Reconstruction for Tibial-Peroneal Arterial Occlusive Disease

- Indications include rest pain, ischemic ulcerations, gangrene of the foot, and highly selected patients with short-distance claudication.
- Selection of conduit is most important. Autogenous vein should be used if possible. In general, adequate vein is larger than 3 mm.
- Ipsilateral vein is preferred over contralateral if possible.
- Inflow should be chosen based on preoperative imaging as well as available conduit length.
- Inflow vessels include common femoral, profunda femoris, superficial femoral artery, and above-knee popliteal artery.
- Outflow vessel chosen for bypass should be the one with in-line flow to the pedal vessels. However, peroneal can also be used despite lack of direct communication.

Anterior Tibial Artery Exposure

- Longitudinal incision lateral aspect of leg between the anterior tibialis and the extensor digitorum longus muscles.
- Dissection should be continued on the lateral aspect of the anterior tibialis muscle rotating it anterior Land medial.

The neurovascular bundle will be identified posterior to this muscle.
- Tunneling can be performed from a medial or a lateral approach.
- For a medial approach, a medial incision is made to expose the popliteal fossa. This is followed by an incision of the interosseous membrane to cross the conduit into appropriate position.
- If a lateral approach is used, then the graft is initially brought subsartorius from the femoral position and lateral through the tensor fascia lata. The tensor fascia will need to be incised to allow the conduit to come through. The graft will then lie in the subcutaneous tissue of the lateral thigh and calf.[6]
- Care should be taken with the lateral tunneling away from the fibular head to avoid injury to the peroneal nerve.

Posterior Tibial Artery Exposure

- Longitudinal incision is made 2 cm below the medial edge of the tibia.
- The gastrocnemius muscle is kept posterior until the soleus muscle is identified.

- Careful dissection is then performed with electro-cautery dissecting the soleus off of the posterior tibia aponeurosis.
- Crossing tibial veins will need to be identified and ligated to allow the posterior tibial artery to be exposed.
- Tunneling for a posterior tibial bypass will be in the same anatomic position as a femoral popliteal artery bypass but extended down to the location of the distal exposure.

Peroneal Artery Exposure

- Longitudinal incision on the medial leg 2 cm below the medial edge of the tibia
- The gastrocnemius and soleus are dissected posteriorly to expose the flexor digitorum longus muscle, which lies on the posterior aspect of the tibia.
- The fascia of the flexor digitorum longus is opened to enter the deep compartment. Dissection is carried until

the peroneal vascular bundle is identified on the anterior aspect of the fibula on the flexor hallucis longus muscle.

Pedal Artery Exposure

- Exposure of the pedal vessels can be accurately identified with the assistance of ultrasound or handheld Doppler prior to making an incision.
- The dorsalis pedis artery will be on the dorsum of the foot just lateral to the extensor hallucis longus tendon.
- A longitudinal incision is made directly over the artery. Dissection will go through the dorsal sheath, and retracting the tendon medially should expose the dorsalis pedis.
- For the posterior tibial artery distally, a longitudinal incision is made half way between the medial malleolus and the Achilles tendon (**TECH FIG 4**).

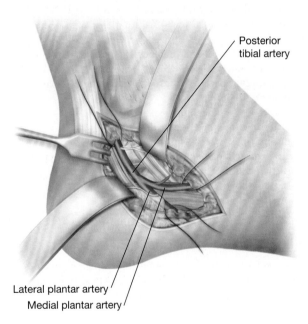

Posterior tibial artery

Lateral plantar artery
Medial plantar artery

TECH FIG 4 • Plantar exposure of the posterior tibial artery. Incision is made posterior to the medial malleolus. As the artery starts to cross the arch of the foot, it will branch into the medial and lateral plantar arteries.

PEARLS AND PITFALLS

Conduit condition	▪ If performing a vein bypass, always ensure careful handling of the venous conduit. If there is an area that appears sclerotic or injured, it is better to remove that segment.
Conduit length	▪ Obtain exposure of the proximal and distal location of your bypass prior to performing the vein harvest, as you want to make sure you have adequate length vein as well as an appropriate location for your proximal and distal anastomosis. ▪ Measure the distance of the bypass with the knee extended to ensure adequate conduit length.
Tourniquet use	▪ A tourniquet can be used for arterial control of the distal anastomosis and is particularly useful if the patient significantly calcified vessels.
Imaging	▪ A completion arteriogram is helpful if there is any question about the patient's outflow.

POSTOPERATIVE CARE

- Average length of stay for a bypass patient is 4 to 6 days.
- Leg elevation postoperatively is important as the patient will have swelling to the limb from both reperfusion and resection of the superficial venous system.
- All patients should be started on a daily 81 mg aspirin following surgery. Patients should also be restarted on their statin and beta-blocker if on them preoperatively.[1,7]
- Dual therapy with antiplatelet and anticoagulation has demonstrated improved patency, particularly in patients who have a prosthetic conduit. However, these patients are also at increased risk of bleeding.
- Repeat ABIs with graft duplex can be performed at the first postoperative clinic visit in 2 to 4 weeks.

OUTCOMES

- Open surgical bypass is accepted as the most durable treatment for critical limb ischemia.
- Five-year overall patency rates range from 60% to 80% and limb salvage rate of 80% to 90% in patients with critical limb ischemia.
- Venous conduits have better patency than using prosthetic graft below the knee.
- Five-year expected patency rates for infrainguinal bypass a vein conduit[4,8]
  - Femoral to above-knee popliteal—75%
  - Femoral to below-knee popliteal—70%
  - Femoral to tibial artery—65%
- Five-year expected patency rates for infrainguinal bypass with prosthetic graft[5,8]
  - Femoral to above-knee popliteal—50%
  - Femoral to below-knee popliteal—35%
  - Femoral to tibial artery—20%

COMPLICATIONS

- Patients with vascular disease often have other comorbid conditions. Systemic complications such as MI, stroke, renal failure, and pneumonia are all potential risks.
- Wound complications can occur with either incision but are particularly higher at the groin incision. Femoral incision complications occur in about 15% to 30% of patients, with underlying graft infection ranging from 1% to 7% depending on if autogenous vein or prosthetic graft were used.
- Early graft failures could be multifactorial.[9]
  - Technical failure due to imperfect anastomosis, or kinking of the conduit due to compression or graft redundancy.
  - Patients may have an undiagnosed hypercoagulable state.
  - Poor inflow. If depressed velocities with poor waveforms are seen in the conduit, further evaluation prior to the graft failing should be performed.

REFERENCES

1. Ardati AK, Kaufman SR, Aronow HD, et al. The quality and impact of risk factor control in patients with stable claudication presenting for peripheral vascular interventions. *Circ Cardiovasc Interv.* 2013;5:850-855.
2. Chen DKW, Conte MS, Belkin M, et al. Arterial reconstruction for lower limb ischemia. *Acta Chir Belg.* 2001;101:106-115.
3. Taylor LM, Hamre D, Dalman RL, et al. Limb salvage vs amputation for critical ischemia: the role of vascular surgery. *Arch Surg.* 1991;126:1251-1258.
4. Belkin M, Know J, Donaldson MC, et al. Infrainguinal arterial reconstruction with nonreversed greater saphenous vein. *J Vasc Surg.* 1996;24:957-962.
5. Klinkert P, Schepers A, Burger DHC, et al. Vein versus polytetrafluoroethylene in above-knee femoropopliteal bypass grafting: five year results of a randomized controlled trial. *J Vasc Surg.* 2003;37:149-155.
6. Dardik H, Dardik I, With FJ. Exposure of the tibioperoneal arteries by the single lateral approach. *Surgery.* 1974;75:377-382.
7. Schanzer A, Hevelone N, Owens CD, et al. Statins are independently associated with reduced mortality in patients undergoing infrainguinal bypass graft surgery for critical limb ischemia. *J Vasc Surg.* 2008;47:774-781.
8. Twine CP, McLain AD. Graft type for femoropopliteal bypass surgery. *Cochrane Database Syst Rev.* 2010;12:CD001487.
9. Schanzer A, Hevelone N, Owens CD, et al. Technical factors affecting autogenous vein graft failure: observations from a large multicenter trial. *J Vasc Surg.* 2007;46:1180-1190.

Management of Diabetic Foot Ulcers

Rahim Nazerali

DEFINITION

- Foot ulcers are the most common complication affecting patients with diabetes mellitus.[1]
- A result of lower extremity neuropathic disease, trauma, and deformity.
  - May be compounded by ischemia, callus formation, and edema.

ANATOMY

- Resembles laceration, puncture, or blister with round or oblong shape.
- May be necrotic, pink, or pale with well-defined smooth edges.
- Periwound often presents with callus.

PATHOGENESIS

- Origin and development have several components.
- Thirty-two unique casual pathways for developing foot ulcers.[2]
  - Peripheral neuropathy, structural foot problems, and minor trauma are present in the majority (63%).
  - Other less prevalent causes include edema, callus, and peripheral ischemia.
- Major common pathways involve pressure/trauma, ischemia/hypoxia, infection, cellular failure, and chronic inflammation.

NATURAL HISTORY

- 12.5% individuals with diabetes will develop lower extremity ulceration.[3]

PATIENT HISTORY AND PHYSICAL FINDINGS

- Basic history, including state of health, record of diabetic complications, shoe problems, pain in extremity, medications, glycated hemoglobin level.
- Risk factor assessment involving absence of protective sensation due to peripheral neuropathy, vascular insufficiency, structural deformities/callus formation, autonomic neuropathy, limited joint mobility, long duration of diabetes, long history of smoking, poor glucose control, obesity, impaired vision, past history, increased age, male gender, poor footwear.
- The Wagner scale for foot wound classification based on depth and presence of osteomyelitis and gangrene is the most widely accepted classification scheme[4] (**FIG 1**) but does not address the critically important parameters of ischemia and infection.
  - Grade 0: intact skin
  - Grade 1: superficial without penetration of deep layers
  - Grade 2: deeper reaching tendon, bone, or joint capsule
  - Grade 3: deeper with abscess, osteomyelitis, or tendonitis extending to those structures
  - Grade 4: gangrene of some portion of the toe, toes, and/or forefoot
  - Grade 5: gangrene involving the whole foot or enough of the foot that no local procedures are possible
- Physical exam:
  - Adequate description of ulcer characteristics such as size, depth, appearance, location, etc.
  - Examine with blunt sterile probe to detect sinus tract, undermining and dissection into tendon, bone or joints

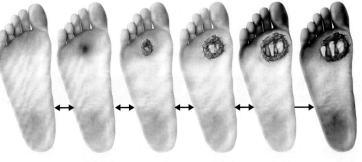

| No open lesion | Superficial ulcer | Deep ulcer | Abscess osteitis | Gangrene of forefoot | Gangrene of entire foot |

FIG 1 • Wagner scale for foot wound classification showing the natural history of dysvascular foot breakdown.

- Identify limb-threatening infection defined by cellulitis extending beyond 2 cm from perimeter, abscesses, or osteomyelitis
- Protective sensation testing with Semmes-Weinstein 5.07 (10-g) monofilament test or vibration tuning fork test (128 cycles per second) with on-off method
- Evaluate for musculoskeletal abnormalities that lead to focal areas of high pressure
- Vascular status evaluation via segmental pressures, toe pressures, or transcutaneous oxygen readings
- Evaluate skin and nail condition of the affected extremity
- Footwear evaluation including bulges on outside of shoes, wear patterns on soles, wearing down heels, worn lining, shoe cushion, and foreign object in shoe

IMAGING

- Duplex studies: ABI/TBI (ABI can be falsely elevated due to atherosclerotic hardened vessels.)
- X-ray, MRI, or bone biopsy to rule out osteomyelitis
- Lower extremity angiography

DIFFERENTIAL DIAGNOSIS

- Peripheral neuropathy

NONOPERATIVE MANAGEMENT

- Early prevention through careful and frequent inspection is important.

- Key therapeutic objectives include addressing global factors (glycemic control and nutritional support) and local factors.
- Aggressive treatment of infection through targeted antibiotic treatment from tissue cultures.
- Establishing if ischemia is present and revascularization is required.
- Topical wound care by optimizing wound bed moisture balance and exudate/odor control.
- Off-loading and redistribution of pressure involving bed rest, wheelchairs, crutches, surgical shoes, custom sandals, healing shoes, cast shoes, and foam dressings.
  - Pressure relief of plantar ulcers utilizing orthotics and total contact casting, which is considered the "standard" treatment for off-loading
- Adjunctive hyperbaric oxygen treatment can be an important aspect of the treatment armamentarium. Cochrane Review supported a 95% reduction in major amputations when adjunctive HBOT (Hyperbaric Oxygen Therapy) was used to treat chronic diabetic foot ulcers.[5]
  - Patient has type 1 or type 2 diabetes and has a lower extremity wound.
  - Wound is classified as Wagner grade 3 or higher.
  - Failed adequate course of standard wound therapy.

SURGICAL MANAGEMENT

- Ensure appropriate blood flow prior to surgical management.
  - Stenting vs bypass coordinated with vascular surgery

TECHNIQUES

- ■ **Aggressive Wound Debridement**
- Initial surgical debridement
  - Removal of free-living bacteria and biofilms
  - Stimulation of growth factors, removal of senescent cells, and removal of hyperproliferative nonmigratory tissue

- Maintenance of surgical debridement
  - Weekly debridement depending on the formation of new necrotic tissue.
  - First 4 weeks of treatment reduces median wound area by 54%.

- ■ **Flaps and Grafts**
- Local flaps and grafts described elsewhere in this text can be used for definitive soft tissue coverage.

PEARLS AND PITFALLS

Blood flow	■ It is critical prior to any surgical intervention that blood flow/perfusion be determined and optimized.
Adequate debridement	■ Ensuring adequate debridement of soft tissue and bone is critical to minimize biofilm and senescent cells.
Off-loading	■ Minimizing pressure to the area of a diabetic foot ulcer helps ensure adequate perfusion.
Infection control	■ It is important to address subclinical infections as well as ensure that the underlying osteomyelitis is appropriately treated for the successful long-term treatment of diabetic foot ulcers.
Consideration for hyperbaric oxygen	■ Studies indicate that Wagner grade 3 wounds benefit from hyperbaric oxygen therapy.

OUTCOMES

- 85% of lower limb amputations in diabetics are preceded by unhealed ulceration.
- 50% to 75% of lower extremity amputations are caused by nontraumatic amputations.
- Five-year mortality after amputation in diabetics is 45%.

REFERENCES

1. Jeffcoate WJ, Harding KG. Diabetic foot ulcers. *Lancet.* 2013; 361(9368):1545-1551.
2. Reiber GE, Vileikyte L, Boyko EJ, et al. Causal pathways for incident lower-extremity ulcers in patients with diabetes from two settings. *Diabetes Care.* 1999;22(1):157-162.
3. Kalish J, Hamdan A. Management of diabetic foot problems. *J Vasc Surg.* 2010;51(2):476-486.
4. Wagner FW. The diabetic foot. *Orthopedics.* 1987;10(1):163-172.
5. Kranke P, Bennett MH, Martyn-St James M, et al. Hyperbaric oxygen therapy for chronic wounds. *Cochrane Database Syst Rev.* 2015;(6):CD004123.

19 CHAPTER

Nerve Repair and Reconstruction—Peroneal Nerve

Shawn Moshrefi and Catherine Curtin

DEFINITION

Peroneal Nerve Injury

- Peroneal nerve injuries vary in severity, mechanism, and needed treatment.
- The nerve injury type dictates the treatment and prognosis.
  - Types of nerve injury[1]
    - Neuropraxia: conduction delay with no axonal injury. These injuries will recover spontaneously without intervention.
    - Axonotmesis: axonal injury resulting in disruption of the axons; however, the supporting nerve scaffolding is intact. In these injuries, distal nerve segment will undergo Wallerian degeneration and proximal fibers will regenerate. Spontaneous recovery is possible.
    - Neurotmesis: complete disruption of the nerve. In these injuries, spontaneous regeneration will *not* occur.
    - Neuroma in continuity: disruption of the axons though the scaffolding seems to be intact. However, at the injury site, there is internal fibrosis, which prevents axons from regeneration. In these injuries, spontaneous regeneration will *not* occur.
    - Mixture of injury types: nerve patterns can be complex, and one nerve can have several different levels of injury.

ANATOMY

- The common peroneal nerve fibers originate from L4 to S3 nerve roots (**FIG 1**).
- The common peroneal nerve branches from the sciatic nerve in the popliteal fossa.
- The motor component of the peroneal nerve innervates the anterior and lateral lower leg compartment muscles as well as some intrinsic muscles of the foot.
- The sensory component of the peroneal nerve supplies the first dorsal web space of the foot and the top of the foot.
- The peroneal gives off the lateral sural cutaneous branch, which joints the medial sural cutaneous branch (contributed from tibial nerve) to form the sural nerve.
- The common peroneal nerve crosses from posterior to anterolateral around the neck of the fibula.
  - The peroneal nerve is susceptible to compression as it wraps around the fibula.
- Once the nerve crosses anterior to the fibula, it branches into the superficial peroneal and deep peroneal nerves.
- The superficial peroneal nerve passes straight down the lateral compartment.
  - The superficial peroneal nerve supplies motor to the lateral compartment (peroneus longus and peroneus brevis).

- The superficial peroneal nerve supplies sensation to the top/lateral portion of the foot.
- The nerve transitions from within the muscle to a more superficial subcutaneous position at the junction of the middle and distal thirds of the lower leg. This transition site can be a point of compression.
- The deep peroneal nerve turns acutely around the fibular neck to enter the anterior compartment of the leg. The deep peroneal nerve then passes under the intermuscular septum between the anterior and lateral compartments to eventually course down between the tibialis anterior and extensor hallucis longus alongside the anterior tibial artery.
- The deep peroneal motor nerve supplies the anterior compartment of the leg as well as some of the small foot extensor muscles: tibialis anterior, extensor digitorum longus, peroneus tertius, extensor hallucis longus, extensor digitorum brevis, and extensor hallucis brevis.
- The deep peroneal nerve supplies sensation to the first web space of the foot.

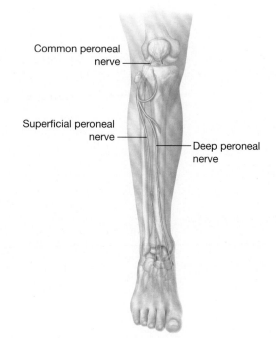

FIG 1 • Anatomy of the peroneal nerve.

PATHOGENESIS

- Direct trauma can injure the nerve along its course.
  - Fibular fracture can lacerate the nerve or result in neuropraxia.
  - Knee dislocation can result in a stretch injury or even a rupture of the peroneal nerve.[2]
  - Iatrogenic injuries that occur include prolonged tourniquet time, laceration of nerve during hardware placement, and compression of nerve from operative positioning.
- Swelling and compression can cause injury along the course of the peroneal nerve.
  - Ankle swelling can cause superficial peroneal nerve entrapment and resulting pain.
  - Compression from tight splints or casts can result in common peroneal nerve injury.
- Soft tissue masses
  - Cysts, especially Bakers cysts, or other nerve compressing structures can result in peroneal nerve injury.
  - Neural tumors such as schwannomas can result in nerve deficits.

PATIENT HISTORY AND PHYSICAL FINDINGS

- A complete and thorough history detailing patient's history of present illness, current injuries, history of prior injuries, prior surgeries (including spinal, buttock, and lower extremity procedures), comorbidities, occupation, and other case-by-case considerations should be obtained.
- Inspection
  - Is the leg/foot swollen?
  - Are there vascular changes?
  - Is there atrophy?
  - Is there a gait abnormality or foot drop?
- Vascular exam should assess for palpable pulses distally, temperature, and capillary refill of the foot.
- Sensory exam
  - Ten test: this quick test uses the contralateral area of normal sensation as a reference. The patient is lightly touched in the contralateral healthy distribution, and this normal sensation is a "ten." Then, both the healthy and affected side are lightly touched at the same time, and the patient is asked to grade the affected side using the scale 0 to 10.[3]
- Motor exam
  - Consists of testing the respective muscles that the peroneal nerve: extension of the foot and ankle.
  - Each muscle can be tested individually and compared to the contralateral side. Comparing to the healthy side allows for identification of subtle motor deficits seen in compression.
  - Motor examination remember mnemonic PED = **P**eroneal **E**verts and **D**orsiflexes or more correctly noted, Extends.
- Scratch collapse test[4]
  - This test can identify site of nerve entrapment.

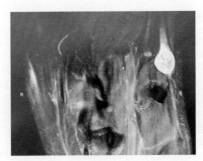

FIG 2 • Large peroneal nerve schwannoma.

  - Directly over the suspected nerve compression, the examiner gently scratches the skin. Then, the examiner immediately tests *arm* external rotation by applying force to the patient's dorsal forearm. The patient attempts to resist.
  - A positive test on the scratch collapse test is when the patient briefly has decreased external rotation strength and "collapses" under the examiner's pressure.
- Tinel test

IMAGING

- X-rays are useful for suspected bony injury.
- Angiography may be required in complex trauma patients.
  - This is particularly important as the deep peroneal nerve runs intimately with anterior tibial artery.
- MRI
  - Standard MRI can assess for soft tissue masses such as Baker cysts, schwannomas, or tumors.
    - **FIG 2** shows a large peroneal nerve schwannoma with its typical smooth bright appearance.
  - MRI neurogram can identify areas of nerve compression and enhancement (**FIG 3**).
- Nerve conduction studies and electromyelography.
  - For acute injuries, perform the first nerve testing at least 1 month after injury.
  - Studies can be repeated at 12 weeks, if there is no signs of recovery on physical examination.
  - Nerve conduction studies may be normal for nerve compression that has not resulted in any axonal injury.

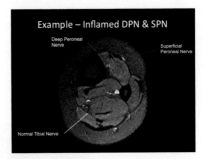

FIG 3 • MRI showing inflamed deep peroneal nerve and superficial peroneal nerve.

DIFFERENTIAL DIAGNOSIS

- Lumbar spinal pathology
- Sciatic pathology
  - If on physical examination, both peroneal nerve and tibial nerve distributions are involved, then sciatic pathology should be suspected.
  - Nerve studies should help differentiate.
- Neurologic problem
  - Peripheral neuropathy
  - Motor neuron disease
- Double crush[5]
  - A nerve may have more than one site of entrapment: for example, common peroneal at the fibular head and superficial peroneal at middle third of lower leg.
  - The theory is that an axon injured in one area may be more susceptible to secondary sites of injury.
  - Missing secondary sites of pathology will result in limitation of recovery if only one site is treated.

NONOPERATIVE MANAGEMENT

- For closed nerve injuries, nonoperative management is appropriate initially.
- Physical modalities
  - Edema prevention with lightly compressive wraps/garments and direct hands on physical therapy can be helpful.
  - Strategic splinting to prevent contractures.
  - Ankle-foot orthoses help improve mobility and stability in patients with a foot drop.
  - Gentle range of motion exercises to allow the nerve to glide and limit potential scarring in an injured soft tissue bed.
  - Desensitization to minimize pain and reeducate the nociceptive pathways.

SURGICAL MANAGEMENT

- Exploration and repair is indicated for open nerve injuries or closed injuries that are not showing signs of recovery.
- Nerve laceration
  - Urgent repair is indicated.
- Blast injuries should be explored no sooner than 6 weeks.
  - These injuries can have a surprising amount of recovery and should be followed until recovery plateaus before surgery.
  - Intraoperative nerve monitoring is critical to define the zone of injury.
- Traction injury should be explored if no signs of recovery at 3 months.

- Intraoperative nerve monitoring is critical to define the zone of injury.
- Be prepared for the need for long nerve grafts.
- Release of compressed common peroneal nerve (or branches) can be performed after thorough workup and no signs of recovery at 3 months.
- If injured superficial peroneal nerve resulting in painful neuroma in ankle or foot region, consider resection of nerve at junction of middle/distal third of the leg.
  - This will trade numbness for pain.
  - It will allow the surgeon to be out of the zone of injury.
  - Allows new placement of the neuroma deep in muscle and not crossing a joint.

Preoperative Planning

- Definitive fracture fixation should be performed prior to nerve repair.
- Arterial injury should be addressed prior to nerve repair.
- If possible, use a lower extremity tourniquet to aid in visualization of the nerve.
- If intraoperative nerve monitoring to be utilized, inform anesthesia team to not use paralytics.
- If pain is a concern, consider a more aggressive perioperative pain strategy.
  - 900 mg of gabapentin preoperatively[6]
  - Intraoperative ketamine
  - Regional block
  - Multimodal postsurgical pain management strategy
- If planning nerve resection of superficial peroneal nerve
  - Preoperative diagnostic block of the nerve at planned level of resection.
  - Ensure patient has significant relief of pain for hour after block.
  - Ensure patient will tolerate the numbness felt at the time of the block for the decrease in pain.

Positioning

- Positioning depends on level of injury (above knee, at level of knee, or below knee).
- Access to popliteal area is easiest when the patient is in the prone position.
- Access to the lateral leg is managed either supine with a hip bump or a "sloppy" lateral with the unaffected side down. **FIG 4** shows positioning for decompression of common peroneal and superficial peroneal nerves.
- Access to compression sites at the extensor retinaculum is managed with the patient supine.

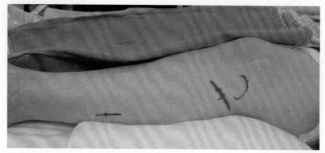

FIG 4 • Patient positioning for decompression of common peroneal and superficial peroneal nerves.

■ Common Peroneal Nerve Decompression

- Regional or general anesthesia
  - If no intraoperative nerve monitoring is required, regional anesthesia with a pain pump can provide several days of pain relief reducing opioid use.
- Thigh tourniquet is placed.
- Hip bump or slight lateral decubitus positioning to internally rotate the leg.
- Oblique incision 2 cm distal to the fibular head (on thin patients, you can palpate the nerve and design your incision above the nerve).
- Skin and subcutaneous tissue are divided down to the overlying fascia of the anterior lower leg muscles. Careful hemostasis is obtained as the dissection proceeds.
- Begin proximal and identify the nerve just posterior to the biceps femoris tendon.
  - The nerve is visualized with gentle longitudinal spread with a dissecting scissor.
- A vessel loop is placed around the nerve.
- The dissection proceeds distally releasing the fascia overlying the nerve. The fascia that overlies the muscles in the lateral muscle compartment is released. Then, the muscle fibers are spread/retracted allowing visualization of the thick fascia overlying the nerve, which is released (**TECH FIG 1**).

- The nerve will start dividing at the level of the fibular neck. In addition to the superficial and peroneal branches, the genicular branch that loops back proximal to the joint.
- Under direct visualization, follow the branches distally to ensure there are no unreleased fascial bands. The intermuscular septum can cause compression so inspect for any overlying compressive bands.
- This dissection can be performed with an incision that only goes about 2 cm anterior to the fibular head.
- Release tourniquet, achieve hemostasis, and close skin.
- Soft bulky dressing is placed.

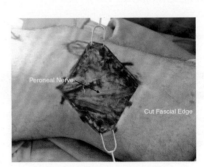

TECH FIG 1 • Visualization of the peroneal nerve.

■ Common Peroneal Nerve Traction Injury (Knee Dislocation)

- General anesthesia is required as patient will be prone and intraoperative nerve monitoring will be used.
- Thigh tourniquet.
- Prone positioning.
- Intraoperative nerve monitoring available.
- Incision is angled from the center of popliteal fossa laterally toward the fibular head.
- The dissection is taken down to the level of the muscle fascia.
- The common peroneal nerve is identified as it branches off the sciatic nerve.
- A vessel loop is placed on the nerve, and the dissection is taken distally.
- The nerve is released from the overlying scar (often a very challenging dissection). The dissection is taken

around the fibular head releasing the anterior muscle fascia.
- Intraoperative nerve monitoring is performed. Start with somatosensory evoked potentials can help establish the proximal level of intact nerve. Nerve-to-nerve monitoring can identify neuroma in continuity.
- If the nerve is ruptured or neuroma in continuity is identified, resect damaged nerve until two healthy nerve ends are revealed.
- Ensure that the proximal nerve is healthy by using the assistance of your neuromonitoring.
- For the nerve gap, harvest sural nerve graft.
- Cable the graft and suture in place with a few 9-0 sutures using microscopic technique. The repair should be tension free to allow for knee motion.
- Augment repair by sealing coaptation site with fibrin glue.
- Close wound.

■ Superficial Peroneal Nerve Compression Release and/or Neurectomy

- Thigh tourniquet.
- Regional anesthesia.
- Supine position.
- Approximately 3 cm longitudinal incision over seam between anterior and lateral compartments at juncture of middle and distal third of the leg.

- The dissection is taken down to the level of the muscle fascia.
- Identify the thin raphe located between the lateral and anterior compartments of the lower leg.
- Of note, there is a wide fat stripe anterior to the superficial peroneal nerve. If you find this first, look about a 1 cm posterior and you will find the seam that contains the nerve.
- Release overlying fascia proximally and distally.

- If performing neurectomy for damaged superficial peroneal nerve, the approach to the nerve is the same.
  - Once the nerve is identified, divide nerve distally and free up the proximal nerve for several centimeters.

- Place nerve stump deep within peroneus longus muscle. Bury the nerve stump in the muscle bed without tension.
- Close wound and place bulky dressing.

■ Nerve Laceration

- The nerve is identified using the existing wounds or the approaches described above.
- The nerve can be directly coapted using microsurgical technique if a tension-free repair is possible.
- If there is tension, a bridging nerve graft is required.
- Nerve repair is done using microsurgical technique and should be tension free.

- Use 9-0 suture and the minimal amount of sutures needed.
- Fibrin glue can be used to seal the repair site and to hold cabled nerve grafts together.
- The wounds are closed.
- Repairs are protected for 3 weeks if concern about the repair with splints/braces to limit mobility at adjacent joints.

PEARLS AND PITFALLS

Nerve repair	■ Nerve coaptation must be without tension. If a 9-0 suture cannot hold the repair, there is too much tension and a graft is required.
Diagnosis of entrapment site	■ Confident location of entrapment can be made if the patient has a positive Tinel sign, positive scratch collapse, and sensory changes in the appropriate distribution. ■ Double crush is a risk so assess if nerve entrapped at both the superficial and common peroneal entrapment sites.
Intraoperative monitoring	■ Communication between neurology and anesthesia team is critical to ensure that patient does not receive medications that will hinder intraoperative monitoring. ■ SCD machine and warming machines can cause background that interferes with intraoperative monitoring. ■ Do not use prolonged tourniquet if planning intraoperative monitoring.
Meticulous hemostasis	■ If not using a tourniquet, preinject incision with bupivacaine with epinephrine before prepping. ■ To improve visualization, a mix of 1 ampule of epinephrine with 100 cc of saline can be used to moisten gauze pads. These can be dabbed in the wound and improve visualization and minimize the need for cautery adjacent to the nerve.

POSTOPERATIVE CARE

- Medications
  - If neuropathic pain is a significant concern, consider multimodal pain control, which can include acetaminophen, NSAIDs, gabapentin, and opioids.[6]
- Therapy
  - At 2 to 3 weeks, consider therapy for scar management, nerve gliding, and desensitization.
- Nerve repair
  - Nerve repairs with slight tension need to be protected from disrupting forces for 3 weeks postoperatively. This can be performed through an immobilizer or splint. However, if reconstructed with a graft with some redundancy, early mobilization is possible.
- Nerve decompression

- Soft dressing and early mobilization will prevent scarring and tethering of the nerve.

OUTCOMES

- Studies show approximate 80% functional nerve recovery in patients with a multitude of methods of common peroneal nerve injuries.[7]
- Other studies indicate a vastly significant difference in prognosis from incomplete nerve palsy (highly favorable functional outcome) to complete peroneal nerve palsy (less than 40% functional recovery).[2]
- Complete peroneal nerve injuries after knee dislocation still have poor functional outcomes with less than 40% recovering extension despite treatment.[2]
- Release of the superficial peroneal nerve has resulted in high rates of pain resolution.[8,9]

COMPLICATIONS

- Most severe complication is iatrogenic nerve injury though this is very rare
- Bleeding
- Infection
- Fibrosis of the release site requiring revisionary surgery

REFERENCES

1. Seddon HJ. A classification of nerve injuries. *Br Med J*. 1942;2:237-239.
2. Woodmass JM, Romatowski NP, Esposito JG, et al. A systematic review of peroneal nerve palsy and recovery following traumatic knee dislocation. *Knee Surg Sports Traumatol Arthrosc*. 2015;23(10):2992-3002.
3. Strauch B, Lang A, Ferder M, et al. The ten test. *Plast Reconstr Surg*. 1997;99(4):1074-1078.
4. Gillenwater J, Cheng J, Mackinnon SE. Evaluation of the scratch collapse test in peroneal nerve compression. *Plast Reconstr Surg*. 2011;128(4):933-939.
5. Upton AR, McComas AJ. The double crush in nerve entrapment syndromes. *Lancet*. 1973;2(7825):359-362.
6. Carroll I, Hah J, Mackey S, et al. Perioperative interventions to reduce chronic postsurgical pain. *J Reconstr Microsurg*. 2013;29(4):213-222.
7. Emamhadi M, Bakhshayesh B, Andalib S. Surgical outcome of foot drop caused by common peroneal nerve injuries; is the glass half full or half empty? *Acta Neurochir*. 2016;158(6):1133-1138.
8. Styf J, Morberg P. The superficial peroneal tunnel syndrome. Results of treatment by decompression. *J Bone Joint Surg Br*. 1997;79(5):801-803.
9. Franco MJ, Phillips BZ, Lalchandani GR, et al. Decompression of the superficial peroneal nerve: clinical outcomes and anatomical study. *J Neurosurg*. 2017;126(1):330-335.

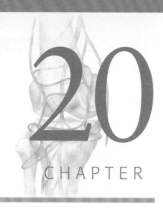

Achilles Tendon Reconstruction

Hani Sbitany

DEFINITION

- Achilles tendon is the most frequently ruptured tendon in the body, with incidence reported as high as 34/100 000, most commonly seen in males in their 30s.[1]
- The male-to-female ratio of this injury is 20:1.
- Classically seen when less active males engage in a new sport, without significant previous experience.

ANATOMY

- Most common site of rupture is 3 to 6 cm above the os calcis (ie, the calcaneus):
  - This area is a watershed zone in terms of blood supply.
- Achilles tendon is made up of gastrocnemius and soleus muscles, along with the plantaris tendon (**FIG 1**).
- This tendon begins in the midportion of the calf (superficial posterior compartment) and narrows to approximately 4 cm width at its insertion on the calcaneus bone.
- Achilles tendon helps to produce plantar flexion of the foot, which is powered through associated muscle innervation by the tibial nerve.

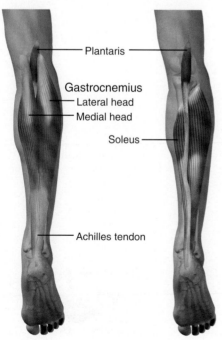

FIG 1 • The Achilles tendon is formed by the convergence of the medial, lateral gastrocnemius, and soleus muscles.

PATHOGENESIS

- With aging, there is an increase in type 3 collagen content on the Achilles tendon and a reduction in type 1 collagen content.[2]
- Increasing age is also accompanied by decreased orderly collagen cross-linking.
- All this results in reduced tensile strength of the tendon.

NATURAL HISTORY

- In addition to aging, there are numerous other risk factors associated with Achilles tendon rupture:
  - Hypercholesterolemia
  - Rheumatoid arthritis
  - Hypercholesterolemia
  - Long-term dialysis
  - Renal transplantation
  - Chronic steroid use

PATIENT HISTORY AND PHYSICAL FINDINGS

- A history of pain and weakening on plantar flexion is usually indicative of Achilles tendon rupture.
- On physical exam, there is usually a palpable defect in the tendon, in 75% of patients.
  - Up to 25% of tendon injuries can be missed when only clinical assessment is used for diagnosis.
- Simmonds/Thompson test: the patient lies face down with feet hanging off the edge of the bed. If there is no plantar flexion of the foot on squeezing the calf, then there is likely rupture of the Achilles tendon.
- O'Brien test: insert 25-gauge needle at right angle through the skin of calf muscle just medial to midline at a point 10 cm proximal to superior border of calcaneus. The needle should be within the substance of the tendon. Movement of the needle in a direction opposite that of the tendon during passive extension and flexion of the foot confirms an intact tendon distal to the level of needle insertion.
- Copeland test: the patient is prone with the feet hanging off of the exam table. A sphygmomanometer is placed around the calf with the foot in plantar flexion and inflated to 100 mm Hg. If the tendon is intact, then extension of the foot will lead to a pressure increase to 140 mm Hg. If the tendon is ruptured, then the pressure does not change.

IMAGING

- Imaging is always recommended when there is clinical concern for Achilles tendon rupture.

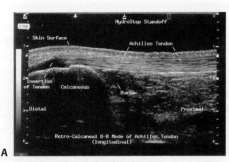
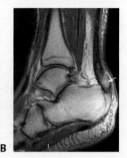

FIG 2 • A. Normal Achilles ultrasound image. **B.** Ankle MRI (T1-weighted image) showing a distal Achilles tendon rupture. (From Labib S. Open Achilles tendon repair. In: Wiesel S, ed. *Operative Techniques in Orthopaedic Surgery*. 2nd ed. Vol. 4. Philadelphia, PA: Wolters Kluwer Health; 2015:4967-4973.)

- Ultrasound is a useful first-line imaging technique, with sensitivity of 100% (**FIG 2A**).
  - Ultrasound tendon gap greater than 4 mm with patient in equinus (plantar flexion) indicates the need for surgical repair.
  - Ultrasound can differentiate partial vs complete tear:
    - This is more difficult with a tear at the proximal musculotendinous junction, in which sensitivity is much lower.
- MRI is the best imaging modality for Achilles tendon rupture, with sensitivity of 100% (**FIG 2B**).
  - MRI should always be obtained if any uncertainty exists regarding location, completeness, or length of tear.

DIFFERENTIAL DIAGNOSIS

- Achilles tendon peritendinitis
- Gastrocnemius tear or strain
- Calcaneus fracture
- Posterior tibialis tendon injury
- Posterior tibialis stress syndrome

NONOPERATIVE MANAGEMENT

- Nonoperative treatment of Achilles rupture is only an option in cases of acute rupture, with immediate diagnosis.
  - In cases of delayed diagnosis, scarring and retraction of tendon ends make conservative management less effective and unlikely to heal properly.
- The purpose of nonoperative management is to appose the ruptured Achilles ends, in stable fashion, such that healing can occur.
- Treatment regimen consists of immobilizing the extremity below the knee, with a brace or rigid cast.
  - The foot is initially placed in full plantar flexion.
  - Ankle is slowly brought into neutral position over 8 to 12 weeks.
- Knee immobilization is not necessary for reapproximation of the tendon edges.
- Early, gradual weight bearing has also been shown to confer protection against repeat rupture in the future.
- Many nonoperative regimens now advocate early weight bearing in a custom or Sheffield splint.
  - This is particularly beneficial in frail patients for whom joint contracture is at high risk.
  - The Sheffield splint is a specialized device worn on the lower leg and foot that allows for early controlled mobilization of the Achilles tendon.
- Early weight bearing also facilitates faster resumption of mobility after complete healing.
- One preferred conservative regimen:
  - Patient in full equinus (30 degrees) with touch weight bearing for 2 weeks

- Ankle then placed in partial equinus (15–20 degrees) with partial weight bearing for 2 weeks
- Finally, placed in neutral (0 degrees) with full weight bearing for 2 weeks

SURGICAL MANAGEMENT

- Operative treatment is used for the majority of acute tendon ruptures in younger patients, as well as in all patients with chronic rupture or delayed diagnosis.
- This is the only treatment option when there has been scarring and retraction of the tendon ends, resulting in a lack of apposition.

Preoperative Planning

- As previously mentioned, ultrasound and MRI assessment of the injury is important, to identify the location of the rupture relative to the musculotendinous junction and the length of the gap.
- The patient's physical examination should also include a workup of mobility potential and strength, to ensure that early mobilization and weight bearing will be possible.

Positioning

- Surgical repair is commonly performed with the patient in the supine position, the hips abducted, and the knees flexed (frog leg position) (**FIG 3**).
- The operation can also be performed with the patient in the prone position, for easier, direct access to the posterior ankle.

Approach

- Open surgical repair is performed with a direct longitudinal incision, directly over the Achilles to expose the entire tendon.

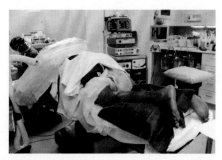

FIG 3 • Patient is placed in the prone position with both legs prepared and draped for surgery. (From Labib S. Open Achilles tendon repair. In: Wiesel S, ed. *Operative Techniques in Orthopaedic Surgery*. 2nd ed. Vol. 4. Philadelphia, PA: Wolters Kluwer Health; 2015:4967-4973.)

■ Percutaneous Repair

- Performed with patient in prone position.
- Skin incision is first made over site of rupture.
- Second skin incision made 4 cm proximal to initial incision.
- Third incision made 4 cm distal to rupture (**TECH FIG 1A**).
- The track of the entire tendon is defined under the skin and spread open.
- For this repair, a suture is first passed on a needle through middle incision and through tendon at this point (**TECH FIG 1B**).
  - A monofilament, permanent suture is used for this.

- Needle is then passed proximal and brought out through proximal incision (see **TECH FIG 1B**).
  - At this proximal incision, the suture is then passed through the proximal cut edge of the Achilles tendon.
- The needle is then passed back through the tunnel, brought out the middle incision, passed through the distal stump of the tendon, and brought out the distal end (**TECH FIG 1C**).
- Traction is then applied to ensure proper tension (**TECH FIG 1D**).

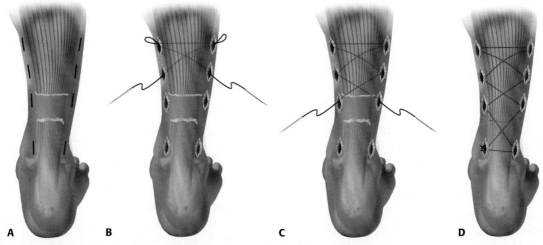

A　　　**B**　　　**C**　　　**D**

TECH FIG 1 • A–D. Pattern for suture passage for percutaneous repair of Achilles tendon rupture.

■ Open Direct (End-to-End) Suture Repair

- Performed in cases of acute rupture, less than 6 weeks old.
- Achilles tendon exposed along the entire length through vertical skin incision.
- Multiple figure-of-8 sutures are used to repair tendon at proper tension (**TECH FIG 2**).
  - Similar to percutaneous, a large monofilament, permanent suture is used for repair.

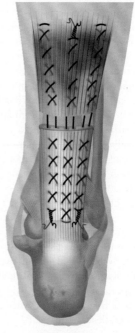

TECH FIG 2 • End-to-end suture repair of Achilles tendon rupture.

■ Reconstruction With VY Advancement

- Used to repair chronic ruptures with defect less than 3 cm between tendon ends.
- The entire posterior compartment, from the calcaneus to the midportion of the calf, is exposed with the incision.
- The gastrocnemius/soleus/Achilles junction is exposed posteriorly from the prone position.
- An inverted V incision is planned along the posterior superficial surface of the muscular complex, with the apex of the V placed at the proximal portion of the myo-tendinous junction.

- The medial and lateral limbs of the V exit through the sides of the Achilles tendon.
- The inverted V is incised through the tendinous, superficial portions of the tissue, leaving underlying muscle intact.
- Then, the tendon ends are sutured to each other across the rupture, using permanent suture.
  - Can use monofilament or braided suture.
  - Done with locking knots, at least five suggested.
- Tension is set with gentle traction, such that the muscle is not disrupted.
- Finally, the limbs of the inverted V are rerepaired with suture.

■ Flexor Hallucis Longus Transfer

- Used to repair chronic ruptures with defect greater than 3 cm between tendon ends.[3]
- Requires a functional tibial nerve.
- The flexor hallucis longus (FHL) tendon can be harvested through the same posterior Achilles incision used for injury exposure.
- The dissection is carried down into the deep posterior compartment fascia, and underneath this, the FHL muscle and tendon sit.
- The FHL muscle belly extends more distal than others in this compartment, usually to the level of tibiotalar joint, which is the method of identification:
  - The muscle is confirmed by retracting manually and seeing flexion of the hallux.
- Medial to the FHL tendon, the neurovascular bundle of tibial nerve and posterior tibial artery is identified.
- The muscle is dissected distally, around the medial malleolus, taking care not to injury the neurovascular bundle.
- Then, the FHL is transected as distal as possible, along its tendinous portion, with the ankle held in flexion and muscle under traction.
- Based on FHL tendon diameter, a bone tunnel is drilled into the calcaneus (posterior tubercle), just anterior to the area of Achilles tendon insertion on the bone.

- The length of the FHL muscle and tendon is set, after the tendon is passed through the tunnel using a suture and passer (**TECH FIG 3**).
  - At this length, the tendon is fixed into the calcaneus after passing through the tunnel, with an interference screw.
- The final resting tension, after repair, is compared to the contralateral uninjured side.
- Gentle extension is applied to test the repair, and then the skin is closed.[4]

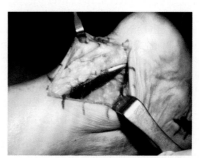

TECH FIG 3 • Flexor hallucis longus tendon used to augment Achilles tendon repair. (From Labib S. Open Achilles tendon repair. In: Wiesel S, ed. *Operative Techniques in Orthopaedic Surgery*. 2nd ed. Vol. 4. Philadelphia, PA: Wolters Kluwer Health; 2015:4967-4973.)

POSTOPERATIVE CARE

- For most repair techniques, the ankle is splinted in equinus for 2 weeks.
- Strict nonweight bearing is employed for 6 to 8 weeks.
- After 2 weeks, once the healing skin is confirmed on examination, the patient is converted to postsurgical boot that gradually allows for passive extension in increasing increments over the next 4 weeks.
- At 6 to 8 weeks, patient is examined and tested for Achilles repair persistence, and weight bearing is started in ankle boot brace.
  - Physical therapy also started at this point.
  - Three sessions of PT for 8 weeks.
  - PT focuses on passive Achilles stretching and gait training.
- At 12 weeks, if the ankle is neutral alignment on exam, the patient is allowed to resume activity slowly.

COMPLICATIONS

- Bleeding
- Infection
- Tendon rerupture

REFERENCES

1. Heckman DS, Gluck GS, Parekh SG. Tendon disorders of the foot and ankle, part 2: Achilles tendon disorders. *Am J Sports Med.* 2009;37(6):1223-1234.
2. Padanilam TG. Chronic Achilles tendon ruptures. *Foot Ankle Clin.* 2009;14(4):711-728.
3. Worth N, Ghosh S, Maffulli N. Management of acute Achilles tendon ruptures in the United Kingdom. *J Orthop Surg (Hong Kong).* 2007;15(3):311-314.
4. Den Hartog BD. Flexor hallucis longus transfer for chronic Achilles tendonosis. *Foot Ankle Int.* 2003;24(3):233-237.

21
CHAPTER

Excision of Soft Tissue Tumors of the Lower Leg

Raffi S. Avedian and Robert J. Steffner

DEFINITION

- Soft tissue tumors of the lower leg may be benign or malignant (soft tissue sarcoma) and exhibit a variable natural history ranging from latency to rapid growth.
- Tumors located entirely above the muscle fascia are considered superficial, whereas tumors involving the fascia or deep to it are considered deep.

ANATOMY

- The lower leg is made up of the tibia and fibula and four muscle compartments: anterior, lateral, deep posterior, and superficial posterior (**FIG 1**).
- Three principal arteries travel in the lower leg.
  - The posterior tibial artery is located in the deep posterior compartment on the surface of the tibialis posterior.
  - The anterior tibial artery is in the anterior compartment located deep to the muscles on the surface of the interosseous membrane.
  - The fibular artery travels in the deep posterior compartment medial to the fibula under the flexor hallucis longus;

it sends branches to the lateral and anterior compartments and a nutrient vessel to the fibula.
- The deep peroneal nerve travels with the anterior tibial artery. The superficial peroneal nerve is located in the lateral compartment; in the distal one-third of the leg, it travels between the peroneus muscles and extensor digitorum longus and pierces the deep fascia to become a cutaneous nerve.

PATHOGENESIS

- The mechanism for soft tissue tumor formation is not known.
- Risk factors for sarcoma development include radiation exposure, radiotherapy, pesticide exposure, and hereditary conditions including Li-Fraumeni syndrome and retinoblastoma gene mutation.

NATURAL HISTORY

- All soft tissue sarcomas have the potential for local recurrence and metastasis.[1]

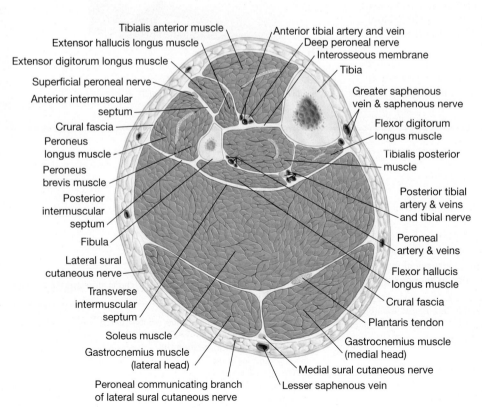

FIG 1 • Cross-sectional anatomy of lower leg showing the contents of the anterior, lateral, superficial posterior, and deep posterior compartments.

- Soft tissue sarcomas exhibit a spectrum of natural history from slow-growing low-grade tumors with low risk of metastasis to high-grade sarcoma that may grow rapidly and pose a high risk of metastasis.
- Lungs are the most common site of metastasis. Lymph node involvement is rare.
- Angiosarcoma, clear cell sarcoma, epithelioid sarcoma, rhabdomyosarcoma, myxofibrosarcoma, and synovial sarcoma are associated with increased risk of lymph node spread compared to other sarcomas.[2]
- Benign tumors by definition do not have metastatic potential but can grow to large sizes and cause symptoms.

PATIENT HISTORY AND PHYSICAL FINDINGS

- A thorough history and examination are important to assess duration of symptoms, comorbidities, physical dysfunction, organ involvement, overall health, and patient expectations in order to best tailor treatment strategy for the individual patient.
- Many sarcomas may be asymptomatic with the only patient complaint being the presence of a mass.
- Neurovascular examination is mandatory for any extremity tumor.

IMAGING

- Magnetic resonance imaging is the principal imaging modality used to characterize tumors, formulate differential diagnosis, define local tissue infiltration, and formulate surgical plan.
- Plain radiographs are used if there is concern for bone involvement or to demonstrate mineralization within a tumor such as vascular malformations.
- Staging for soft tissue sarcomas consists primarily of lung imaging.

DIFFERENTIAL DIAGNOSIS

- The differential diagnosis for a soft tissue tumor includes benign tumors, sarcomas, lymphoma, infection, and inflammatory lesions (eg, rheumatoid nodules).
- There are over 50 sarcoma subtypes. Common histology types include pleomorphic undifferentiated sarcoma, synovial sarcoma, leiomyosarcoma, malignant peripheral nerve sheath tumor, liposarcoma.

SURGICAL MANAGEMENT

- The appropriate treatment for any musculoskeletal tumor is based on its diagnosis and natural history.
- Biopsy incisions are considered contaminated and must be resected at the time of definitive surgery. Care should be taken to place the biopsy in a location that does not interfere with the final surgical plan.[3]
- Simple marginal excision is appropriate for most benign tumors, and wide resection with a clean margin is performed for soft tissue sarcomas.
- Given the relatively low volume of tissue in the lower leg and ankle, soft tissue reconstruction with local or free flaps is often needed.

Preoperative Planning

- A patient is considered ready for surgery after completion of staging and multidisciplinary review of pertinent imaging, pathology, and treatment strategy.
- The surgical plan is created by thorough study of the preoperative MRI scan. Fluid-sensitive sequences and fat-suppressed contrast images show the extent of disease that must be accounted in the excision. T1 fat-sensitive images show the normal anatomy best including fat planes between tumor and critical structures such as nerves and vessels.
- When tumor abuts, but does not encase blood vessels or nerves, they can be dissected free by leaving adventitia and epineurium on the tumor as the margin.[4]

Positioning

- Patient positioning is based on the surgeon's assessment of the critical anatomy of the surgery and how best to visualize it during surgery.
- Supine is the most common position for tumor excision of the lower leg. A hip bump may be used to access more lateral tumors; conversely, frog legging the extremity facilitates medial and posterior visualization.
- If a flap is to be used, the harvest must be performed using a separate back table and instruments and the surgical sites completely isolated to avoid contamination.

Approach

- The surgical approach varies based on location of the tumor.
- Previous biopsy and surgical scars are considered contaminated and must be excised en bloc with the tumor.

■ Excision of Soft Tissue Tumor of the Lower Leg

- Tourniquet is used at the discretion of the surgeon by using gravity exsanguination rather than Esmarch to avoid tumor compression and potential risk of tumor spreading.
- A skin incision is used to approach the tumor.
- Superficial sarcomas require a large paddle of skin to be excised on top of the tumor to serve as the superficial margin and the deep fascia with a small cuff of deep muscle to serve as the deep margin. Deep sarcomas can often

be approached with a longitudinal incision, but more extensive soft tissue excision is done in the deeper layers.

- A unique consideration for the lower leg is the relatively smaller volume of soft tissue compared to the thigh. Even a medium-sized sarcoma, eg, 5 cm, will occupy a large proportion of the leg. After excision, there is typically a relatively large defect that will require free tissue transfer for soft tissue reconstruction.
- Benign tumors may be excised through a longitudinal skin incision and simple dissection along the margin of the tumor by leaving most of the native tissues in place (**TECH FIG 1**).

T
E
C
H
N
I
Q
U
E
S

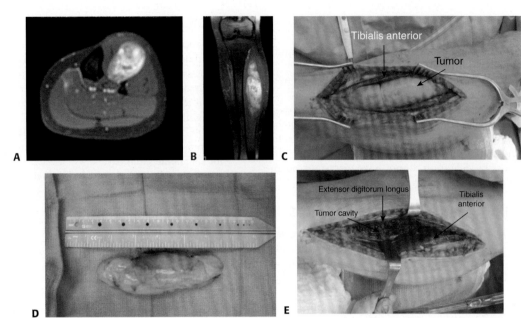

TECH FIG 1 • **A.** Axial T1 fat-suppressed contrast MRI showing a tumor in the anterior compartment of the lower leg between the tibialis anterior and extensor digitorum longus. Biopsy confirmed benign schwannoma. **B.** Coronal view demonstrating craniocaudal extent of tumor. **C.** Intraoperative photograph showing dissection through deep fascia and separation of the tibialis anterior and extensor digitorum. Simple dissection around the tumor capsule was performed to deliver the tumor. **D.** Excised specimen on the back table. **E.** Photograph showing the defect after excision. Because the native muscles were not excised, a primary closure was possible.

PEARLS AND PITFALLS

Wound breakdown	■ Dead space after tumor removal should be managed with drains, muscle flap, free tissue transfer, or a combination of these techniques. ■ Have low threshold for aggressive soft tissue coverage.
Positive margins (sarcoma excision)	■ Appropriate preoperative planning is important to minimize risk of unplanned positive margins. ■ Inability to primarily close a wound should not interfere with decision to remove a tumor with a clean margin. Plan on soft tissue reconstruction. ■ Planned positive margins around critical structures such as nerves and vessels may be appropriate in certain settings.

POSTOPERATIVE CARE

■ Mobilization and weight bearing depend on the extent of surgery. Activity with no restriction may begin after simple tumor excision, whereas bed rest may be desired after free tissue transfer.
■ Extremity elevation is recommended while the patient is in bed.
■ May administer antibiotics in the perioperative period.

OUTCOMES

■ Oncological outcomes include local recurrence and metastasis. Surveillance for recurrence should be managed by a multidisciplinary sarcoma team. Local recurrence is higher when margins are positive.
■ Functional outcomes depend on the extent of tissue resection and patient overall health status. Most patients will experience some form of disability that is proportional to the volume of muscle and bone resected.

COMPLICATIONS

■ Local recurrence occurs in a minority of patients with sarcoma and is more common in patients with positive margins.

■ Deep infection can occur at any time after surgery and requires aggressive therapy including surgical debridement and antibiotic therapy to achieve limb salvage.
■ Weakness with ankle and foot motion is not uncommon given the proximity of the nerves to most leg tumors and the need for extensive muscle excision.

REFERENCES

1. Christie-Large M, James SL, Tiessen L, et al. Imaging strategy for detecting lung metastases at presentation in patients with soft tissue sarcomas. *Eur J Cancer.* 2008;44(13):1841.
2. Johannesmeyer D, Smith V, Cole DJ, et al. The impact of lymph node disease in extremity soft-tissue sarcomas: a population-based analysis. *Am J Surg.* 2013;206(3):289-295.
3. Mankin HJ, Mankin CJ, Simon MA. The hazards of the biopsy, revisited. Members of the Musculoskeletal Tumor Society. *J Bone Joint Surg Am.* 1996;78(5):656-663.
4. O'Donnell PW, Griffin AM, Eward WC, et al. The effect of the setting of a positive surgical margin in soft tissue sarcoma. *Cancer.* 2014;120(18):2866-2875.

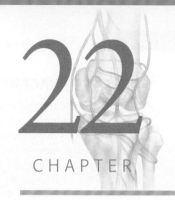
Excision of Bone Tumors of the Lower Leg

Raffi S. Avedian and Rohit Khosla

DEFINITION

- Bone tumors of the tibia and fibula may be benign or malignant (bone sarcoma) and exhibit a variable natural history ranging from latent to rapid growth. Aggressive benign tumors and malignant tumors typically cause pain, dysfunction, and fracture.
- A bone tumor located in the tibia or fibula such that definitive treatment requires excision of an intercalary segment of bone, sparing the ankle and knee joints, is discussed in this chapter.

ANATOMY

- The lower leg is made up of the tibia and fibula and four muscle compartments: anterior, lateral, deep posterior, and superficial posterior (**FIG 1**).
- Three principal arteries travel in the lower leg. The posterior tibial artery is located in the deep posterior compartment on the surface of the tibialis posterior. The anterior tibial artery is in the anterior compartment located deep to the muscles on the surface of the interosseous membrane. The fibular artery travels in the deep posterior compartment medial to the fibula under the flexor hallucis longus; it sends branches to the lateral and anterior compartments and a nutrient vessel to the fibula.
- The deep peroneal nerve travels with the anterior tibial artery. The superficial peroneal nerve is located in the lateral compartment; in the distal one-third of the leg, it travels between the peroneus muscles and extensor digitorum longus and pierces the deep fascia to become a cutaneous nerve.

PATHOGENESIS

- The mechanism for bone tumor formation is not known.
- Risk factors for sarcoma development include radiation exposure, radiotherapy, pesticide exposure, and hereditary conditions including Li-Fraumeni syndrome and retinoblastoma gene mutation.

NATURAL HISTORY

- Active benign tumors such as giant cell tumor of bone, chondroblastoma, and aneurysmal bone cyst will progress over time and may recur after excision but are not lethal.
- All bone sarcomas have the potential for local recurrence and metastasis.
- Some bone sarcomas such as low-grade chondrosarcoma exhibit a slow rate of growth and low risk of metastasis, whereas aggressive tumors like high-grade osteosarcoma and dedifferentiated chondrosarcoma grow rapidly and have a relatively high risk of metastasis.
- Tumor variables that are associated with increased risk of metastasis include high grade and large size (greater than 8 cm).

- Lungs and other osseous sites are the most and second most common location of metastasis, respectively.

PATIENT HISTORY AND PHYSICAL FINDINGS

- Pain is a common presenting symptom for aggressive bone tumors.
- A thorough history and examination are important to assess duration of symptoms, comorbidities, physical dysfunction, organ involvement, overall health, and patient expectations to best tailor treatment strategy for the individual patient.
- Neurovascular examination is mandatory for any extremity tumor.

IMAGING

- Plain radiographs are used to formulate a differential diagnosis and a preoperative plan.
- Magnetic resonance imaging is routinely used to determine the extent of intramedullary tumor involvement, presence of soft tissue extension, status of the neurovascular structures, and preoperative planning.

DIFFERENTIAL DIAGNOSIS

- The differential diagnosis for a bone tumor includes benign tumors, sarcomas, lymphoma of bone, infection, and metabolic lesions (eg, hyperparathyroidism).
- The most common bone sarcomas are osteosarcoma, chondrosarcoma, and Ewing sarcoma.

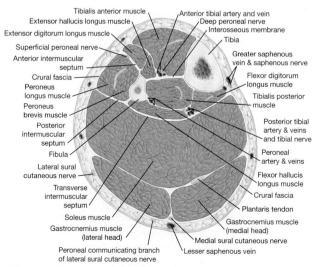

FIG 1 • Cross-sectional anatomy of the lower leg showing the contents of the anterior, lateral, superficial posterior, and deep posterior compartments.

SURGICAL MANAGEMENT

- The appropriate treatment for any musculoskeletal tumor is based on its diagnosis and natural history.
- Biopsy incisions are considered contaminated and must be resected at the time of definitive surgery. Care should be taken to place the biopsy in a location that does not interfere with the final surgical plan.
- Intralesional curettage is the preferred treatment for benign tumors. Radical resection with a clean margin is required for bone sarcomas.
- Reconstruction depends on the extent of bone excision and may include simple bone grafting, endoprosthetic implants, structural allografts, vascularized fibula (ipsilateral centralized or contralateral free transplant), or combined allograft and vascularized fibula.
- The goal of surgery is to remove the tumor adequately to minimize recurrence and restore the mechanical integrity of the bone and joints so that the patient may have sufficient function to perform activities of daily living with minimal pain.

Preoperative Planning

- A patient is considered ready for surgery after completion of staging and multidisciplinary review of pertinent imaging, pathology, and treatment strategy.
- The surgical plan is created by thorough study of the preoperative radiographs and MR imaging.
- Bone cuts are planned by measuring on preoperative imaging the distance from an intraoperatively identifiable landmark (eg, medial malleolus or tibial condyle) to the desired osteotomy site (**FIG 2A,B**).
- The soft tissue margin depends on the size and location of a soft tissue component to the tumor.

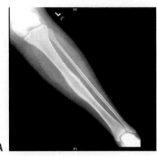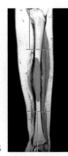

FIG 2 • A. Anteroposterior radiograph of a 16-year-old girl with a midtibia Ewing sarcoma. **B.** Sagittal T1-weighted MRI demonstrating the intramedullary extent of the tumor and measurements for bone resection.

- When tumor abuts, but does not encase blood vessels or nerves, they can be dissected free by leaving the adventitia and epineurium on the tumor as the margin.

Positioning

- Patient positioning is based on the surgeon's assessment of the critical anatomy of the surgery and how best to visualize it during surgery.
- Supine is the most common position for tumor excision of the lower leg. A hip bump may be used to access more lateral tumors; conversely, frog legging the extremity facilitates medial and posterior visualization.
- If a flap is to be used, the harvest must be performed using a separate back table and instruments and the surgical sites completely isolated to avoid contamination.

Approach

- The surgical approach varies based on location of the tumor.
- Previous biopsy and surgical scars are considered contaminated and must be excised en bloc with the tumor.

TECHNIQUES

■ Diaphyseal Tibia Tumor Resection and Reconstruction

- Tourniquet is used at discretion of the surgeon by using gravity exsanguination rather than Esmarch to avoid tumor dissemination.
- A longitudinal incision is created that ellipses out the biopsy site. Skin flaps are created as needed to ensure adequate visualization of the tumor and critical anatomy (**TECH FIG 1A,B**).
- Soft tissue dissection around the tumor is performed with the following principles:
  - Adequate visualization must be achieved.
  - Margin of healthy tissue is kept on the tumor.
  - Nerves must be moved away from tumor. The epineurium may be used as margin if tumor abuts the nerve.
  - Vessels must be moved away from tumor; the adventitia may be used as margin if tumor abuts the vessels.
  - Single-vessel runoff to the foot may be acceptable depending on the extent of soft tissue and collateral circulation excision.
- Bone cuts are performed based on preoperative planning and measurements to ensure complete tumor removal. Steinman pins may be inserted proximal and distal to bone cuts prior to osteotomy for the purpose creating reference points for leg length and rotation restoration (**TECH FIG 1C,D**).

- Alternatively, an external fixator may be applied prior to osteotomy to facilitate leg length and rotation restoration.
- Fluoroscopy may be used at the discretion of the surgeon.
- Hemicortical resection is an option if the tumor does not involve the entire diameter of the bone.
- Reconstruction is performed to restore mechanical stability of the extremity using one of the following options:
  - Endoprosthetic implants may be cemented or press fit into native bone.[1]
  - Allografts are fashioned to fit the defect and secured in place with internal fixation.
  - Vascularized fibula may be inserted end-to-end to the native tibia or telescoped into the tibial canal to increase contact surface area (**TECH FIG 2A–C**).
  - A composite graft using vascularized fibula inserted into a structure allograft (Capanna technique) has the theoretical advantage of combing the structural support of a large allograft with the healing potential of a vascularized graft.[2]
  - Ilizarov technique for bone lengthening.[3]
- Allografts and endoprosthesis are at increased risk for infection; thus, aggressive soft tissue reconstruction is recommended to minimize risk of wound dehiscence resulting in exposed hardware.
- Often, primary closure is not possible, and a local rotational flap or free tissue transfer is used to reconstruct the soft tissues.

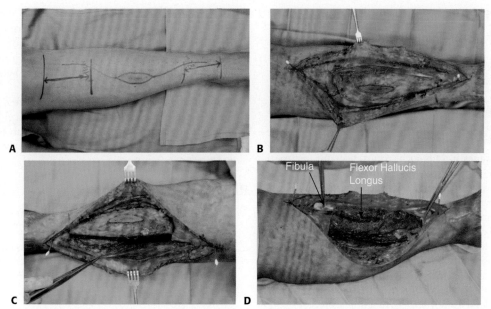

TECH FIG 1 • **A.** Intraoperative photograph of planned incision incorporating biopsy site. **B.** Dissection through skin and elevation of full-thickness flaps to visualize the extent of tumor. Steinmann pins are placed proximal and distal away from tumor as references for leg length and rotation. **C.** Bone cuts are made and muscle attachments released to allow excision of the tumor in its entirety. **D.** The ipsilateral fibula is dissected free keeping the flexor hallucis longus muscle and associated nutrient vessels attached. Notice that additional fibula length relative to defect is harvested to allow for intramedullary insertion.

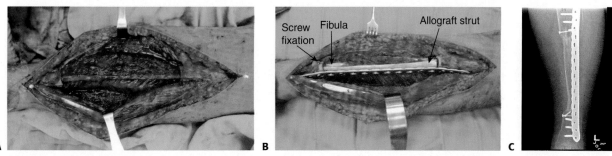

TECH FIG 2 • **A.** Photograph showing fibula inserted into the proximal and distal ends of the tibia. **B.** The fibula is stabilized to the native tibia with internal fixation, and allograft strut is placed for additional support. **C.** Radiograph 14 months after surgery showing incorporation of the fibula and allograft to the native tibia.

PEARLS AND PITFALLS

Wound breakdown	■ Dead space after tumor removal should be managed with drains, muscle flap, free tissue transfer, or a combination of these techniques. ■ Have low threshold for aggressive soft tissue coverage.
Positive margins	■ Appropriate preoperative planning is important to minimize risk of unplanned positive margins. ■ Planned positive margins around critical structures such as nerves and vessels may be appropriate in certain settings
Allograft nonunion/ fracture	■ May be minimized by good cortical apposition of graft to the native bone. ■ Restrict weight bearing until evidence of bone healing is observed. ■ Counsel patients that reoperation for nonunion is possible.
Malrotation/ malalignment	■ Provisional placement of internal fixation, reference pins, or external fixation away from tumor may be used to maintain anatomic alignment.

POSTOPERATIVE CARE

- Mobilization and weight bearing depend on the extent of surgery.
- Extremity elevation is recommended while the patient is in bed.
- Range of motion and therapy may begin after wound healing is sufficient.
- May administer antibiotics while drains are in place.

OUTCOMES

- Oncological outcomes include local recurrence and metastasis. Surveillance for recurrence should be managed by a multidisciplinary sarcoma team. Local recurrence is higher when margins are positive.
- Functional outcomes depend on the extent of tissue resection and patient overall health status. Most patients will experience some form of disability that is proportional to the volume of muscle and bone resected.
- Benevenia et al. showed an overall 27% nononcological complication rate for intercalary prosthesis and average 77% Musculoskeletal Tumor Society function score.[4]

COMPLICATIONS

- Allograft nonunion and fracture, endoprosthesis loosening, and infection are known complications and typically require additional surgery to achieve a limb salvage.

- Local recurrence occurs in a minority of patients and is more common in patients with positive margins.
- Malalignment of the reconstruction may occur and can be avoided by the use of provisional fixation prior to making bone cuts and intraoperative radiographs to ensure restoration of alignment and rotation.
- Deep infection can occur at any time after surgery and requires aggressive therapy including surgical debridement and antibiotic therapy to achieve limb salvage. Removal of implants and allografts is often necessary to eradicate infection.

REFERENCES

1. Ahlmann ER, Menendez LR. Intercalary endoprosthetic reconstruction for diaphyseal bone tumours. *J Bone Joint Surg Br.* 2006;88(11):1487-1491.
2. Bakri K, Stans AA, Mardini S, Moran SL. Combined massive allograft and intramedullary vascularized fibula transfer: the Capanna technique for lower-limb reconstruction. *Semin Plast Surg.* 2008;22(3):234-241.
3. McCoy TH Jr, Kim HJ, Cross MB, et al. Bone tumor reconstruction with the Ilizarov method. *J Surg Oncol.* 2013;107(4):343-352.
4. Benevenia J, Kirchner R, Patterson F, et al. Outcomes of a modular intercalary endoprosthesis as treatment for segmental defects of the femur, tibia, and humerus. *Clin Orthop Relat Res.* 2016;474(2):539-548.

Debridement of Soft Tissue Infections of the Lower Leg

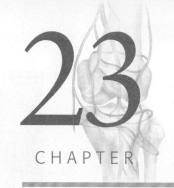

CHAPTER 23

L. Scott Levin and Paulo Piccolo

DEFINITION

- The term *debridement* was coined by Joseph Pierre DeSault in the 18th century. The French term implies the removal of soft tissues and bone that are nonviable, with the goal of preventing infection. It is defined by the Oxford medical dictionary as the process of cleaning an open wound by removal of foreign material and nonviable tissue, so that healing may occur without hindrance.[1]
- By removing molecular, physical, and microbiologic barriers to healing, debridement facilitates endogenous wound healing.

ANATOMY

- The lower extremity consists of four major regions: the hip, thigh, leg, and foot. It is specialized for support of body weight, adaptation to gravity, and locomotion.
- The thigh is divided in three compartments (anterior, posterior, and medial), and the leg is divided in four compartments (anterior, deep, superficial posterior, and lateral).

PATHOGENESIS

- Wounds may originate through a variety of causes, such as soft tissue infection (acute or chronic), trauma (thermal, electric, chemical, penetrating, or blunt), vascular issues (arterial, venous, or lymphatic), neuropathic (eg, diabetes), or malignancy.
- The pathogenesis of the wound will play a key role in the treatment plan. A wound from necrotizing fasciitis needs emergent attention and wide debridement, as opposed to one caused by venous stasis, which can be dealt with in an ambulatory setting and may be amenable to a more conservative treatment approach.

PATIENT HISTORY AND PHYSICAL FINDINGS

- A thorough history of present illness must be obtained. This is paramount in establishing the cause, timing, and clinical implications of that wound, the potential level of disability caused by it, and to plan further treatment.
- Patient's comorbidities such as obesity, diabetes, peripheral vascular disease, surgical history, nutritional status, previous trauma and, nicotine use should all be taken into account.
- A thorough physical exam of the extremity in question must be performed preoperatively, and many times, it should be completed in the operating room under anesthesia to minimize patient's discomfort and allow for a precise and thorough analysis of the area.
- Nerve integrity must be assessed before the patient is under anesthesia—both motor and sensory aspects must be checked from the proximal thigh to the distal toe.

- Peripheral pulses are of extreme importance when treating lower extremity wounds, as this will give vital information regarding limb perfusion, wound pathogenesis, and options for future reconstruction.
- Size and appearance of the wound, characteristics of the surrounding soft tissue, and skeletal stability of the extremity should also not be overlooked. The presence of exposed vital structures, including nerves, vessels, bones, and joints, must be appreciated and well documented on the patient's chart. The presence of foreign body on the wound bed must be ruled out (eg, a chronic wound caused by a retained piece of packing/dressing material).

IMAGING

- Preoperative imaging studies are not always mandatory but often provide valuable information to the reconstructive surgeon.
- Plain films are important to assess proper bony alignment in the setting of trauma or in acute infections to quickly assess for the presence of subcutaneous gas.
- Computed tomography (CT) with the aid of intravenous contrast (computed tomography angiography [CTA]) may determine proper vascularization to the extremity when there is any question regarding distal blood flow, be that acute or chronic.
- Bone scans and magnetic resonance imaging (MRI) to assess for bone viability or osteomyelitis are important adjuncts when planning for debridement of a lower extremity wound with exposed bone.
- Other imaging modalities may aid the operating surgeon in evaluating vascularity of the bone such as PET scans.[2]

SURGICAL MANAGEMENT

- The decision to perform a surgical debridement of a lower extremity wound lies in the hands of the reconstructive surgeon.
- Before the era of free tissue transfer, debridement was often limited because removing questionable tissue could lead to exposure of vital structures, such as tendon devoid of paratenon, vessels, or nerves, and bone devoid of the periosteum. Surgeons were reluctant to make the traumatic defects larger by radical debridement. Subsequently, surgical techniques were more conservative, and healing by secondary intention with wound contracture, scar, and unstable soft tissues was the rule. Currently, free tissue transfer using large well-perfused flaps facilitates radical debridement and necrectomy (removal of dead tissue).

Preoperative Planning

- General anesthesia is preferred. If patient is not a suitable candidate for general anesthesia due to comorbidities, spinal anesthesia or regional block can be considered.

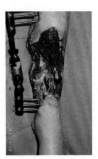

FIG 1 • Left lower extremity wound following high-energy trauma resulting in severe wound involving soft tissue and bone. An external fixator was necessary for skeletal support due to severe bony comminution.

- As mentioned previously, a more thorough physical exam can be performed with the patient under anesthesia.
- Debridement should be performed with the use of the tourniquet. The tourniquet is inflated to 350 mm Hg after an Esmarch bandage is used to exsanguinate the limb. In cases of malignancy or infection, the use of the tourniquet is contraindicated. In these cases, elevating the leg for 5 minutes before inflating the tourniquet aids in limb exsanguination.
- In an ischemic operative field, it is simpler to distinguish between healthy and damaged tissues. The basic elements of this judgment are the appearance and consistency of the tissues. Healthy tissue in the exsanguinated field is bright and homogeneous in color. Subcutaneous tissue is yellow, muscles are bright red, and the tendons and fascia have a white and shiny appearance.
- Damaged tissues are recognized by the presence of foreign bodies, irregular tissue consistency, and irregular distribution of dark red stains, caused by hematomas or hemosiderin (**FIG 1**).
- Evaluating muscle viability may propose a challenge in some cases. Classically, the so-called 4 Cs—muscle color, consistency, contractility, and capacity to bleed—are generally used to assess muscle viability and guide debridement. Recent studies, however, show a potential tendency for normal muscle resection[3] as the surgeon's impression of muscle viability does not correlate with histological findings of the debrided muscle in the majority of cases. Therefore, when large amounts of muscle

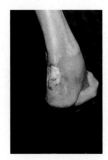

FIG 2 • Chronic right posterior ankle wound. One can appreciate the surrounding scarring and the exposed Achilles tendon with marked desiccation from prolonged exposure. Undermining may not be immediately appreciated, but further debridement may demonstrate tissue undermining and small pockets of fluid and nonviable tissue.

appear of questionable viability in the first stage of debridement, a second trip to the operating room may be necessary to avoid over resection of viable muscle. This is in contrast with clearly necrotic muscle, which will be discussed further.
- Chronic wound
  - A: Chronic wounds present a different challenge to the surgeon. The presence of scarring in the wound bed may impair the surgeon's ability to appreciate important aspects of the wound such as occult infection, its true area and depth, and potential undermining and tunneling (**FIG 2**).
  - B: Due to the fact that these wounds remain open for a prolonged period of time, in addition to other factors such as poor blood flow and hypoxia, they are prone to become heavily colonized with bacterial or fungal organisms, leading to biofilm formation (glycocalyx).

Positioning

- The patient is positioned supine on the operating room table.

Approach

- A "top-down" or "outside-in" approach to the debridement should be undertaken, starting with the skin and subcutaneous tissue, followed by the fascia and muscle, neurovascular structures, and bone.

T E C H N I Q U E S

■ Sharp Debridement of the Acute Wound

- The patient is prepped with antiseptic solution and draped. The extremity is elevated (as described above), and the tourniquet is inflated to 350 mm Hg.
- Next, the wound is superficially washed gently with irrigating solution usually attached to a cystoscopy tubing or through a bulb syringe to eliminate blood clots or superficial debris. Pulsed irrigation systems are advocated by some, but if used too vigorously with too high pressure or too close to tissue planes, particularly around tendons, nerves, and vessels, it can insufflate fascial planes, causing excessive tissue damage and increased edema. Furthermore, it may not be productive in removing bacterial contamination.[4]
- First, a no. 10 or no. 15 scalpel or sharp scissors are used to excise the skin and dermis, particularly around the edge of the wound, back to the normal tissue.

- Next, the subcutaneous layer is inspected, debrided sharply with a no. 10 or no. 15 scalpel to the level of the fascia. All fascia that is ripped, avulsed, or contaminated is then removed.
- The next layer encountered is the muscle. Necrotic muscle should be excised and removed from the wound bed regardless of the volume. Leaving unhealthy, necrotic muscle is most likely to result in subsequent infection. This is often difficult to assess in a crush injury or gunshot blasts where the zone of injury is less clearly defined (**TECH FIG 1**).
- Denuded tendon, if not frayed, should be cleaned or fixed with a suture to the surrounding tissue for later reconstruction.
- Severed vessels are ligated, provided they are of no significance in the viability of the injured extremity. If vessels are vital, they are excised to normal-looking margins, and continuity is restored with interposition vein grafts.

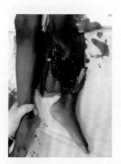

TECH FIG 1 • Left lower extremity wound caused by a gunshot resulting in severe soft tissue and bony trauma. There is a large amount of injured muscle evidenced by the dark red stains, in contrast with likely viable muscle superiorly.

- The nerves are the only structures in which debridement is not radical. Those parts that are destroyed without any doubt are removed, and nerve stumps are tagged and anchored in the wound so as to avoid traction and allow later reconstruction with nerve grafts. We prefer that a large cystoclip or hemoclip be applied to the nerve stump so this can be seen on radiograph and appropriate secondary planning can be done in terms of surgical approach and location of the neuroma stump.
- The periosteum that is elevated from the bone should be excised to the level from which it is elevated. Small bone fragments devoid of the periosteum or free-floating large segments, although they may be of structural significance, should be removed for fear of colonization, contamination, and latent infection.
- At the conclusion of debridement, the wound is again irrigated and tourniquet is let down, and then all tissue planes, particularly muscle, are observed for bleeding as the arterial pressure increases in the limb.
- Areas that are persistently nonviable, particularly the dermis, skin, and muscle, are excised. Excision then can be done sequentially, watching for punctate bleeding from either the dermis or the muscle. If large flaps have been avulsed, excision is carried out through the skin to the level of bright red blood coming from dermis on incision.
- No attempt should be made to close the wound defect under any undue tension for fear of further ischemic damage to already compromised tissues.
- In cases of degloving injuries, the sequence of debridement remains the same; however, in the end of the procedure, the portions of the avulsed skin that appear viable may be used as a full-thickness graft after thorough in situ defatting with sharp scissors or blade and bolstered to the wound. Special attention is warranted in the postoperative period to ascertain skin graft take.[5]
- Avulsed flaps with impaired venous outflow may be salvaged with microsurgical venous anastomosis to more proximal veins.

■ Debridement of the Chronic Wound

- Debridement of a chronic wound is also done with the limb exsanguinated with aid of a tourniquet.
- Superficial scar is excised completely so that the wound margins are in healthy skin and subcutaneous tissue appears normal. The goals are to treat the chronic wound like a tumor and excise it in its entirety down to normal tissue planes. All scar in the wound should be removed in the same manner as tumor surgeons operate; that is, the knife should always cut through healthy tissues.
- If a sinus tract is present or suspected, methylene blue dye may be injected to identify its limits and its course. This way the entirety of the sinus tract can be excised to its origin.
- If functionally important structures are entrapped in the scar, the dissection should commence in the healthy surrounding tissue, passing toward the scar entrapment, where the structures such as nerves or tendons are carefully dissected.
- All areas of the bone not covered with the periosteum are removed, and those that are exposed are burred with an iced saline bur. If punctate bleeding is encountered from the cortical bone, the bone is left behind. If not, the bone is removed until the so-called paprika sign, is identified. This is punctate bleeding from the Haversian canals and indicates bone viability.
- If there is sequestrum in the medullary canal, the anterior part of the bone cortex, such as in the anterior tibia, should be removed even if it is well perfused, to allow access to the medullary canal for placement of muscle flaps that eliminate dead space and help control infection.

■ Hydrosurgery System

- Recently, new modalities for wound debridement have emerged such as the use of hydrosurgery systems (VERSAJET, Smith & Nephew, London, UK). This novel modality allows accurate debridement of only unwanted tissue while precisely conserving viable structures for eventual repair. It employs a high-pressure water jet at 15 000 psi to create a Venturi effect, which eliminates debrided tissues in the water stream, extricating it from the underlying tissue (**TECH FIG 2**).[6]
- The cost-effectiveness of such systems is still controversial, and it may not be superior to conventional debridement so its use is left up to the surgeon's preference and the capabilities of the facility in which he/she operates.

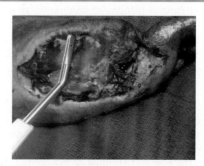

TECH FIG 2 • VERSAJET system for wound debridement.

TECHNIQUES

■ Other Forms of Wound Debridement

- Many other forms and mechanisms for debridement have been described but are beyond the scope of this chapter such as biodebridement using maggots, enzymatic debridement using topical products such as collagenase, newer technologies such as ultrasound therapy, and plasma-mediated bipolar radiofrequency ablation.[7]

- These methods are measured against the current reference standard, which is the sharp debridement technique described, and the method of choice for a particular wound depends on various factors such as type, size and position of wound, quantity and character of the exudate, patient tolerance, cost-effectiveness and available equipment, and expertise of the treatment team.

PEARLS AND PITFALLS

Use of tourniquet	■ The use of tourniquet decreases the amount of blood loss during the procedure. ■ The use of Esmarch bandage is not necessary and sometimes discouraged (eg, presence of infection or malignancy) as elevating the extremity for approximately 5 minutes should exsanguinate the extremity satisfactorily.
Hemostasis	■ Thorough hemostasis is performed after tourniquet is let down and arterial pressure rises.
Necrotic muscle	■ Muscle that appears clearly necrotic should be excised. Leaving necrotic muscle behind is the surest way to acquire an infection.
Loupe magnification	■ Use of loupe magnification helps the operating surgeon better identify structures during the debridement. It also aids in differentiating between viable and nonviable tissues.
Technique	■ The surgeon should approach the debridement as one would a tumor, ie, excise its entirety down to healthy tissue.

POSTOPERATIVE CARE

- An occlusive dressing is applied according to the surgeon's preference. Dressing changes should be performed on a daily or every-other-day basis.
- Patient's comfort is of paramount importance, so proper postoperative pain control should be optimized and depending on size and location of the wound; dressing changes have to be performed in the operating room under sedation or general anesthesia.
- Wound surfaces must be continually moistened and tissue desiccation must be prevented.
- The use of splints may aid in postoperative comfort and should be considered for the postoperative period.
- Elevation of the limb is of upmost importance to decrease the amount of edema and aid in limb circulation.
- Finally, one should take care of the "whole patient, not the hole in the patient"—proper medical optimization, nutrition assessment, and physical rehabilitation must be arranged as part of the postoperative regimen.

OUTCOMES

- The primary outcome is wound healing. This may not be achieved by debridement and closure alone.
- Depending on the size and etiology of the wound, further treatment may be warranted. Frequent dressing changes, application of biomaterials, or coverage with a skin graft or flap may be necessary and are used at the discretion of the treatment team.

COMPLICATIONS

- Nonhealing wound. This may be caused by inadequate debridement of necrotic tissues or foreign bodies, persistent contamination, underlying metabolic disorder, noncompliance with postoperative care, or any other number of factors.
- Secondary infections. This is caused mainly by failure to debride necrotic tissue or to remove colonized foreign body from the wound bed, which serves as substrate for microorganism superinfection.

REFERENCES

1. "debridement". In Concise Medical Dictionary. Oxford University Press, 2010. http://www.oxfordreference.com/view/10.1093/acref/9780199557141.001.0001/acref-9780199557141-e-2473
2. Dyke JP, Aaron RK. Noninvasive methods of measuring bone blood perfusion. *Ann N Y Acad Sci.* 2010;1192:95-102.
3. Sassoon A, Riehl J, Rich A, et al. Muscle viability revisited: are we removing normal muscle? A critical evaluation of dogmatic debridement. *J Orthop Trauma.* 2016;30(1):17-21.
4. Owens BD, White DW, Wenke JC. Comparison of irrigation solutions and devices in a contaminated musculoskeletal wound survival model. *J Bone Joint Surg Am.* 2009;91(1):92-98.
5. Yan H, Gao W, Li Z, et al. The management of degloving injury of lower extremities: technical refinement and classification. *J Trauma Acute Care Surg.* 2013;74(2):604-610.
6. Liu J, Ko JH, Secretov E, et al. Comparing the hydrosurgery system to conventional debridement techniques for the treatment of delayed healing wounds: a prospective, randomised clinical trial to investigate clinical efficacy and cost-effectiveness. *Int Wound J.* 2015;12(4):456-461.
7. Madhok BM, Vowden K, Vowden P. New techniques for wound debridement. *Int Wound J.* 2013;10(3):247-251.

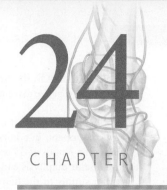

Tibial Reconstruction

Vishwanath R. Chegireddy, Michael J. A. Klebuc, and Anthony Echo

DEFINITION

- Trauma and neoplasia, requiring segmental bone resection, are the most common causes for segmental defects of the tibia.
- Radiation-induced bone necrosis and infection, namely osteomyelitis, is also an indication for resection and possible reconstruction.
- Reconstruction requires technical expertise, careful operative planning, and a detailed understanding of the problem at hand.
- Large commitment by both the patient and the physician is paramount due to long complex rehabilitation period.
- Options for reconstruction include either allograft or autograft material, most commonly a vascularized fibular graft.
- Allografts were initially used but were associated with considerably high rates of complications and failures.
- The concept of reconstruction of the tibial shaft with a vascularized fibular graft was first suggested by Chacha and colleagues in 1981.[1] They used the ipsilateral fibula as a vascularized pedicle graft for nonunion of the tibia.
- It has since been shown to be a viable and reliable technique for tibial reconstruction.
- The main advantage of using a vascularized autograft for tibial reconstruction is the ability to use the normal biology of bone healing for incorporation rather than relying on creeping substitution innate to prosthetic material/nonvascularized graft use.
- The vascularized fibular graft undergoes hypertrophy overtime in response to continuous pressure load, which translates to remarkable long-term durability.[2-4]
- Factors that make the fibula an optimal source for a vascular graft are as follows:
  - Anatomic accessibility
  - Independent blood supply
  - Relatively dispensable in lower extremity function
  - Capability to hypertrophy overtime in response to pressure

ANATOMY

- The tibia is the second largest bone in the human body, after the femur.
- Relevant leg anatomy includes four compartments (anterior, posterior, superficial, and deep posterior) (**FIG 1**).
- The tibia is the stronger of the two bones in the lower leg. It is found on the medial side and is connected to the fibula by the interosseous membrane. It forms a type of fibrous joint called syndesmosis with very little movement.

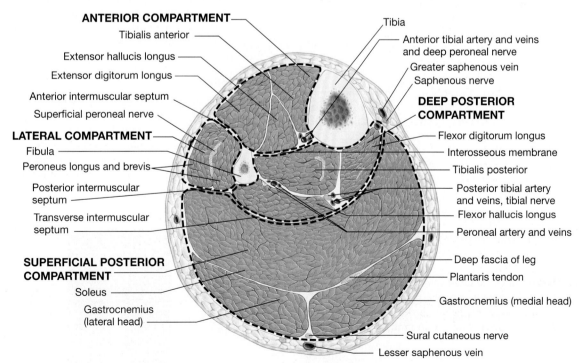

ANTERIOR COMPARTMENT
- Tibialis anterior
- Extensor hallucis longus
- Extensor digitorum longus
- Anterior intermuscular septum
- Superficial peroneal nerve

LATERAL COMPARTMENT
- Fibula
- Peroneus longus and brevis
- Posterior intermuscular septum
- Transverse intermuscular septum

SUPERFICIAL POSTERIOR COMPARTMENT
- Soleus
- Gastrocnemius (lateral head)

Tibia
- Anterior tibial artery and veins and deep peroneal nerve
- Greater saphenous vein
- Saphenous nerve

DEEP POSTERIOR COMPARTMENT
- Flexor digitorum longus
- Interosseous membrane
- Tibialis posterior
- Posterior tibial artery and veins, tibial nerve
- Flexor hallucis longus
- Peroneal artery and veins
- Deep fascia of leg
- Plantaris tendon
- Gastrocnemius (medial head)
- Sural cutaneous nerve
- Lesser saphenous vein

FIG 1 • Cross-sectional anatomy of four compartments at the midtibial level.

- The blood supply to the tibia is derived from a main nutrient artery and periosteal branches derived from the anterior tibial artery.
- The fibula is a long and thin cortical bone with a small medullary component. In adults, the width of the fibula is 1.5 to 2 cm with a length of 35 cm of which approximately 25 cm of the fibular diaphysis can be harvested for free grafting.
- Vascular supply to the diaphysis of the fibula is via a dominant nutrient endosteal artery and minor musculoperiosteal branches from the peroneal artery and veins. These vessels run parallel to the fibula and course between the flexor hallucis longus (FHL) and tibialis posterior muscle group.
- The dominant nutrient artery branches 6 to 14 cm from the peroneal artery bifurcation and enters the fibula posterior to the interosseous membrane. It then courses into the nutrient foramen located in the middle third of the diaphysis and further divides into an ascending and descending branch.
- Musculoperiosteal vessels are derived from the peroneal artery and travel within the posterolateral septum, through the flexor hallucis longus and tibialis posterior muscle, giving segmental rise to four to eight branches that supply the muscles in the anterior compartment, soleus muscle, and lateral leg skin territory. The majority of the periosteal branches are located in the middle third of the fibula.
- Soft tissue defect coverage is achieved with a skin paddle supplied by perforators traversing through the posterior crural septum with the majority concentrating at the proximal and distal ends of the fibula. These fasciocutaneous perforators supply a skin paddle up to 10 × 20 cm in size.[5]

PATIENT HISTORY AND PHYSICAL FINDINGS

- Detailed preoperative evaluation is required for patients undergoing extensive long bone resection and intercalary bone defect reconstruction.
- Determination should first be made as to whether reconstruction or salvage is a viable option.
- General health status should be carefully evaluated. An extensive reconstructive effort should not be undertaken on a patient with an overall poor health status.
- The patient should have the ability to be compliant with both treatment and rehabilitation.
- Pertinent history includes the presence of significant comorbidities such as deep venous thrombosis, peripheral vascular disease, lymphedema, trauma, venous insufficiency, diabetes, or social history such as smoking.
- Special attention should be to consider cardiovascular, surgical, or hematologic diseases that may affect peripheral blood flow.
  - Physical exam should include a lower extremity and vascular examination. This includes an evaluation of knee and ankle joints for range of motion and laxity and a foot Allen test with a Doppler probe to assess dorsalis pedis and posterior tibial arteries.
- Peronea arteria magna is a congenital variant of the arterial inflow to the foot that affects about 1% to 8% of the population, where both the anterior and posterior tibial arteries are hypoplastic or absent with the peroneal artery serving as the single arterial supply below the knee. The artery may need to be reconstructed with a vein graft, or the other leg should be inspected.
- Patients with an abnormal vascular exam or a history of trauma to the affected extremity will need additional preoperative imaging such as computed tomography angiogram

(CTA), duplex ultrasound, or magnetic resonance angiography (MRA) to identify atherosclerotic occlusive disease or congenital anomalies.

IMAGING

- Preoperative imaging of both the recipient and donor sites should include an evaluation of:
- Recipient site:
  - The extent of bone resection, length and diameter of the intercalary defect, and potential soft tissue defect (**FIG 2**). This allows the surgeon to determine the extent of the tumor burden, traumatic bone loss, or chronic osteomyelitis and plan for reconstructive options.
- Donor site:
  - Evaluate vascular supply with Doppler ultrasound (anterior tibial, posterior tibial, and dorsalis pedis arteries), and exclude any fibular deformities.
  - Angiogram to look for vessel patency and flow to the foot

SURGICAL MANAGEMENT

Preoperative Planning

- Determination must be made as to whether limb salvage is a viable option.
- Taking into account patient factors and the extent of disease and/or resection is imperative in determining the need for tibial reconstruction vs amputation.
- Assessment of defect must include the need for bone, muscle, and skin; all of which free fibular graft can provide.
- Four centimeters of bone must be left proximally, whereas 6 cm must be left at the distal portions of the fibula for knee and ankle stabilization, respectively. Therefore, the maximum length of the graft obtainable will be the length of the donor tibia less 10 cm.
- Donor site should be the contralateral leg if used as a free flap. This allows for simultaneous preparation of recipient site during fibula harvest and avoids the use of potentially injured/involved donor site where the fibula may have been fractured in the setting of trauma.

Positioning

- Positioning depends mainly on the recipient site, as the fibula can be harvested in both supine and lateral positions.
- For contralateral free fibula flap harvest, the proper positioning facilitates two teams to work together for recipient preparation and donor dissection simultaneously (**FIG 3**).
- In a supine position, a roll is placed under the ipsilateral hip, and the patient's knee is bent to 90 degrees.

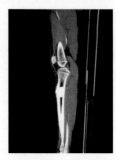

FIG 2 • Preoperative MRI showing left proximal tibial osteosarcoma.

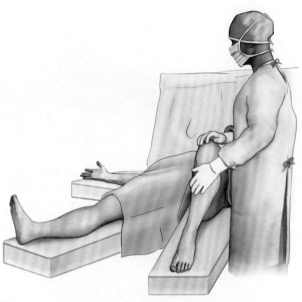

FIG 3 • If the contralateral fibula flap is desired, the patient can be placed in a supine position, which allows two teams to work simultaneously for recipient preparation and donor site harvest.

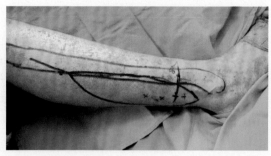

FIG 4 • Intraoperative marking of anatomical landmarks for a contralateral fibula harvest: head of the fibula, lateral malleolus, anteroposterior fibular border, and skin paddle if needed.

- A heel stop can be placed on the operative room table to help knee at 90 degrees when harvesting in the supine position.
- If the patient is in a prone position, a roll is placed under the anterior ipsilateral hip, and bending of the leg is not required.
- All pressure points should be carefully padded and protected.

Approach

- Multidisciplinary team approach is taken involving both plastic surgeons and orthopedic surgical teams to coordinate resection of the involved tibial bone and reconstruction of the ensuing intercalary defect.
- Careful planning of the incision for the exposure is necessary for flap harvest and inset without compromising the skin envelope for coverage.

- Tibial reconstruction can be achieved with free or pedicled fibula graft, in a single- or double-barrelled fashion.
- Reconstruction of smaller intercalary defects up to 13 cm can be achieved with double-barrelled fibular flap, keeping the arterial blood supply intact while performing an osteotomy in the fibula flap.
- If a pedicled flap is desired, the ipsilateral leg will be used for both harvest and inset. The advantages of pedicled flaps are that microvascular anastomosis is unnecessary, and distant donor-site morbidity is avoided, which can occur with free fibula graft.[6]
- Intraoperative preparation of the fibula flap includes marking of anatomical landmarks: head of the fibula, lateral malleolus, and anterior and posterior fibular border (**FIG 4**).
- If a skin deficit is present either in the setting of tumor/chronic osteomyelitis resection or trauma, a skin paddle can be harvested with the fibular flap sharing the same vascular pedicle, which facilitates early detection of flap compromise and provides tension-free skin closure of recipient site.
- A perforator is marked on the proposed skin paddle using intraoperative Doppler localization along the posterior border of the fibula, corresponding to the posterior intramuscular septum.

■ Free Fibula Flap

- After the tibial bone resection is completed by the orthopedic surgical team, the dimensions of the intercalary bone defect are measured (**TECH FIG 1A**).
- Prior to flap harvest, a sterile tourniquet is placed on the midthigh while avoiding compression over the fibular head and common peroneal nerve.
- Using marked anatomical landmarks, a midlateral vertical incision is made over the fibula, and skin flaps are elevated at the level of the fascia.
- Dissection is carried through the investing fascia of the lateral compartment, anterior to the posterior intermuscular septum (**TECH FIG 1B–D**).
  - Care should be taken to preserve fasciocutaneous perforators traveling through the posterior intermuscular septum if a skin island is needed for osteocutaneous flap.
- During proximal dissection, identify and preserve the common peroneal nerve traversing around the head of the fibula to become the superficial peroneal nerve.
- The peroneal muscles are dissected off the anterior surface of the fibula and reflected anteriorly to expose the

anterior intermuscular septum. After incising the septum to gain access to the anterior compartment, reflect the extensor digitorum and hallucis muscles to identify and preserve anterior tibial vessels and deep peroneal nerve.
- The interosseous membrane is incised to enter the deep posterior compartment, and the peroneal vessels are located between tibialis posterior and flexor hallucis longus muscles.
- Next, the peroneal vessels are identified proximally and distally, and dissection is propagated circumferentially around the fibula and staying medial to the vessels using a large right angle clamp. The vascular pedicle should be maintained during dissection.
- After adequate length of the fibula is marked for reconstruction, towel clamps are used to apply lateral traction on the proximal and distal fibula while osteotomizing with an oscillating saw or Gigli saw. A strip of periosteum overlying the osteotomy site should be included to overlap the osteotomy sites at the recipient site.
- Prior to performing osteotomy, a microvascular clamp can be applied to the peroneal artery distal to the osteotomy site to ensure adequate supply to the foot and then divided (**TECH FIG 1E**).

TECHNIQUES

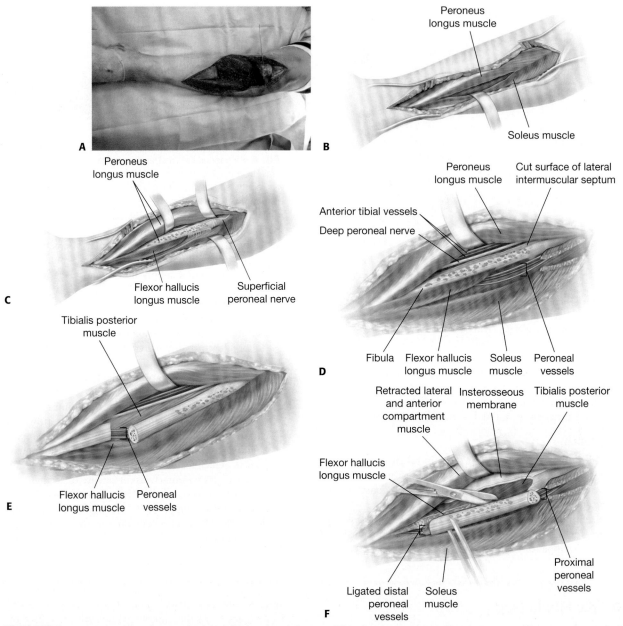

TECH FIG 1 • A. Intraoperative photograph of the left intercalary defect remaining after the tumor resection. **B.** Exposure of peroneus longus and soleus at the midtibial level. **C.** Dissection around the fibula and lateral muscle compartment. Proceed dissection proximally to identify and protect the superficial peroneal nerve. **D.** Dissection proceeds anterior to the fibula through the anterior intermuscular septum and protects the deep peroneal nerve and anterior tibial vessels. **E.** After the distal fibula osteotomy, the peroneal vessels should be ligated distally, which are located between FHL and tibialis posterior muscle groups. **F.** Adequate fibula length is freed, and proximal osteotomy is performed carefully while protecting the pedicle vessels.

- The vascular pedicle is dissected starting distally, carried proximally up to the origin of tibioperoneal trunk, and ligated with approximately 2 to 6 cm of pedicle length.
- After the fibula graft is fully mobilized with the pedicle (**TECH FIG 1F**), the tourniquet is released with robust

arterial inflow and venous outflow and healthy back bleeding from both the periosteum and intramedullary canal.
- An osteomuscular flap can also be harvested in similar fashion to include soleus and flexor hallucis longus muscles. This can aid in filling the dead space in patients with extensive soft tissue defect.

- If the distal osteotomy is close to the lateral malleolus, a screw fixation to the tibia can be utilized to prevent valgus deformity and ankle instability, which is more important in pedicle flap.
- In a clean and well-vascularized recipient bed, the proximal and distal tibial should be stabilized, and the medullary cavities should be prepared to receive the free fibula graft.
- The free fibula graft is then telescoped into the intercalary defect. Next, the graft is anchored to the tibia proximally and distally with long compression plates and screws spanning the bone defect. During this step, care is taken to prevent any damage to the peroneal vessels.
- Standard microvascular anastomosis is performed between the recipient vessels and peroneal artery and accompanying venae comitantes. Additionally, several fat grafts can be placed around the pedicle in an effort to prevent compression.
- After skin closure, a well-padded posterior leg splint is applied to keep the foot in extension to prevent an equinus deformity.

■ Pedicled Fibula Graft

- The recipient site defect is measured to estimate the length of the fibula required for reconstruction (see **TECH FIG 1A**).
- If the fibula flap is to remain pedicled (**TECH FIG 2A**), the flap is raised in standard fashion, but the proximal vascular pedicle is not ligated (**TECH FIG 2B**).
- The vascularized fibula flap is then transported through the space created between the tibialis posterior muscle and the tibialis anterior muscle.

- The distal-most segment of the bone will be used for the reconstruction. It can either be transposed or reversed, but whichever way the flap is oriented, it needs adequate pedicle length.
- If the fibula is reversed and rotated 180 degrees, the pedicle will make a U-turn, and care needs to be taken not to kink the pedicle on inset.
- Additionally, if the length of the vascular pedicle of the graft is expected to be inadequate, it is necessary to harvest the graft as far from the base of the pedicle as possi-

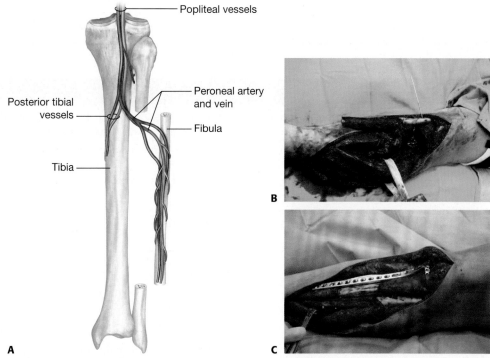

TECH FIG 2 • A. Illustration of pedicled fibula graft with intact peroneal vessels. **B.** Intraoperative photograph of an ipsilateral pedicled fibula graft. **C.** Intraoperative photograph showing an allograft sp anning the defect and an onlay fibula graft being stabilized with long compression plates and screws.

ble and separate the periosteum with the vascular pedicle to make a longer vascular pedicle.

- Once inset as an interposition graft, bone fixation of the fibula graft is achieved with long compression plates and screws traversing the tibial defect.

- Alternatively, an allograft can be used as an interposition graft spanning the intercalary defect with an onlay fibula graft as a buttress, which can provide greater stability (**TECH FIG 2C**).

■ Double-Barrelled Fibula Technique

- Blood supply to the fibula is both endosteal and periosteal.
- This technique is useful for proximal tibial reconstruction when the defect is shorter than 13 cm.
  - Larger defects will not be able to be reconstructed with a single fibula in a double-barrelled fashion; both fibulas would be required, and the second fibula would need to be as a free fibula flap.
  - Additionally, this method provides two segments of bone, which doubles the cross-sectional area of the flap but only requires one anastomosis.
- Following the harvest, the graft is osteotomized at the midpoint, taking care to avoid the peroneal vessels (**TECH FIG 3**).
- At the site of the proposed osteotomy, the vascular pedicle is carefully elevated off the bone flap in the subperiosteal plane with an elevator over a segment of 2 to 3 cm, which will allow a malleable retractor to be placed to protect the pedicle.
- The graft is osteotomized at the midpoint and folded, with care taken to preserve the peroneal vessels.

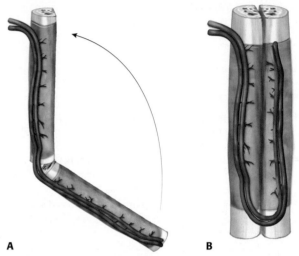

A   **B**

TECH FIG 3 • In the double-barrelled fibula repair, free fibula is harvested with the peroneal vessels intact. The graft is then osteotomized at the midpoint and folded.

PEARLS AND PITFALLS

Peronea arteria magna	▪ A congenital variant of the arterial inflow to the foot, where both the anterior and posterior tibial arteries are hypoplastic or absent with the peroneal artery serving as the single arterial supply below the knee.
Injury to common peroneal nerve	▪ The nerve courses inferior to the head of the fibula and should be identified during proximal dissection to prevent injury.
Careful dissection of skin perforators	▪ Preserve the posterior intermuscular septum, which carries perforators to the skin paddle.
Joint instability	▪ At least 4 cm of fibula bone is preserved proximally to preserve the stability of the knee. ▪ At least 6 cm of fibula bone is preserved distally above lateral malleolus to preserve stability of the ankle.

POSTOPERATIVE CARE

- Recipient and donor sites should be monitored during the postoperative period for vascular insufficiency and signs of free flap compromise, which can be monitored if a skin island is harvested.
- Flap function can be monitored with a combination of clinical exam and a Doppler probe every hour during the first 24 hours. The flap patency should be assessed until patient discharge.
- Initially, patients should be advised no weight bearing on the surgical limb up to 2 weeks. Afterward, partial weight bearing can be resumed with assistance and progressed to full weight-bearing status after bone union.

OUTCOMES

- Union time can range from 3 to 7 months.
- Union rates upward of 75%.
- Ambulation: all patients (100%) at an average 9.5[5] to 14.3 months[7].
- Joint stiffness (40%) and pain (18%) are frequent[8].
- Fibular hypertrophy occurs secondary to microfractures and callous formation.

COMPLICATIONS

- Recipient site
  - Loss of flap primarily caused by vascular thrombosis
  - Nonunion

- Infection
- Hardware malfunction
- Donor site
  - Inability to flex the great toe due to damage to flexor hallucis longus:
    - Knee or ankle joint instability with secondary pseudoarthrosis
  - Common peroneal nerve injury

ACKNOWLEDGMENTS

Thank you to Drs. C. Arroyo-Alonso and A.J. Steinberg, Institute for Reconstructive Surgery, Houston Methodist Hospital and Weill Cornell Medicine, Houston, Texas, for their contributions to the preparation of this chapter.

REFERENCES

1. Chacha PB, Ahmed M, Daruwalla JS. Vascular pedicle graft of the ipsilateral fibula for non-union of the tibia with a large defect: an experimental and clinical study. *J Bone Joint Surg.* 1981;63B:244-253.

2. Capanna R, Campanacci DA, Belot N, et al. A new reconstructive technique for intercalary defects of long bones: the association of massive allograft with vascularized fibular autograft. Long-term results and comparison with alternative techniques. *Orthop Clin North Am.* 2007;38(1):51-60, vi.

3. Malizos KN, Zalavras CG, Soucacos PN, et al. Free vascularized fibular grafts for reconstruction of skeletal defects. *J Am Acad Orthop Surg.* 2004;12(5):360-369.

4. Zaretski A, Amir A, Meller I, et al. Free fibula long bone reconstruction in orthopedic oncology: a surgical algorithm for reconstructive options. *Plast Reconstr Surg.* 2004;113(7):1989-2000.

5. Chen ZW, Yan W. The study and clinical application of the osteocutaneous flap of fibula. *Microsurgery.* 1983;4(1):11-16.

6. Vail TP, Urbaniak JR. Donor-site morbidity with use of vascularized autogenous fibular grafts. *J Bone Joint Surg.* 1996;78A:204-211.

7. Weichman KE, Dec W, Morris CD, et al. Lower extremity osseous oncologic reconstruction with composite microsurgical free fibula inside massive bony allograft. *Plast Reconstr Surg.* 2015;136(2):396-403.

8. Pelissier P, Boireau P, Martin D, Baudet J. Bone reconstruction of the lower extremity: complications and outcomes. *Plast Reconstr Surg.* 2003;111(7):2223-2229.

25 CHAPTER

Soft Tissue Coverage of Lower Leg—Free Flap

Goo-Hyun Mun and Kyong-Je Woo

DEFINITION

- Microvascular free flap transfer is a reliable and often ideal option for soft tissue reconstruction of a complex or large wound of the lower leg.
- The goal of reconstruction is to provide durable soft tissue coverage to maximize bony union in a traumatic wound and functional recovery and to restore the aesthetic contour of the lower leg.

ANATOMY

- Three main arteries branching from the popliteal artery are potential recipient vessels for microvascular free flap transfer for soft tissue coverage of the lower leg: the anterior tibial, posterior tibial, and peroneal arteries (**FIG 1A–E**).
- Apart from the concomitant veins of the named arteries of the lower leg, the two major superficial veins, which are the long (great) and short (small) saphenous veins, may be used as recipient veins. The superficial veins run superficial to the fascia cruris (deep fascia) of the lower leg (**FIG 1F**).
- Sizable perforators to the overlying skin derived from any of the three major vessels can also be recipient vessels when they are found near the defect.[1,2]

- The specific recipient vessels are chosen according to the site of the defect.
  - Upper third of the lower leg: the upper third of the lower leg is technically the most difficult zone for microvascular repairs because of the deep location of major vessels. A long vein graft from the flap passing proximally to the side of the femoral artery was commonly used in the past. However, sural vessels (**FIG 2**) and the reversed descending branch of the lateral circumflex femoral vessels can also be effective recipient options in this region.[3]
  - Middle third of the leg: the anterior tibial vessels are often used because the vessels become more superficial as they descend (**FIG 3**). The posterior tibial arterial and venous system may be easily exposed after retraction of the soleus muscle when the defect is on the medial side of the leg (**FIG 4**).
  - Distal third of the leg: distal branches of all three major vessels are easily accessible in this region because there is less overlying soft tissues, which also makes them more susceptible to injury in traumatic defects. The peroneal artery or its terminating calcaneal artery can also be used in the lateral region of the leg (**FIG 5**). Perforators from the peroneal artery can be used as recipient vessels in the lateral region (**FIG 6**).

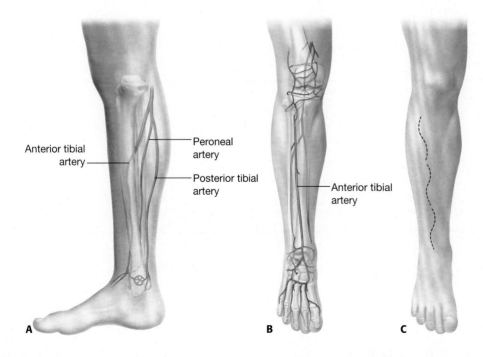

Anterior tibial artery — Peroneal artery

Posterior tibial artery

Anterior tibial artery

A　　　　**B**　　　　**C**

FIG 1 • Main arteries and veins of the lower leg and incisions for exposure of recipient vessels. **A.** Three named arteries of the lower leg. **B.** Anterior tibial artery. **C.** Incisions for exposure of the anterior tibial artery.

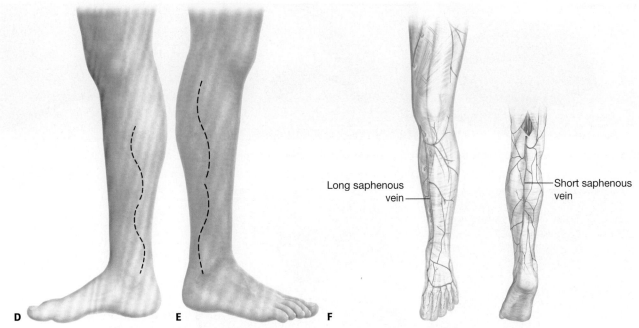

Long saphenous vein

Short saphenous vein

FIG 1 (Continued) • **D.** Incisions for exposure of the posterior tibial artery. **E.** Incisions for exposure of the peroneal artery. **F.** Long and short saphenous veins.

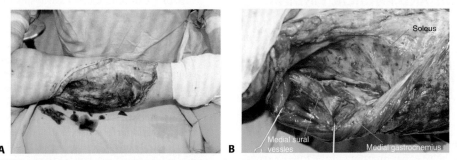

FIG 2 • **A,B.** Medial sural vessels as recipient vessel.

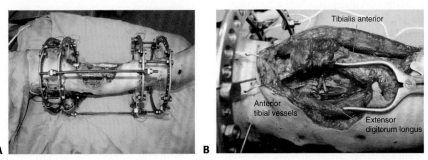

FIG 3 • **A,B.** Anterior tibial vessels for recipient vessel.

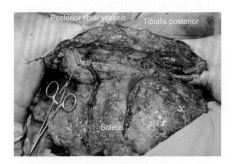

FIG 4 • Posterior tibial vessels for recipient vessel.

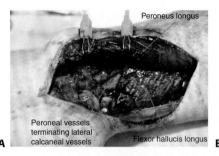
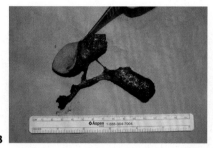
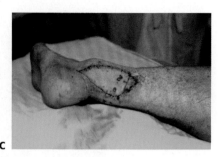

Peroneus longus

Peroneal vessels terminating lateral calcaneal vessels

Flexor hallucis longus

A   B   C

FIG 5 • Peroneal vessels for recipient vessel. **A.** Peroneal vessels. **B.** Muscle chimeric TDAP perforator flap. **C.** After inset of the flap.

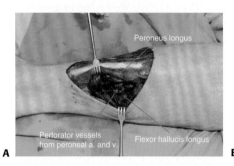
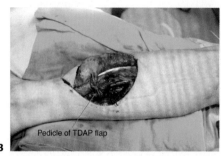

Peroneus longus

Perforator vessels from peroneal a. and v.   Flexor hallucis longus

A   B   Pedicle of TDAP flap

FIG 6 • **A,B.** Peroneal artery perforators for recipient vessel.

PATIENT HISTORY AND PHYSICAL FINDINGS

- A multidisciplinary approach with comprehensive communication between the oncologist and/or orthopedic surgeon will allow better treatment outcomes.[4]
- Preoperative planning should be carried out by considering anticipated defect size, location, vascular anatomy, and comorbid conditions related to the outcomes of reconstruction.

IMAGING

- The authors routinely perform preoperative CT angiography to delineate the vascular anatomy of the lower extremity except when it is contraindicated.
- Detailed information of the vascular status helps determine proper reconstruction options and recipient vessels, which ultimately decreases the risk of reconstruction failure in the free flap transfer.[5]

SURGICAL MANAGEMENT

- Soft tissue stability and long-term durability are of paramount concern in the reconstruction of the lower leg.
- The simple method is not always the best and often, a more complex method of reconstruction, such as the free flap, is initially chosen to obtain better functional and aesthetic outcomes.
- Elaborate preoperative planning regarding recipient vessels, donor site, flap composition (cutaneous, fasciocutaneous, musculocutaneous, chimeric, composite flap), and positioning of the patient during the surgery is crucial for successful soft tissue reconstruction of the lower leg. A muscle chimeric perforator flap is useful for filling dead spaces created by soft tissue loss (see **FIG 5**).[6]
- Vascular complications are significantly higher if anastomoses are carried out in the zone of injury, due to inflammation and trauma to recipient vessels. A sufficiently longer pedicle or vessel graft may be necessary to reach normal suitable vessels.
- Donor site morbidity should also be considered in the preoperative planning. The donor site that permits primary clo-

sure of the donor defect is always favored over the ones that require skin grafting. The exact measurement of the shape and size of the defect is valuable for donor tissue economy and acceptable aesthetic results at the recipient site. A customized flap may be effectively designed by using paper or transparent plastic template based on the final defect shape.
- The flap thickness can be controlled by defatting of the perforator flap at the time of inset, which facilitates aesthetic reconstruction. On the other hand, flap thickness can be controlled secondarily when tissue edema resolves completely.
- Fasciocutaneous flap vs muscle flap in contaminated wounds: A previous animal study demonstrated that muscle flaps have advantages over the fasciocutaneous flap for contaminated wounds.[7] However, recent studies show that there is no difference in bacterial eradication and quality of wound healing between muscle and fasciocutaneous flap use.[8,9]
- There is a controversy regarding how early a soft tissue defect should be closed in lower extremity trauma. Early definitive soft tissue coverage may be necessary where vital structures such as blood vessels and peripheral nerves or hardware are exposed.[10] The recent advent of negative pressure wound therapy has helped provide additional time for better delineation of nonviable tissues before final reconstruction in large, complex open wounds.[11]

Preoperative Planning

- Vascular anatomy and degree of atherosclerosis are evaluated by preoperative CT angiography (**FIG 7**).
- Donor site and components of the flap are often decided preoperatively according to predicted defect size, location, type of tissue requirement, required pedicle length, surgeon's expertise, and patient preference.
- Rectus abdominis, latissimus dorsi, and the gracilis muscle flaps have been commonly used for lower leg reconstruction. Popular cutaneous or fasciocutaneous flaps for lower leg reconstruction are the radial forearm, sural, anterolateral thigh, and thoracodorsal artery perforator (TDAP) flaps.[8,12–14] Each flap has its advantages and disadvantages.

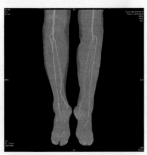

FIG 7 • CT angiography of the patient described in the surgical technique in the text. All three main vessels of lower legs are patent, and no atherosclerosis or vascular occlusion exists in both lower legs.

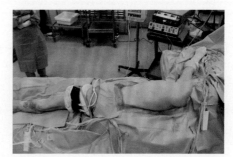

FIG 8 • Positioning of the patient when the flap is to be harvested from the ipsilateral back.

Positioning

- Patient position is influenced by the donor site selection and planned recipient vessel approach. The lateral decubitus position is convenient for harvesting flaps from the back nourished by the subscapular vascular tree. When the medial approach is used for the recipient vessel, such as the posterior tibial vessel or medial sural vessel, the contralateral side

of the back is the favored donor site. When the anterior or lateral approach is to be used for the anterior tibial artery or peroneal artery branches, it is better to harvest the flap from the ipsilateral back, which helps to avoid patient repositioning during the free flap surgery (**FIG 8**).
- A tourniquet is usually applied on the thigh during defect preparation including debridement and recipient vessel approach.

■ Wound Preparation

- Recipient vessel decided on preoperative planning is checked for patency using a handheld audible Doppler.

- The ultimate defect is made by the complete debridement or excision of pathologic, necrotic, or infected tissues under tourniquet control (**TECH FIG 1**).
- Limited undermining of the skin flap around the wound margin is performed to facilitate subsequent flap inset.

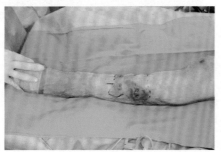
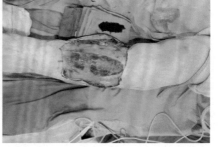

TECH FIG 1 • **A,B.** Wound preparation for free flap reconstruction.

■ Recipient Vessel Preparation

- Approach to recipient vessels
  - When the defect is extensive such as in oncologic resection or located in the distal lower leg over the course of the major vessel, the recipient vessel can be harvested directly inside the wound, which is advantageous for avoiding added incisional scars.
  - An incision extending from the defect may be used when the adjacent recipient vessel is to be utilized. A separate incision with subcutaneous tunneling may be effectively employed for distant recipient vessel approach.
- Anterior tibial vessels are exposed through a dissection through the intermuscular septum between the tibialis anterior and extensor digitorum longus muscles (**TECH FIG 2**).

- The deep peroneal nerve is carefully separated from the anterior tibial artery and veins.

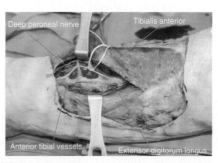

TECH FIG 2 • Recipient vessel preparation. Anterior tibial vessels are exposed through a dissection through the intermuscular septum between the tibialis anterior and extensor digitorum longus muscles.

▪ Assessment of the Defect

- The tourniquet is deflated and meticulous hemostasis is performed. Irrigation with saline solution is carried out.

- Defect size along with its shape can be exactly measured using transparent plastic or paper template, which will be used for flap design in the donor site.
- Dead space that needs to be filled is also marked on the defect template.

▪ Flap Harvest

- Outline of relevant muscles and landmarks are marked on the skin (**TECH FIG 3A**).
- Perforators are located using handheld pencil Doppler and the flap is designed using the template of the defect.
- Once the targeted perforator is identified via a suprafascial dissection through a limited incision on superior border of the flap, then the whole skin paddle is elevated and meticulous intramuscular dissection of the pedicle with bipolar forceps is commenced.
- Motor nerve branches to the muscle are maximally preserved and the pedicle is divided when sufficient length is obtained (**TECH FIG 3B**).
- A closed suction drain is placed, and the donor wound is primarily closed in layers (**TECH FIG 3C,D**).

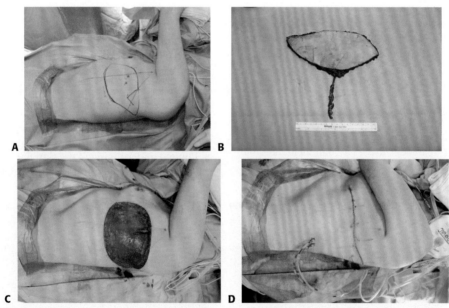

TECH FIG 3 ▪ A. Design of the flap using transparent plastic template. **B.** Elevated TDAP flap. **C.** Defect of the donor site after elevation of the TDAP flap. **D.** Primary closure of the donor site.

▪ Microanastomosis With Temporary Inset (TECH FIG 4)

- Temporary inset of the flap is performed using a skin stapler.
- It is important to avoid twisting or kinking of the pedicle. A useful way to mitigate twisting of the pedicle is to lift and hold the flap in the air and allow the vessels to dangle and unwind. If the pedicle is long, lazy-S–shaped positioning of the pedicle under the flap is performed to avoid kinking of the pedicle.
- Vascular tension should be avoided through prudent planning, harvesting a sufficient length of the pedicle, and judicious use of a vascular graft when needed.
- Wide exposure of the field and ensuring a conducive atmosphere are critical for successful microvascular anastomosis.

- End-to-side anastomosis of the artery is preferred to maintain vascular flow in inherent arteries of the leg and to avoid iatrogenic ischemic complications of the leg.
- The deep vein system (comitantes vein) is usually given the first consideration because of the special convenience with dissection and inset. However, the superficial veins (long saphenous and short saphenous veins) can be used when there is significant size mismatch with the deep veins or if no adequate deep vein is suitable. Regardless of the use of the deep or superficial veins, the quality of the recipient vein should be checked based on intraoperative findings such as the absence of scarring around the vein, existence of backflow, absence of thrombi, and absence of resistance to an intraluminal heparinized saline flush.[15]
- The vascular clamp is removed after completion of the anastomosis. Warm saline is irrigated onto the vessels

and flap, followed by waiting for several minutes to check patent inflow and outflow of the flap.

■ Meticulous hemostasis is performed under the microscope to ensure that branches of the pedicle and recipient vessels are secured as hematoma is known to be one of the main causes of re-exploration after free flap reconstruction in lower extremities.[12]

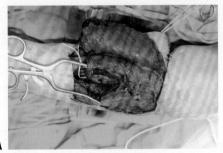
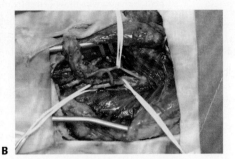

TECH FIG 4 • A. Temporary inset of the flap for microvascular anastomosis. **B.** After completion of microvascular anastomosis. End-to-side anastomosis of the artery and end-to-end anastomosis of the vein were carried out.

■ Final Inset

■ If a flap is too bulky, then meticulous defatting of the perforator flap can be performed at the time of insetting. The deep fat, superficial fascia, and deep layer of superficial fat can be safely removed, but not the area near the perforators (about 2–3 cm diameter), using scissors with or without loupe but microscope magnification is not usually necessary (**TECH FIG 5A**). This is a crucial procedure for obtaining a satisfactory contour of the reconstructed lower leg. However, to completely avoid tissue damage within the flap and risk of ischemic complication at the initial operation, secondary procedure for thinning is an alternative option.

■ The final inset of the flap needs to be carefully performed because the pliability and extensibility of the flap may change after the defatting procedure.[16] Excessive flap tissue is diligently excised to yield a more natural appearance (**TECH FIG 5B,C**).

■ The wound is closed by placing drains under the flap to prevent fluid collection.

■ A leg splint is frequently applied for immobilization. An elastic bandage is loosely applied. Part of the flap is left open for postoperative monitoring of the flap (**TECH FIG 5D**). Excessive compression over the vascular pedicle should be avoided.

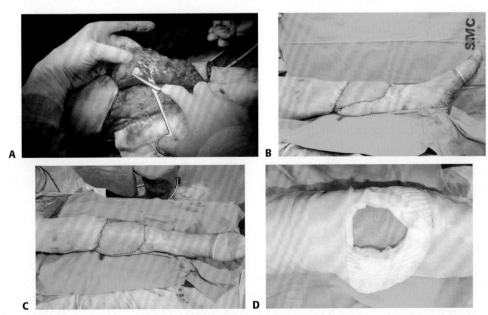

TECH FIG 5 • A. Defatting of the perforator flap. **B,C.** Immediate postoperative photos. **D.** Dressings of the reconstruction site.

PEARLS AND PITFALLS

Planning	■ Elaborate preoperative planning of recipient vessels, donor site, flap composition, and positioning of the patient is important for successful reconstruction. ■ A multidisciplinary approach including comprehensive communication with the oncologist and/or orthopedic surgeon will allow better treatment outcomes.
Flap design	■ The exact template created according to the final defect size and shape is helpful to avoid harvesting an unnecessarily large flap and to obtain an aesthetically pleasing contour of the lower leg.
Placement of the pedicle	■ It is important to avoid twisting of the vascular pedicle. ■ If the pedicle is excessively long, it is placed in a lazy-S–shaped position under the flap to avoid kinking of the pedicle. ■ Minimize tension on the pedicle. Sufficient acquisition of the pedicle can be a safe strategy.
Microanastomosis	■ End-to-side anastomosis of the artery is preferred to maintain distal vascular flow in named arteries of the lower leg and to avoid potential ischemic sequelae of the leg. ■ The deep vein system (venae comitantes) is usually given the first consideration as a source of outflow because of special convenience for dissection and inset and because it is less vulnerable to trauma than the superficial venous system.
Flap inset	■ Defatting of the perforator flap is a valuable technique for obtaining an aesthetic contour at the time of inset, but must be done meticulously to avoid compromising perfusion. ■ Dimensional excess of the flap is diligently corrected by careful trimming.
Hemostasis	■ Meticulous hemostasis needs to be performed during the entire surgical procedure because hematoma is known to be one of the main causes of re-exploration after free flap reconstruction in lower extremities.

POSTOPERATIVE CARE

■ Proper patient positioning and avoidance of vascular pedicle compression (by splinting or inattentive wound dressings) play vital roles in the postoperative period.

■ The leg is elevated for better venous return and to minimize edema while the patient is lying in bed.

■ There is no consensus regarding the use of medications for thromboprophylaxis, such as aspirin, heparin, and dextran. The authors do not routinely use any of these medications.

■ Enoxaparin (low molecular weight heparin) is considered for deep vein thrombosis prophylaxis in lower extremity reconstructions as chemoprophylaxis is recommended for general surgery patients scoring 3 or higher on the Caprini scale.[17] Patients undergoing lower extremity reconstruction with free flap frequently fall into the high-risk group with Caprini scores of 5 or greater.[18]

■ Postoperatively the flap can be monitored every 1 to 3 hours for the first 48 hours, and every 4 to 6 hours for the next 48 hours after the surgery. Monitoring is typically performed by physical examination and handheld pencil Doppler.

■ An oral diet is allowed 24 hours after surgery.

■ Although the duration of immobilization time varies based on the orthopedic and bony injuries, generally progressive weight bearing and ambulation are achieved once the flap maturation is assured, which occurs in 2 to 3 weeks for isolated soft tissue reconstruction.

OUTCOMES

■ Microvascular free flap for lower extremity reconstruction is currently a safe and reliable procedure with a high success rate. Recent advancements in technology and improvement in surgical techniques have led to reported success rates of between 94% and 100%.[5,8,12,19]

■ Microvascular free flap is a reliable reconstructive option for defects of various sizes in various locations of the lower leg, and multiple tissue components such as cutaneous, muscle, and muscle chimeric can be used according to tissue requirements (**FIG 9**).

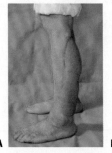 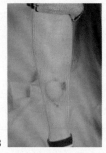 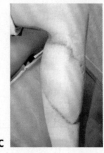 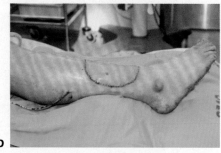

A **B** **C** **D**

FIG 9 • Cases of lower leg reconstruction with free flaps. **A.** Dual-pedicled deep inferior epigastric artery perforator (DIEP) flap for extensive lower leg defect. Dual pedicles were anastomosed to the posterior tibial artery and vein with the end-to-side method. **B.** Reconstruction of small defect with TDAP flap. Anterior tibial vessels were used as recipient vessel. **C.** Reconstruction of extensive defects on the proximal lower leg using the DIEP flap. Medial sural vessels were used for recipient vessels, and the great saphenous vein was used for superdrainage. **D.** Reconstruction of the distal lower leg using the TDAP flap. Anterior tibial vessels were used as recipient vessels.

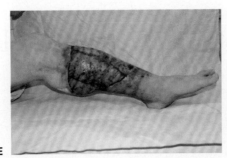
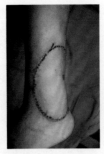

FIG 9 (Continued) • **E.** Free muscle (latissimus dorsi) flap with skin graft. **F.** Muscle chimeric TDAP flap for distal lower leg reconstruction.

COMPLICATIONS

- Vascular-related complications such as venous and arterial thrombosis
- Hematoma: Early diagnosis of a hematoma under the flap is critical so that it can be evacuated promptly to prevent the compression and obstruction of the anastomotic site from the expanding hematoma. In particular, any time a postoperative hematoma is noted, the surgeon must consider venous thrombosis.
- Infection
- Partial flap necrosis

REFERENCES

1. Haddock N, Garfein ES, Reformat D, et al. Perforator vessel recipient options in the lower extremity: an anatomically based approach to safer limb salvage. *J Reconstr Microsurg.* 2010;26:461-469.
2. Tashiro K, Harima M, Yamamoto T, et al. Locating recipient perforators for perforator-to-perforator anastomosis using color Doppler ultrasonography. *J Plast Reconstr Aesthet Surg.* 2014;67:1680-1683.
3. Gao SH, Feng SM, Chen C, et al. A new recipient artery for reconstruction of soft-tissue defects in the lower limb with a free anterolateral thigh flap: the reversed descending branch of the lateral femoral circumflex artery. *Plast Reconstr Surg.* 2012;130:1059-1065.
4. Suh HS, Lee JS, Hong JP. Consideration in lower extremity reconstruction following oncologic surgery: patient selection, surgical techniques, and outcomes. *J Surg Oncol.* 2016;113:955-961.
5. Duymaz A, Karabekmez FE, Vrtiska TJ, et al. Free tissue transfer for lower extremity reconstruction: a study of the role of computed angiography in the planning of free tissue transfer in the posttraumatic setting. *Plast Reconstr Surg.* 2009;124:523-529.
6. Lee KT, Wiraatmadja ES, Mun GH. Free latissimus dorsi muscle-chimeric thoracodorsal artery perforator flaps for reconstruction of complicated defects: does muscle still have a place in the domain of perforator flaps? *Ann Plast Surg.* 2015;74:565-572.
7. Calderon W, Chang N, Mathes SJ. Comparison of the effect of bacterial inoculation in musculocutaneous and fasciocutaneous flaps. *Plast Reconstr Surg.* 1986;77:785-794.

8. Hong JP, Shin HW, Kim JJ, et al. The use of anterolateral thigh perforator flaps in chronic osteomyelitis of the lower extremity. *Plast Reconstr Surg.* 2005;115:142-147.
9. Rodriguez ED, Bluebond-Langner R, Copeland C, et al. Functional outcomes of posttraumatic lower limb salvage: a pilot study of anterolateral thigh perforator flaps versus muscle flaps. *J Trauma.* 2009;66:1311-1314.
10. Medina ND, Kovach SJ III, Levin LS. An evidence-based approach to lower extremity acute trauma. *Plast Reconstr Surg.* 2011;127: 926-931.
11. Soltanian H, Garcia RM, Hollenbeck ST. Current concepts in lower extremity reconstruction. *Plast Reconstr Surg.* 2015;136: 815e-829e.
12. Basheer MH, Wilson SM, Lewis H, Herbert K. Microvascular free tissue transfer in reconstruction of the lower limb. *J Plast Reconstr Aesthet Surg.* 2008;61:525-528.
13. Hallock GG. Medial sural artery perforator free flap: legitimate use as a solution for the ipsilateral distal lower extremity defect. *J Reconstr Microsurg.* 2014;30:187-192.
14. Hwang JH, Lim SY, Pyon JK, et al. Reliable harvesting of a large thoracodorsal artery perforator flap with emphasis on perforator number and spacing. *Plast Reconstr Surg.* 2011;128:140e-50e.
15. Lorenzo AR, Lin C-H, Lin C-H, et al. Selection of the recipient vein in microvascular flap reconstruction of the lower extremity: Analysis of 362 free-tissue transfers. *J Plast Reconstr Aesthet Surg.* 2011;64: 649-655.
16. Jeon BJ, Lim SY, Pyon JK, et al. Secondary extremity reconstruction with free perforator flaps for aesthetic purposes. *J Plast Reconstr Aesthet Surg.* 2011;64:1483-1489.
17. Gould MK, Garcia DA, Wren SM, et al. Prevention of VTE in nonorthopedic surgical patients: Antithrombotic Therapy and Prevention of Thrombosis, 9th ed: American College of Chest Physicians Evidence-Based Clinical Practice Guidelines. *Chest.* 2012;141:e227S-e277S. doi:210.1378/chest.1311-2297.
18. Kim SY, Lee KT, Mun GH. Postoperative venous insufficiency in microsurgical lower extremity reconstruction and deep vein thrombosis potential as assessed by a Caprini risk assessment model. *Plast Reconstr Surg.* 2015;136:1094-1102.
19. Wettstein R, Schurch R, Banic A, et al. Review of 197 consecutive free flap reconstructions in the lower extremity. *J Plast Reconstr Aesthet Surg.* 2008;61:772-776.

26
CHAPTER

Soft Tissue Coverage of Lower Leg–Soleus Flap

Rahim Nazerali and Lee L. Q. Pu

DEFINITION

- Mathes and Nahai type II muscle
- Most commonly proximally based pedicled flap, but a distally based flap has been reported.

ANATOMY

- Broad, large, bipennate muscle
- Deep to the gastrocnemius muscle in the posterior compartment of the leg
- Occupies major portion of superficial posterior compartment of the leg in the middle third tibial level
- Two separate muscle bellies, medial and lateral with separate origins
  - Origin
    - Lateral belly: posterior surface of the fibula
    - Medial belly: middle third of the medial border of the tibia
  - Insertion
    - Lateral belly: dorsal lateral aspect of the Achilles tendon
    - Medial belly: dorsal medial aspect of the Achilles tendon
- Vascular supply (**FIG 1**)
  - Proximal portion of muscle receives independent axial vascular supply to its medial and lateral bellies.
  - Dominant pedicle: muscular branches of the popliteal artery and from proximal two branches of the posterior tibial artery and peroneal artery
  - Distal portion of muscle primarily receives segmental blood supply from two to four segmental branches from the posterior tibial artery.
- Innervation
  - Motor: posterior tibial and medial popliteal nerves
- Function
  - Plantar flexion

PATIENT HISTORY AND PHYSICAL FINDINGS

- Just like any other major flap surgery for the lower extremity, a patient's general medical condition and neurovascular physical examination should be evaluated carefully.
- Previous orthopedic trauma to the leg and ongoing orthopedic procedures should also be taken into a consideration when planning a soleus muscle flap.

IMAGING

- Preoperative angiogram is recommended if using a distally based medial hemisoleus muscle flap to assess the blood supply, which is typically from branches of the posterior tibial vessels.

SURGICAL MANAGEMENT[1-7]

- Soleus is the standard muscle flap of choice for middle third defects of the leg.
- Numerous limitations with bulk, arc of rotation and weakening of plantar flexion when using the entire muscle.
- Medial hemisoleus muscle flap can be elevated based either proximally or distally depending on the location of the soft tissue reconstruction required.
- Medial hemisoleus muscle flaps should be chosen to reconstruct a less extensive wound (less than 50 cm² in most adult patients).
- Proximally based flaps can be used to cover middle third tibial wounds in the leg, whereas distally based flaps can be used for distal third defects. In addition, proximally based flaps can also be used to cover distal third defects if done properly.

Preoperative Planning

- Physical exam including pulse, neurological status, tissue quality

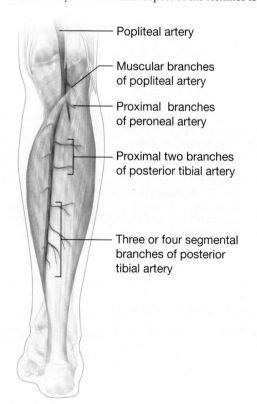

FIG 1 • A schematic diagram shows the vascular anatomy of a soleus muscle.

- Popliteal artery
- Muscular branches of popliteal artery
- Proximal branches of peroneal artery
- Proximal two branches of posterior tibial artery
- Three or four segmental branches of posterior tibial artery

- Ensure that the soleus muscle has not been traumatized from previous injury.
- Standard ABI/TBI exam
- Evaluate and treat concerns for hardware infection or osteomyelitis.

Positioning

- Frog leg positioning

Approach

- Elevate under tourniquet control.
- Longitudinal skin incision made 2 cm medial to the medial border of the tibia and parallel to the tibia.
- Only the muscular portion of the soleus muscle is used as the flap, whereas the tendon portion of the flap is left intact.
- To cover a wound at:
  - Middle and distal third of the leg: medial hemisoleus muscle flap is elevated to the level just below the junction between the proximal and middle third of the leg for a middle third defect or just above the junction between the middle and distal thirds of the leg so that an adjacent perforator from the posterior tibial vessels to the flap can be preserved (**FIG 2A**).
  - Distal third of the leg: medial hemisoleus muscle flap is elevated only to the level just below the junction between the middle and distal thirds of the leg, preserving as many major perforators to the flap as possible, even in the distal third of the leg while allowing adequate arc of flap rotation (**FIG 2B**).

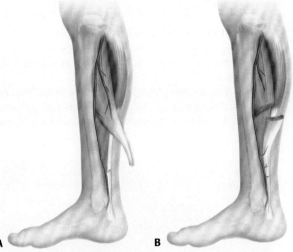

FIG 2 • **A.** Flap dissection and blood supply to the proximally based medial hemisoleus muscle flap. The flap receives its blood supply primarily from the posterior tibial vessels. The flap also receives additional blood supply from one or two perforators from the posterior tibial vessels to its distal portion. **B.** Flap dissection and blood supply to the distally based medial hemisoleus muscle flap. The flap receives its blood supply primarily from the most distal two perforators of the posterior tibial vessels. The flap also receives additional blood supply from the proximal source in a retrograde fashion.

■ Proximally Based Medial Hemisoleus Flap[1-3,5,6]

- Identify and dissect free from medial gastrocnemius muscle.
- Divide distally at the level of the junction between middle and distal thirds of the leg for covering a middle third defect of the leg or at the level close to the Achilles tendon if covering the distal third of defect in the leg.
- Medial half of the muscle is split longitudinally along with a raphe between the bellies of the soleus muscle.
- Only one or two distal perforators from the posterior tibial vessels to the medial hemisoleus muscle are divided

so the flap rotation can be facilitated, but proximal major perforators should be preserved to maximize the blood supply to the flap (**TECH FIG 1A**).
- The spared tendon is approximated to the remaining lateral half of the soleus muscle with nonabsorbable sutures in a figure of eight fashion to help minimize the functional loss of the leg after flap harvested (**TECH FIG 1B**).
- The elevated hemisoleus muscle flap can be rotated to cover the defect and a split-thickness skin graft can be placed after flap transfer.

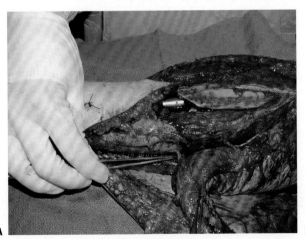

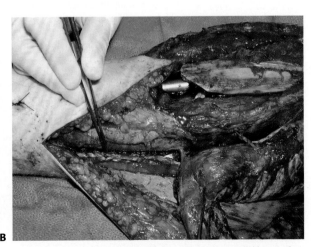

TECH FIG 1 • **A.** Intraoperative view shows an adjacent perforator (indicated by forceps) from the posterior tibial vessels to the medial hemisoleus muscle flap. Preservation of this perforator can be critical to ensure an adequate blood supply to the distal flap. **B.** The spared conjoined tendon is approximated to the remaining lateral half of the soleus muscle with sutures to minimize the functional loss of the leg after flap elevation.

TECHNIQUES

T E C H N I Q U E S

■ Distally Based Medial Hemisoleus Flap[3,4,6]

- Preoperative angiogram can be helpful for determining the presence of major perforators from posterior tibial vessels to the distal portion of the medial soleus muscle.
- Only one or two distal perforators from the posterior tibial vessels to the medial hemisoleus muscle are divided so the flap turnover can be facilitated; however, one adjacent proximal perforator should be preserved to maximize the blood supply to the flap (**TECH FIG 2**).
- The medial hemisoleus muscle flap is transposed or turned over into the defect and inset with absorbable half-buried horizontal mattress sutures. Scoring the fascia over the medial hemisoleus muscle belly can produce a few more centimeters of arc of rotation. The muscle flap is covered immediately with a split-thickness skin graft after flap transfer.

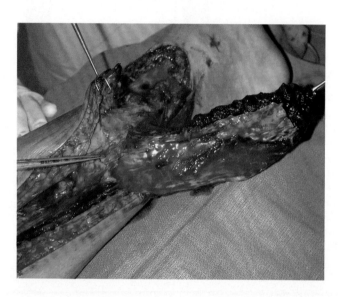

TECH FIG 2 • Intraoperative view shows the first large perforator (indicated by forceps) from the posterior tibial vessels to the distally based medial hemisoleus muscle flap. This perforator serves as a pivot point of the flap turn over and should be well preserved. Preservation of this perforator can be critical to ensure an adequate blood supply to this distally based flap.

PEARLS AND PITFALLS

Muscle damage	■ Before dissecting the medial hemisoleus muscle flap, the surgeon should make sure that the soleus muscle has not been traumatized from the previous injury.
Blood supply	■ When performing a proximally based flap, any perforators from the posterior tibial vessels to the distal medial half of the soleus muscle just at or above the level of a tibial wound should be preserved while allowing adequate arc of flap rotation to cover a wound in the distal third of the leg.
	■ The modifications of surgical techniques emphasize the preservation of an adequate blood supply to the distal portion of the medial hemisoleus muscle flap after the flap is elevated. These techniques would maximize reliability of the medial hemisoleus muscle flap and expand its role in reconstruction of a wound in the distal third of the leg. With the aid of a preoperative angiogram, major perforators in the lower third of the leg can be identified when planning a distally based medial hemisoleus flap.
	■ The most proximal perforators from the posterior tibial vessels to the medial half of the distal soleus muscle within the upper distal third of the leg should be preserved while allowing adequate flap turnover to cover a tibial wound in the distal third of the leg. This perforator will serve as a pivot point for flap turnover and the level of the perforator will determine how far this flap can reach.
	■ The modified surgical techniques in flap dissection emphasize the preservation of an adequate blood supply to the distal portion of the distally based flap and maximize reliability of the medial hemisoleus muscle flap even when it is based distally.
Free tissue transfer[8,9]	■ Free tissue transfer should still be considered for a larger soft tissue wound in the middle or distal third of the leg or for a less extensive wound when either the soleus muscle or those perforators from the posterior tibial vessels are traumatized.

POSTOPERATIVE CARE

- Place patient in knee and ankle immobilizer with minimal pressure on the transposed flap.
- Effective leg elevation to reduce edema
- Placement of a warming unit around leg to maintain a warm temperature
- Monitoring frequently with clinical assessments

OUTCOMES

- Based on the author's experience, the proximally based medial hemisoleus muscle flap can be used for a relatively proximal tibial wound in the junction of the middle and distal thirds or in the distal third of the leg.
- The flap is fairly reliable and can often be done within 2 hours. In addition, the flap can provide just enough muscle bulk for soft tissue coverage of the tibial wound, and thus, reconstructive outcomes are usually quite good (**FIG 3**).
- The distally based flap can be used for a less extensive distal tibial wound (often close to the medial malleolus) in the distal third of the leg. The flap can be reliable in most healthy and compliant patients.
- The initial venous congestion may also become a problem in certain patients such as smokers or those with an inability for leg elevation during the postoperative period.
- In general, the distal flap necrosis occurs infrequently if the flap is proximally based but occurs in about 20% of the patients if the flap is distally based (**FIG 4**).

COMPLICATIONS[3,4,6]

- Like any other pedicled flaps, the distal flap necrosis may occur, but total flap loss should not happen.
- The distal flap necrosis is usually insignificant and can be managed with debridement.
- The flap can then be readvanced adequately to cover the wound, and the final outcome can still be good.
- Further advancement of the flap is possible by dividing the most proximal perforator, which has served as a pivot point since the flap has been "delayed" after initial flap elevation.

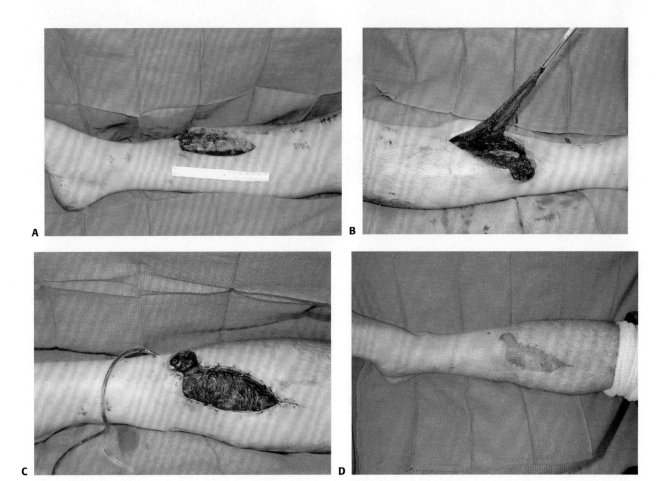

FIG 3 • A. A male patient had a 12 × 6-cm soft tissue defect in the middle third of the leg with exposed fracture site. **B.** A proximally based medial hemisoleus muscle flap was elevated and rotated to cover the defect. **C.** Completion of the muscle flap inset before placement of skin graft. **D.** Result at 3.5-month follow-up.

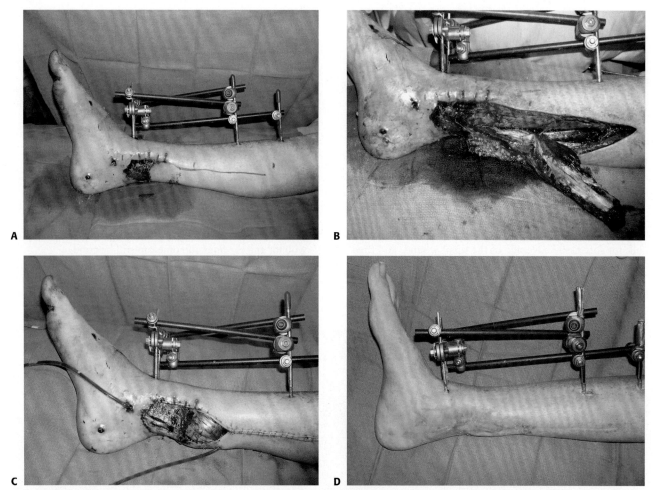

FIG 4 • **A.** A female patient had a 6 × 5-cm soft tissue defect in the distal third of the leg with exposed fracture site. **B.** A distally based medial hemisoleus muscle flap was elevated and turned over to cover the defect. **C.** Completion of the muscle flap inset before placement of skin graft. **D.** Result at 2-month follow-up before subsequent bone grafting.

REFERENCES

1. Pu LLQ. Medial hemisoleus muscle flap: a reliable flap for soft tissue reconstruction of the middle-third tibial wound. *Int Surg.* 2006;91:194.
2. Pu LLQ. Soft-tissue coverage of an open tibial wound in the junction of the middle and distal thirds of the leg with the medial hemisoleus muscle flap. *Ann Plast Surg.* 2006;56:639.
3. Pu LLQ. Successful soft-tissue coverage of a tibial wound in the distal third of the leg with a medial hemisoleus flap. *Plast Reconstr Surg.* 2005;115:245.
4. Pu LLQ. The reversed medial hemisoleus muscle flap and its role in reconstruction of an open tibial wound in the lower third of the leg. *Ann Plast Surg.* 2006;56:59.
5. Pu LLQ. The laterally extended medial hemisoleus flap for reconstruction of a tibial wound in the distal third of the leg. *Eur J Plast Surg.* 2007;30:19.
6. Pu LLQ. Further experience with the medial hemisoleus muscle flap for soft-tissue coverage of a tibial wound in the distal third of the leg. *Plast Reconstr Surg.* 2008;121:2024.
7. Tobin GR. Hemisoleus and reversed hemisoleus flaps. *Plast Reconstr Surg.* 1985;76:87.
8. Pu LLQ. Soft-tissue reconstruction of an open tibial wound in the distal third of the leg: a new treatment algorithm. *Ann Plast Surg.* 2007;58:78.
9. Thornton BP, Rosenblum WJ, Pu LLQ. Reconstruction of limited soft-tissue defect with open tibial fracture in the distal third of the leg. *Ann Plast Surg.* 2005;54:276.

Nerve Repair and Reconstruction—Tibial Nerve

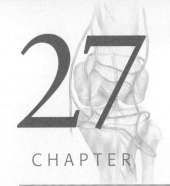

Shawn Moshrefi and Catherine Curtin

DEFINITION

- Tibial nerve injuries can vary in severity, mechanism, and treatment.
- Nerve injury categories[1]
  - Neurapraxia: conduction delay with no axonal injury. These injuries will recover spontaneously without intervention.
  - Axonotmesis: axonal injury resulting in disruption of the axons, but the supporting nerve scaffolding is intact. In these injuries, distal nerve segment will undergo Wallerian degeneration and proximal fibers will regenerate. Spontaneous recovery is possible.
  - Neurotmesis: complete disruption of the nerve. In these injuries, spontaneous regeneration will *not* occur.
  - Neuroma in continuity: disruption of the axons though the scaffolding seems to be intact. However, at the injury site, there is internal fibrosis, which prevents axons from regenerating. In these injuries, spontaneous regeneration will *not* occur.
  - Mixture of injury types: nerve patterns can be complex and one nerve can have several different types of injury.

ANATOMY (FIG 1)

- Tibial nerve originates from L4 through S3 nerve roots.
- The motor branches innervate the posterior calf compartment muscles and the majority of small muscles in the foot.
- The sensory branches supply the knee joint, part of the sural nerve distribution, and the sole of the foot.
- Tibial nerve branches from the sciatic nerve in the popliteal fossa.
- The first branch off the tibial nerve is a sensory contribution to the sural nerve.
- The next branches are the motor nerves to the gastrocnemius muscles.
- Then, the tibial nerve passes through popliteal fossa under arch of soleus. (This area is a potential area of tibial nerve entrapment called the *soleal sling*.)
- The tibial nerve courses distally adjacent to the tibia on undersurface of soleus in the leg running with the peroneal artery and vein.
- At the ankle, tibial nerve is posterior to the medial malleolus adjacent to posterior tibial artery beneath the flexor retinaculum (This is a potential area of entrapment known as the *tarsal tunnel*.) (**FIG 2**).

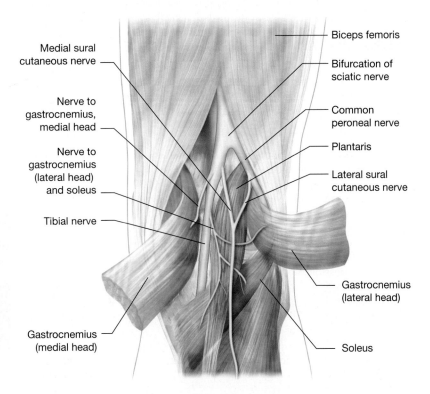

Medial sural
cutaneous nerve

Nerve to
gastrocnemius,
medial head

Nerve to
gastrocnemius
(lateral head)
and soleus

Tibial nerve

Gastrocnemius
(medial head)

Biceps femoris

Bifurcation of
sciatic nerve

Common
peroneal nerve

Plantaris

Lateral sural
cutaneous nerve

Gastrocnemius
(lateral head)

Soleus

FIG 1 • Anatomy of the proximal tibial nerve.

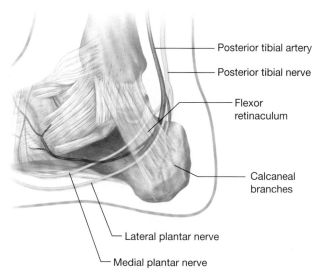

FIG 2 • Anatomy of the tarsal tunnel.

- At the medial malleolus, the tibial nerve branches into the calcaneal, medial plantar, and lateral plantar nerves. The anatomy of the branching is highly variable between patients.[2]

PATHOGENESIS

- Tibial nerves can be injured in many ways and in any location along its course. Listed below are some of the more common causes of tibial nerve injury.
  - Traumatic knee dislocation
  - Direct trauma to the popliteal area, both blunt or sharp
  - Iatrogenic prolonged tourniquet, hardware, or limb lengthening procedures
  - Ankle swelling or compression
  - Cysts or other nerve compressing structures (both in the popliteal fossa as well as at the medial malleolus)

PATIENT HISTORY AND PHYSICAL FINDINGS

- A complete and thorough history detailing patient's history of present illness, current injuries, history of prior injuries, prior surgeries (including spinal, buttock, and lower extremity procedures), comorbidities, occupation, and other case-by-case considerations should be obtained.
- Inspection
  - Is the calf or foot swollen?
  - Are there vascular changes?
  - Is there atrophy?
- Vascular exam—palpable pulses distally, temperature, and capillary refill of the toes and foot.
- Sensory exam—Ten test: an area of normal or baseline sensation is compared to an area of concern for sensory loss and the difference is rated from 1 to 10 with 10 being the best score possible.[3]
- Motor exam
  - Test the respective muscles that the tibial nerve and its branches supply (tibial nerve controls plantar flexion and inversion of the foot and ankle).
  - Each individual movement tested should be compared to the contralateral side. This allows the examiner to identify subtle weakness.

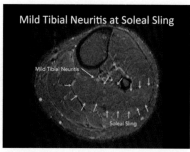

FIG 3 • MRI of tibial nerve at soleal sling. Note that the tibial nerve is bright like the surrounding vessels, and normal nerve is isointense with the muscle. (Courtesy of Sandip Biswal, Stanford University.)

- Motor examination remember mnemonic TIP = *T*ibial *I*nverts and *P*lantar flexes.
- Scratch collapse test.[4] This tool originally described for the upper limb is also useful for assessing nerve entrapment in the lower limb. For this test, the examiner is testing external rotation of the arm.
  - To do this, the examiner has the patient sitting straight with arms adducted to their side and elbows bent to 90 degrees. The patient is told to keep the arm in this position.
  - The examiner then gently scratches the skin directly over the area of suspected nerve compression (eg, posterior to the medial malleolus for suspected tarsal tunnel).
  - After scratching the skin, the examiner then directly applies internal rotation force to the patient's dorsal forearm while the patient actively attempts to resist. The test is positive for nerve pathology if the patient is briefly unable to resist your force of internal rotation.
- Tinel sign
- Point tenderness: the tibial nerve can be compressed at the level of the soleal sling. Patients are often tender to direct pressure over the site (posterior midline of the calf about 10 cm distal to the posterior knee crease).

IMAGING/STUDIES

- X-rays are obtained if there is a suspected bony injury.
- MRI can assess for soft tissue masses such as Baker cysts and also provide information on the nerve.
  - Enhancement of fascicles on MRI can help identify tibial neuritis (**FIG 3**).
  - MRI is increasing in resolution and is taking an increasing role in identifying nerve pathology (**FIG 4**).

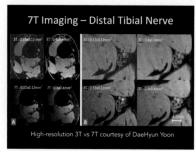

FIG 4 • Comparison of 3T and 7T MRI of tibial nerve. (Courtesy of Daehyun Yoon, Stanford University.)

- Nerve conduction studies and electromyelography (NCS/EMG) are a mainstay in the workup of nerve injury.
  - NCS/EMG useful for closed nerve injury
    - Studies are performed at 4 to 6 weeks to achieve a baseline and assess type and severity of the injury.
    - If there is no recovery on physical exam, the nerve studies are repeated at 3 months.
- If there is evidence of recovery, close follow-up is continued. If no signs of recovery at three months, operative intervention should be considered. Motor endplates begin to permanently degenerate at 3 months; thus, if surgery is required, earlier intervention improves functional outcomes.

DIFFERENTIAL DIAGNOSIS

- Spinal pathology
- Sciatic pathology
  - If on physical exam there are deficits in both peroneal nerve and tibial nerve distributions, then suspect possible sciatic pathology.
- Neurologic problems
  - Peripheral neuropathy
  - Motor neuron disease

NONOPERATIVE MANAGEMENT

- For closed nerve injuries, treatment starts with nonoperative management.
- Therapy
  - Edema prevention with lightly compressive wraps/garments and physical therapy with massage may be helpful.
  - Range of motion exercises to maintain supple joints and prevent the nerve from scarring.
  - Desensitization to decrease areas of sensitivity.
- Orthotics
  - Custom splint that keeps the hindfoot in the neutral position in order to maintain function and minimize discomfort.
  - Shoe inserts are a first step in people with suspected tarsal tunnel.

SURGICAL MANAGEMENT

- Surgical treatment is used for open nerve injuries, closed nerve injuries that are not showing any signs of recovery at 3 months, and nerve compressions that did not respond to conservative measures.

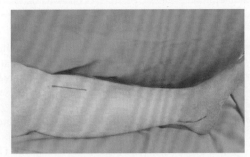

FIG 5 • Incisions for soleal sling and tarsal tunnel release.

Preoperative Planning

- Definitive fracture fixation should be performed prior to nerve repair.
- Arterial injury should be treated prior to nerve repair.
- If possible, use of a lower extremity tourniquet is advisable to aid in visualization of injury.
- If intraoperative nerve monitoring is planned, inform anesthesia team to not use paralytics.

Positioning

- Positioning depends on level of injury (above knee, at level of the knee, or below knee).
- Access to popliteal area is easiest with the patient in the prone position.
- Access to the soleal sling is managed with the patient supine, hip externally rotated, and knee bent.
- Access to tarsal tunnel is managed with the patient supine.

Approach

- For the posterior knee approach, a curved incision rather than a straight incision across the joint is required to prevent scar contracture that can limit mobility.
- For access to the soleal sling, a medial incision on the posterior border of the tibia starting just distal to the tibial plateau (**FIG 5**).
- The tarsal tunnel is accessed posterior to the medial malleolus.

- ## ■ Repair of Acute Traumatic Injury to Tibial Nerve

- Patient positioned supine.
- Tourniquet placed above the knee.
- If a wound is present, incorporate wound into exposure.
- If wound orientation or access is inadequate, then either extend wound incision to match standard approach or create counter incisions.
- Resect any damaged or scarred nerve until two healthy nerve ends are revealed. (The proximal healthy end should have fascicles clearly seen bulging out the end of the nerve.)

- Use microsurgical technique to handle the nerve and align the internal fascicle anatomy.
- Perform a tensionless repair. (If the 9-0 nylon suture cannot hold the repair, there is too much tension).
- If there is a nerve gap, harvest a sural nerve graft.
  - Cable the graft and suture in place with a few 9-0 nylon sutures using microscopic technique.
- Augment repair by sealing coaptation site with fibrin glue.
- Closure of wound.
- Place in a leg splint or knee immobilizer to protect repair.

TECHNIQUES

■ Release of Soleal Sling[5]

- Anesthesia options: regional anesthetic (popliteal/distal sciatic block and saphenous block) or general anesthesia
- Patient is supine and the hip is externally rotated, exposing the medial side of the leg.
- A thigh tourniquet is placed.
- The incision is placed at the medial tibial plateau and runs distally for about 10 cm and is placed about 1 cm posterior to the medial edge of the tibia (**TECH FIG 1A**).
- The subcutaneous tissue is carefully dissected, preserving the saphenous nerve and vein.

- The fascia over the gastrocnemius is opened and the plane between the soleus is identified.
- The gastrocnemius is retracted out of the way.
- The soleal sling can be palpated with a finger as a fascial notch in the proximal border of the muscle.
- The medial soleal muscle is reflected and perforating vessels are clipped.
- The tibial nerve is identified and a vessel loop is placed.
- Constricting fascial bands are released over about a 5 cm length.
- Skin is closed and a bulky dressing placed.
- Early ambulation is encouraged.

■ Release of Tarsal Tunnel

- Patient is placed supine.
- Regional block of the popliteal and saphenous nerve is performed.
- Tourniquet is placed on the calf.
- A bent incision is placed posterior to medial malleolus.
- Skin and subcutaneous tissue are divided.
- Care is taken to preserve the overlying sensory nerves.
- The flexor retinaculum is incised proximally and the posterior tibial vessels are visualized below. Small crossing vessels are clipped.
- The nerve is identified deep to the vessels and a loop is placed around the nerve.

- The dissection is taken distally and the branches are identified. (Note the calcaneal branches have variable anatomy and number) (**TECH FIG 1B**).
- The medial and lateral plantar nerves are identified and loops placed.
- The fascia overlying the medial and lateral plantar nerves is divided including the fascia overlying the abductor hallucis.
- All fascia must be released distally and the dissecting scissors can easily fit in the tunnels over the medial and lateral plantar nerves.
- Meticulous hemostasis is required.
- Closure and placement of a bulky dressing
- Early ambulation is encouraged.

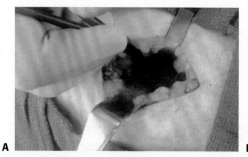 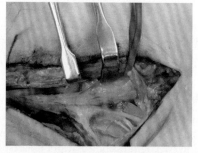

TECH FIG 1 • A. Tibial nerve exposed through soleal sling. Note the deep exposure required. The tibial nerve is at the base of the wound identified by the forceps. **B.** Tibial nerve exposed in a tarsal tunnel release. Note the multiple calcaneal branches going posteriorly.

■ Tibial Nerve Traction Injury

- General anesthesia
- Thigh tourniquet (to obtain optimal nerve monitoring results the tourniquet needs to be released for 20 minutes). If tourniquet is not used, preinject with bupivacaine with epinephrine prior to prepping the patient.
- Prone positioning
- Intraoperative nerve monitoring should be available.
- Incision is angled from the center of popliteal fossa.

- The dissection is taken down to the level of the muscle fascia.
- The tibial nerve is identified as it branches off the sciatic nerve.
- A vessel loop is placed on the nerve and the dissection is taken distally.
- The nerve is released from the overlying scar (often a very challenging dissection). The dissection is taken posterior to the gastrocnemius muscles to release the soleal sling.

- Intraoperative nerve monitoring is performed. Starting with somatosensory evoked potentials can help establish the proximal level of intact nerve. Nerve to nerve monitoring can identify neuroma in continuity.
- If the nerve is ruptured or neuroma in continuity is identified, resect damaged or scarred nerve until two healthy nerve ends are revealed.
- Ensure that the proximal nerve is healthy by using the assistance of your neurologist performing the intraoperative nerve monitoring.

- If there is a nerve gap, harvest a sural nerve graft.
- Cable the graft and suture in place with 9-0 nylon sutures using microscopic technique.
- Augment repair by sealing coaptation site with fibrin glue.
- Closure of wound
- Place in a leg splint or knee immobilizer to protect repair.

PEARLS AND PITFALLS

Hemostasis (if no tourniquet)	▪ Preinject incision with bupivacaine with epinephrine. ▪ A solution of 1 amp of epinephrine diluted in 100 cc of saline can be used to moisten a gauze that is then dabbed in the wound to help with visualization.
Technique	▪ To ensure complete release of the tarsal tunnel, the distal compression of the medial and lateral plantar nerves must be released. The distal dissection is challenging due to the overlying vessels. Clip crossing vessels as needed to adequately expose the nerves.
Intraoperative monitoring	▪ Communication between neurology and anesthesia team is critical to ensure that patient does not receive medications that will hinder intraoperative monitoring. ▪ Sequential compression device machine and warming machines can cause background that interferes with intraoperative monitoring. ▪ Do not use tourniquet if planning intraoperative monitoring. The nerve can suffer neuropraxia after 30 minutes of ischemia.
Diagnosis	▪ MRI imaging can help if proximal nerve entrapment suspected.

POSTOPERATIVE CARE

- Postoperative splint utilized for 3 weeks if there is a nerve repair to protect
- Early mobilization for neurolysis patients
- Affected lower extremity should be elevated at all times initially to aid in reduction of swelling.
- Multimodal pain management for postoperative pain
- Early therapy for desensitization, scar management, and nerve gliding

OUTCOMES

- The literature on results from tibial nerve surgery is sparse.
- Tarsal tunnel release is an effective procedure when performed properly. A case series found that patients improved their Maryland Foot Score from 61 to 80, 3 months after tarsal tunnel release.[6]
- Tarsal tunnel release can fail for several reasons including incorrect diagnosis, proximal compression, and intrinsic nerve damage.[7]

COMPLICATIONS

- Neuropathic pain
- Inadequate release
- Bleeding/hematoma

REFERENCES

1. Seddon HJ. A classification of nerve injuries. *Br Med J.* 1942;2:237-239.
2. Havel PE, Ebraheim NA, Clark SE, et al. Tibial nerve branching in the tarsal tunnel. *Foot Ankle.* 1988;9(3):117-119.
3. Strauch B, Lang A, Ferder M, et al. The ten test. *Plast Reconstr Surg.* 1997;99:1074-1078.
4. Cheng CJ, Mackinnon-Patterson B, Beck JL, Mackinnon SE. Scratch collapse test for evaluation of carpal and cubital tunnel syndrome. *J Hand Surg [Am].* 2008;33(9):1518-1524.
5. Williams EH, Rosson GD, Hagan RR, et al. Soleal sling syndrome (proximal tibial nerve compression): results of surgical decompression. *Plast Reconstr Surg.* 2012;129(2):454-462.
6. Sammarco GJ, Chang L. Outcome of surgical treatment of tarsal tunnel syndrome. *Foot Ankle Int.* 2003;24(2):125-131.
7. Gould JS. Recurrent tarsal tunnel syndrome. *Foot Ankle Clin.* 2014;19(3):451-467.

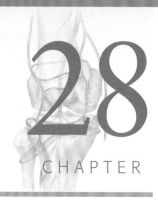

28

CHAPTER

Excision of Soft Tissue Tumors of the Knee

Raffi S. Avedian

DEFINITION

- Soft tissue sarcomas are malignant tumors that arise from mesenchymal cells and are classified according to their cell of origin such as muscle, tendon, or fat.
  - Peripheral nerve sheath tumors arise from neural crest cells but are typically grouped with sarcomas because of similarities in location, natural history, and treatment.
  - The World Health Organization groups soft tissue sarcomas into 10 categories based on the tissue of origin.
- Most sarcomas occur in a deep location, meaning below the muscle and fascia, whereas one-third of sarcomas occur in a subcutaneous location.
- Patients with soft tissue sarcomas and patients with benign tumors often present with the same chief complaint of having a soft tissue mass.
  - Rendering an accurate diagnosis prior to surgery is important because the treatment plan may vary based on the nature of the diagnosis. For example, a benign tumor may be monitored or removed with a simple excision, whereas in the case of a sarcoma, the goal of surgery is to remove the tumor with a wide margin. With appropriate planning, radiotherapy and/or chemotherapy is often incorporated into the treatment plan either before or after definitive surgery.

ANATOMY

- The knee is the largest joint in the body. It is made up of the patellofemoral, lateral, and medial compartments.
- Knee motion is primarily flexion and extension; however, bending and rotation are important components of knee kinematics.
- The primary stabilizers of the knee are the extra-articular medial and lateral cruciate ligaments and intra-articular anterior and posterior cruciate ligaments.
- The knee has several layers of covering including the capsule and retinacular tissues. During tumor resection, superficial layers may be used as the deep margin for the tumor, whereas the deeper capsule may be preserved to keep the joint closed.[1]
- The popliteal artery travels along the back of the knee and along with the tibial nerve travels between the lateral and medial head of the gastrocnemius. It branches into the posterior tibial artery, which travels deep to the soleus muscles; the anterior tibial artery, which passes from posterior to the anterior compartment distal to the tibia-fibula joint; and the peroneal artery, which branches off the tibiofibular trunk and is located medial to the fibula next to the flexor hallucis longus.
- The geniculate vessels branch off from the popliteal vessels and are often all ligated during tumor resection of the distal femur.

- The tibial nerve is located next to the popliteal vessels. The common peroneal nerve travels medial and deep to the biceps femoris muscle, a constant relationship that facilitates finding and protecting the nerve during tumor dissection.
- The common peroneal nerve wraps around the neck of the fibula and divides into the deep branch that innervates the anterior muscle compartment and the superficial branch that innervates the lateral compartment.
- The lateral sural cutaneous nerve, which branches off the common peroneal nerve, may be large in some patients and be confused with the common peroneal nerve.

PATHOGENESIS

- The mechanism for sarcoma formation is not known.
- Risk factors for sarcoma development include radiation exposure such as medical radiotherapy, pesticide exposure, and hereditary conditions including Li-Fraumeni syndrome and neurofibromatosis.

NATURAL HISTORY

- All sarcomas have the potential for local recurrence and metastasis.
- Tumor variables that are associated with increased risk of metastasis include high grade and large size (greater than 5 cm).
- Lungs are the most common location of metastasis.

PATIENT HISTORY AND PHYSICAL FINDINGS

- Determining when the mass was first noticed and how rapidly it is growing can help the clinician differentiate between benign and malignant tumors.
- The presence of pain is often associated with a benign tumor, such as a schwannoma or vascular malformation, and may not be present with sarcomas until late in the disease course.[2]
- Determining the size of the tumor, manual muscle strength testing, and sensory examination are useful to determine if there is a neurological compromise. Limb edema assessment and pulse examination can help determine if the tumor is causing vascular or lymphatic compromise.
- Range of motion testing and gait assessment are helpful in assessing a patient's mobility and functional status to guide perioperative and postoperative counseling.

IMAGING

- Plain radiographs can help diagnose joint degeneration or joint-based lesions such as gout and synovial osteochondromatosis.

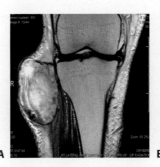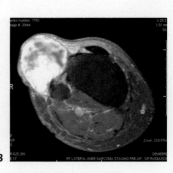

FIG 1 • **A.** Coronal and axial (**B**) MRIs demonstrating a high-grade soft tissue sarcoma abutting the proximal tibia and knee joint.

- Magnetic resonance imaging is the modality of choice for soft tissue tumor evaluation (**FIG 1A,B**).
- Fat-sensitive images such as T1-weighted sequences are best for identifying critical anatomic structures such as nerves and vessels.
- Fluid-sensitive images including T2-weighted and STIR sequences highlight pathology very well.
- Contrast-enhanced sequences are used to differentiated cystic from solid areas in tumors and identify reactive peritumoral edema, which will be high signal on fluid sequences but not enhance with contrast.
- Some benign tumors such as lipoma, lipoma arborescens, and schwannoma may be diagnosed on MRI; however, most soft tissue tumors require a biopsy for diagnosis.[3]

DIFFERENTIAL DIAGNOSIS

- Giant cell tumor of tendon sheath
- Synovial chondromatosis
- Lipoma arborescens
- Other benign tumors
- Sarcoma
- Reactive and inflammatory lesions such as gout or infection

SURGICAL MANAGEMENT

- The appropriate treatment for any musculoskeletal tumor is based on its diagnosis and natural history.
- Performing a surgery without consideration of the diagnosis and the appropriate margin may cause harm to patients.[4]
- In cases where MR imaging is not diagnostic, a biopsy should be performed.

- Treatment strategy including the use of preoperative radiation and specific surgical plan should be formulated by a multidisciplinary team specializing in sarcoma care.[5]
- Treatment of knee tumors may require resection of the joint capsule, extensor mechanism, and/or stabilizing structures such as the collateral ligaments. Reconstruction of these structures should be accounted in the operative plan.

Preoperative Planning

- A patient is considered ready for surgery after completion of staging and multidisciplinary review of pertinent imaging, pathology, and treatment strategy.
- The surgical plan is created by thorough study of the preoperative MR scan. A plane of surgical dissection is planned to remove the tumor in its entirety while maintain a clean margin around it.
- If the tumor encases important vascular structures, a plan for vascular reconstruction is made with a vascular surgeon.
- Anticipated soft tissue coverage needs are assessed such as skin graft, local rotation flap, or free tissue transfer.

Positioning

- The patient is placed in the supine position unless the tumor is in the posterior compartment in which case the patient is placed in the prone position.
- The site of a flap harvest must be completely isolated from the tumor site to avoid contamination and tumor spread. A separate back table and clean instruments should be used.

Approach

- The surgical approach varies based on location of the tumor.
- Previous biopsy and surgical scars are considered contaminated and must be excised en bloc with the tumor.

■ Wide Resection of a Knee Sarcoma

- Most knee tumors are subcutaneous and require a paddle of skin to be removed as the superficial margin.
- An incision is made 2 to 3 cm peripheral to the edge of the tumor as determined by palpation and preoperative MRI (**TECH FIG 1A**).
- The dissection is carried through the subcutaneous fat angling away from the tumor (**TECH FIG 1B**).
- The deep fascia is identified and cut circumferentially around the tumor (**TECH FIG 1C**).
- For tumors abutting the joint capsule, the surgeon must assess if the tumor is adherent to the capsule, in which

case the entire capsule must be removed, or if the tumor only abuts the capsule in which case only the retinaculum needs to be removed.
- Sutures may be used to secure the deep layer to the skin to prevent the tumor from "leaking out" of the superficial layer.
- Take care not to shear off the fat from the fascia during dissection.
- Avoid retractors on the tumor side of the dissection.
- Do not sacrifice margin in order to save tissue for a primary closure (**TECH FIG 1D**).
- Most surgeries require a skin graft or muscle flap for closure (**TECH FIG 1E,F**).

TECHNIQUES

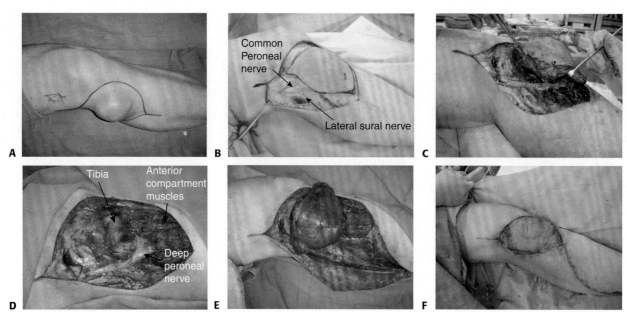

TECH FIG 1 • **A.** Planned skin incision. Notice the margin of skin around the palpable tumor. **B.** Superficial dissection of skin and subcutaneous tissue and identification of the common peroneal and lateral sural cutaneous nerves. **C.** The deep fascia is cut peripherally and a small cuff of muscle and retinacular tissue is removed as the deep margin. The muscular branches of the peroneal nerve are preserved. **D.** Defect after tumor removal. **E,F.** Lateral gastrocnemius muscle flap is rotated to cover the defect and split-thickness skin graft applied.

PEARLS AND PITFALLS

Hematoma	▪ Dead space after tumor removal should be managed with drains, muscle flap, free tissue transfer, or a combination of these techniques. ▪ Seroma drainage in the clinic may be necessary.
Wound breakdown	▪ Negative pressure dressings, aggressive dead space management, and maximizing patients' nutrition may reduce wound problems. ▪ Patients should be counseled about potential need for reoperation for wound management.
Positive margins	▪ Appropriate preoperative planning is important to minimize risk of unplanned positive margins. ▪ Planned positive margins around critical structures such as nerves and vessels may be appropriate in certain settings.

POSTOPERATIVE CARE

- Mobilization and weight bearing depend on the extent of surgery.
- Extremity elevation is recommended while patient is in bed.
- Range of motion and therapy may begin after wound healing is sufficient.
- Postoperative radiotherapy, if needed, may be take place 4 to 6 weeks after surgery.

OUTCOMES

- Oncological outcomes include local recurrence and metastasis. Surveillance for recurrence should be managed by a multidisciplinary sarcoma team.
- Functional outcomes depend on the extent of tissue resection, patient overall health status, and late effects of radia-

tion. Aggressive wound care and physical therapy may help maximize patient function.

COMPLICATIONS

- Wound healing problems that require operative intervention can occur in up to 33% of patients who undergo preoperative radiotherapy and 17% of patients who undergo postoperative radiotherapy.[6]
- Local recurrence occurs in a minority of patients and is more common in patients with positive margins. Radiotherapy decreases the risk of local recurrence.

REFERENCES

1. Dye SF, Campagna-Pinto D, Dye CC, et al. Soft-tissue anatomy anterior to the human patella. *J Bone Joint Surg Am.* 2003;85-A(6):1012-1017.

2. George A, Grimer R. Early symptoms of bone and soft tissue sarcomas: could they be diagnosed earlier? *Ann R Coll Surg Engl.* 2012;94(4):261-266.

3. Jim S, Wu MD, Mary G, Hochman MD. Soft-tissue tumors and tumorlike lesions: a systematic imaging approach. *Radiology.* 2009;253(2):297-316.

4. Jones DA, Shideman C, Yuan J, et al. Management of unplanned excision for soft-tissue sarcoma with preoperative radiotherapy followed by definitive resection. *Am J Clin Oncol.* 2016;39(6):586-592.

5. Siegel GW, Biermann JS, Chugh R, et al. The multidisciplinary management of bone and soft tissue sarcoma: an essential organizational framework. *J Multidiscip Healthc.* 2015;8:109-115.

6. O'Sullivan B, Davis AM, Turcotte R, et al. Preoperative versus postoperative radiotherapy in soft-tissue sarcoma of the limbs: a randomised trial. *Lancet.* 2002;359(9325):2235-2241.

Excision of Bone Tumors of the Knee

Raffi S. Avedian

DEFINITION

- Bone tumors of the knee may be benign or malignant (bone sarcoma) and exhibit a variable natural history ranging from latent to rapid growth.
- A bone tumor located in the distal femur or proximal tibia such that definitive treatment requires excision of part or all of the knee is discussed in this chapter.
- Treatment for a bone tumor of the knee requires reconstruction of the knee articulation.

ANATOMY

- The knee is the largest joint in the body. It is made up of the patellofemoral, lateral, and medial compartments.
- Knee motion is primarily flexion and extension; however, bending and rotation are important components of knee kinematics.
- The primary stabilizers of the knee are the extra-articular medial and lateral cruciate ligaments and intra-articular anterior and posterior cruciate ligaments.
- The popliteal artery travels along the back of the knee and along with the tibial nerve travels between the lateral and medial head of the gastrocnemius. It branches into the posterior tibial artery, which travels deep to the soleus muscles; the anterior tibial artery, which passes from posterior to the anterior compartment distal to the tibia-fibula joint; and the peroneal artery, which branches off the tibiofibular trunk and is located medial to the fibula next to the flexor hallucis longus.
- The geniculate vessels branch off from the popliteal vessels and are often all ligated during tumor resection of the distal femur.
- The tibial nerve is located next to the popliteal vessels. The common peroneal nerve travels medial and deep to the biceps femoris muscle; a constant relationship that facilitates finding and protecting the nerve during tumor dissection.

PATHOGENESIS

- The mechanism for bone tumor formation is not known.
- Risk factors for sarcoma development include radiation exposure, radiotherapy, pesticide exposure, and hereditary conditions including Li-Fraumeni syndrome and retinoblastoma gene mutation.[1]

NATURAL HISTORY

- Active benign tumors, such as giant cell tumor of bone, chondroblastoma, and aneurysmal bone cyst, will progress over time, may recur after excision, but are not lethal.
- All bone sarcomas have the potential for local recurrence and metastasis.

- Bones sarcomas have an *estimated incidence of 3260* in the United States.
- Lungs and other osseous sites are the most and second most common location of metastasis, respectively.

PATIENT HISTORY AND PHYSICAL FINDINGS

- Pain is a common presenting symptom for aggressive bone tumors.
- A thorough history and examination are important to assess duration of symptoms, comorbidities, physical dysfunction, organ involvement, overall health, and patient expectations in order to best tailor treatment strategy for the individual patient.
- Neurovascular examination is mandatory for any extremity tumor.

IMAGING

- Plain radiographs are used to formulate a differential diagnosis and a preoperative plan.
- Magnetic resonance imaging is routinely used to determine extent of intramedullary tumor involvement, presence of soft tissue extension, status of the neurovascular structures, and presence of tumor within the joint space.

DIFFERENTIAL DIAGNOSIS

- The differential diagnosis for a bone tumor includes benign tumors, sarcomas, lymphoma of bone, infection, and metabolic lesions (eg, hyperparathyroidism).
- The most common bone sarcomas are osteosarcoma, chondrosarcoma, and Ewing sarcoma.

SURGICAL MANAGEMENT

- The appropriate treatment for any musculoskeletal tumor is based on its diagnosis and natural history.
- Biopsy incisions are considered contaminated and must be resected at the time of definitive surgery. Care should be taken to place the biopsy in a location that does not interfere with the final surgical plan.[2]
- If a bone sarcoma extends into the knee joint space by direct growth, pathological fracture, or iatrogenic contamination, an extra-articular resection (keeping the knee joint closed) should be performed.
- Reconstruction depends on the extent of bone excision and may include simple bone grafting, endoprosthetic implants, bulk allografts, osteoarticular implants, or vascularized fibula.
- The goal of surgery is to remove the tumor adequately to minimize recurrence and restore the mechanical integrity

of the bone and joints so that the patient may have sufficient function to perform activities of daily living with minimal pain.

Preoperative Planning

- A patient is considered ready for surgery after completion of staging and multidisciplinary review of pertinent imaging, pathology, and treatment strategy.
- The surgical plan is created by thorough study of the preoperative radiographs and MR scan.
- Bone cuts are planned by measuring on preoperative imaging the distance from an intraoperatively identifiable landmark (eg, femoral condyle, epicondyle) to the desired osteotomy site.
- The soft tissue margin depends on the size and location of a soft tissue component to the tumor. For example, an anterior soft tissue mass long the distal femur can be safely resected by incorporating a portion of the vastus intermedius as the margin.

- When tumor abuts but does not encase blood vessels or nerves, they can be dissected free by leaving adventitia and epineurium on the tumor as the margin.

Positioning

- The patient is placed in the supine position; a hip bump may be placed if more lateral exposure is desired.
- A sterile or nonsterile tourniquet may be used.
- A leg holder may be used in cases where an endoprosthetic knee replacement is being performed.

Approach

- The surgical approach varies based on location of the tumor.
- The guiding principles for the approach to the knee in the setting of a bone sarcoma are to maintain a sufficient margin around the tumor and preserve as much normal tissue as possible without sacrificing cancer treatment.
- Previous biopsy and surgical scars are considered contaminated and must be excised en bloc with the tumor.

■ Distal Femur Resection and Endoprosthetic Reconstruction

- Tourniquet is used at the discretion of the surgeon by using gravity exsanguination rather than Esmarch to avoid tumor compression
- A longitudinal incision is made that includes a fusiform skin excision of the biopsy site. Skin flaps are created as needed to ensure adequate visualization of the tumor and critical anatomy.
- Soft tissue dissection around the tumor is performed with the following principles:
  - Adequate visualization must be achieved.
  - Margin of healthy tissue is kept on the tumor.
  - Nerves are dissected free; epineurium may be used as margin if tumor abuts the nerve. Sciatic nerve branches to hamstring muscles may be cut as needed to adequately mobilize the nerve away from the tumor.
  - Vessels are mobilized; adventitia may be used as margin if tumor abuts the vessels.
- Tumor removal may be broken down into four steps:
  - *Knee disarticulation*: perform an arthrotomy and cut collateral and cruciate ligaments, joint capsule, gastrocnemius origins, and popliteus tendon.
  - *Neurovascular mobilization*: the popliteal vessels must be mobilized by dividing the geniculate branches and dissecting the vessels free from the adductor canal. The tibial nerve is located next to the vessels and the common peroneal nerve is located medial to the biceps femoris. They should be identified and mobilized away from the tumor as needed.
  - *Muscle dissection*: often bone sarcomas of the distal femur or proximal tibia will have a soft tissue component. The muscle layer immediately covering the tumor is removed as the margin. For example, the vastus

intermedius serves as good margin for anterior soft tissue masses. The lateral and medial intermuscular septa must be divided as close to the bone as tumor margin permits.
  - *Osteotomy*: Measure the length of bone to be resected on preoperative MRI and translate that to intraoperative landmarks such as a measurement from the femoral condyle to the femoral diaphysis above the tumor. Bennett or Hohmann retractors are placed around the bone to prevent iatrogenic neurovascular injury and an oscillating saw is used to complete the osteotomy.
- The remaining posterior soft tissue attachments are cut, and the specimen is removed.
- Leg length can be restored by measuring the contralateral leg from the anterior superior iliac spine to the medial malleolus and recreating this on the operative side or measuring and recreating the length of bone removed from the affected side (**TECH FIG 1**).

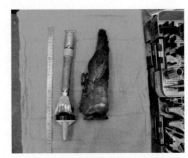

TECH FIG 1 • Intraoperative photograph demonstrating technique for leg length recreation. Trial implants are measured side by side with femur and tibial plateau to ensure what goes into patient matches exactly what was taken out.

■ Reconstruction

- The femur is prepared for endoprosthetic reconstruction using one of the currently available fixation techniques: a cemented stem, uncemented stem, or compress compliant prestress device (**TECH FIG 2**).
- Rotational alignment can be achieved by using the linea aspera as a posterior landmark. Also, trial implants may

be placed and the knee taken through a range of motion check to ensure proper rotation of implants and patellar tracking. Once the surgeon is satisfied with the rotation, a mark is placed on the bone denoting anterior. This mark is used as a guide for correct insertion of the final implant.

- Deep drains are placed, and the deep fascia is closed over drains, followed by a subcutaneous fascia and dermal layer.

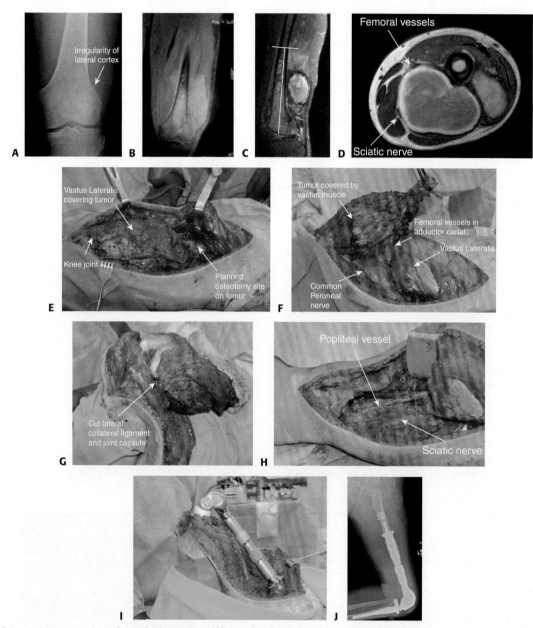

TECH FIG 2 • A. Anteroposterior radiograph of a 14-year-old boy with a distal femur osteosarcoma. **B.** Coronal MRI demonstrating large intramedullary extension and soft tissue mass. **C.** Sagittal MRI after induction chemotherapy demonstrating tumor extent and measurement for planned osteotomy. **D.** Axial MRI demonstrating soft tissue mass in vastus lateralis and popliteal fossa abutting sciatic nerve and vessels. **E.** Intraoperative photograph after initial dissection around tumor, note a portion of the vastus lateralis is left on the tumor as a margin and the femur is exposed proximal to the tumor in anticipation of osteotomy. **F.** After osteotomy, the femur is lifted out of the wound to facilitated dissection of the posterior anatomy including the sciatic nerve and femoral vessels as they pass through the adductor canal. **G.** Photograph showing that the ligamentous structures of the knee including the capsule are identified and cut. **H.** Photograph of defect after tumor removal. **I.** Endoprosthetic reconstruction is performed including large metal segment to replace bone and a hinged total knee arthroplasty. **J.** Lateral radiograph 4 months after surgery.

TECHNIQUES

■ Endoprosthetic Reconstruction of the Proximal Tibia

- The principles of distal femur tumor resection outlined in the previous section apply to resection of tumors of the proximal tibia.
- Unique aspects of proximal tibia resection include the following (**TECH FIG 3**):
  - Large skin flaps must be raised to visualize critical anatomy.
  - Patellar tendon must be detached from the tibial tubercle and subsequently reconstructed.
  - The popliteus muscle can be used as the margin covering posterior soft tissue masses.
  - The anterior tibial artery often must be ligated and divided as it branches from the popliteal artery at the lower order of the popliteus muscle.

- The proximal fibula may be excised along with the tibia depending on the lateral extent of the tumor.
- The patellar tendon may be repaired using 5-mm Mersilene tape sewed into the tendon using Krackow stitches, the ends of which are then tied into the endoprosthesis.
- The repair may be reinforced using no. 5 nonabsorbable to sew the tendon down into additional holes in the endoprosthesis either directly or after cerclage around the patella.
- A gastrocnemius flap is elevated and rotated to cover the prosthesis and provide biological augmentation to the patellar tendon repair.
- A deep drain is placed, and the wound is closed in layers. A split-thickness skin graft is often needed to cover a portion of the gastrocnemius flap.

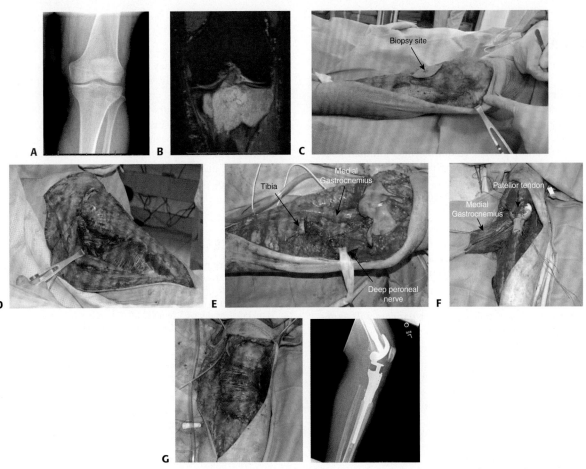

TECH FIG 3 • **A.** Anteroposterior radiograph of a 61-year-old man with a proximal tibia chondrosarcoma. **B.** MRI demonstrating tumor extent. **C.** Intraoperative photograph showing initial dissection including large skin flaps to enable adequate visualization. **D.** Deep dissection is performed by identifying the popliteal vessels and tibial nerve and mobilizing healthy muscle away from the tumor. The soleus muscle is eventually detached along its insertion on the tibia and the gastrocnemius muscle is isolated in anticipation of rotational flap. **E.** Defect after tumor removal, notice the deep peroneal nerve has been preserved. **F.** The patellar tendon is secured to the implant with a 5-mm Mersilene tape using Krackow stitches and reinforced with no. 5 FiberWire. **G.** The gastrocnemius flap is brought over and secured in place making sure to cover the prosthesis and anchoring into the patellar tendon and joint capsule to maximize healing of the extensor mechanism. The wound was otherwise closed in layers over drains and a small skin graft was applied to the portion of the flap that remained exposed after skin closure.

PEARLS AND PITFALLS

Hematoma	▪ Dead space after tumor removal should be managed with drains, muscle flap, free tissue transfer, or a combination of these techniques.
Wound breakdown	▪ *Incisional negative pressure dressings*, aggressive dead space management, and maximizing patients' nutrition may reduce wound problems. ▪ Low threshold to debride draining wounds to minimize risk of prosthetic joint infection.
Positive margins	▪ Appropriate preoperative planning is important to minimize risk of unplanned positive margins. ▪ Planned positive margins around critical structures such as nerves and vessels may be appropriate in certain settings.
Venous thromboembolic events	▪ Risk of VTE compared to risk of hemorrhage into dead space should be balanced and patient counseled regarding risks. ▪ Aspirin and low molecular weight heparin are options for chemical prophylaxis. ▪ Mechanical compression is routinely used.
Prosthetic infection	▪ Most common mode of failure in the long term. ▪ May coat prosthesis with high doses of antibiotic bone cement at time of revision for local antibiotic delivery.

POSTOPERATIVE CARE

- Mobilization and weight bearing depend on the extent of surgery.
- Extremity elevation is recommended while patient is in bed.
- Range of motion and therapy may begin the first 1 to 2 weeks for distal femur reconstructions.
- Proximal tibia reconstructions require strict knee extension for 6 weeks to allow patellar tendon healing. Gradual knee flexion is begun at 6 weeks and progresses under the supervision of a physical therapist.
- May administer antibiotics while drains are in place.

OUTCOMES

- Oncological outcomes include local recurrence and metastasis. Surveillance for recurrence should be managed by a multidisciplinary sarcoma team. Local recurrence is higher when margins are positive.[1]
- Functional outcomes depend on the extent of tissue resection and patient overall health status. Most patients will experience some form of disability that is proportional to the volume of muscle and bone resected.[3]
- Distal femur reconstructions do not require extensor mechanism reattachment and therefore generally function better than proximal tibia reconstructions.

COMPLICATIONS

- Prosthetic loosening may occur over time necessitating revision surgery. Generally, implant survival is approximately 80% at 20 years.
- Local recurrence occurs in a minority of patients and is more common in patients with positive margins.
- Deep infection can occur at any time after surgery and requires aggressive therapy including surgical debridement and antibiotic therapy to achieve limb salvage. Removal of implants may be necessary to eradicate infection.

REFERENCES

1. Bielack SS, Kempf-Bielack B, Delling G, et al. Prognostic factors in high-grade osteosarcoma of the extremities or trunk: an analysis of 1,702 patients treated on neoadjuvant cooperative osteosarcoma study group protocols. *J Clin Oncol.* 2002;20(3):776-790.
2. Mankin HJ, Mankin CJ, Simon MA. The hazards of the biopsy, revisited. Members of the Musculoskeletal Tumor Society. *J Bone Joint Surg Am.* 1996;78(5):656-663.
3. van Egmond-van Dam JC, Bekkering WP, Bramer JAM, et al. Functional outcome after surgery in patients with bone sarcoma around the knee; results from a long-term prospective study. *J Surg Oncol.* 2017;115(8):1028-1032.

Bony and Soft Tissue Debridement Around the Knee

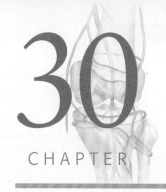

30

CHAPTER

Derek F. Amanatullah, Michael J. Chen, Sahitya K. Denduluri, and James I. Huddleston

DEFINITION

- Several conditions affect the knee that requires meticulous soft tissue and bony debridement for treatment: these include open fractures, osteomyelitis, and infected total knee arthroplasty (TKA).
- The expertise of plastic surgeons is frequently needed for soft tissue management and coverage as the knee is relatively devoid of surrounding soft tissues in comparison to the muscle bound femur.

ANATOMY

- The knee is a complex synovial joint composed of two joints: the tibiofemoral and patellofemoral articulations.
    - The tibiofemoral articulation functions as a hinge joint allowing for flexion and extension with minimal rotation.
        - It transfers body weight from the femur to the tibia and can experience high joint reaction forces.
    - The patella is the largest sesamoid bone in the human body and transmits tensile forces from the quadriceps tendon to the patellar ligament.
        - By increasing the lever arm of the extensor mechanism from the center of rotation of the tibiofemoral joint, the patella reduces the amount of work the quadriceps have to perform to extend the knee.
- The distal femur is trapezoidal in shape with two condyles that articulate with the two condyles of the tibial plateau, forming the medial and lateral compartments of the knee. The majority of the weight is borne through the medial compartment in a native healthy knee.
    - The mechanical axis of the lower extremity is characterized by a straight line that passes from the center of the hip through the center of the ankle. Ideally, this line passes through the center of the knee.
- Compared to the hip, which is a ball and socket joint, the knee is a relatively incongruent and relies on both static and dynamic forces for rotational, sagittal, and coronal stability.
- The dynamic stabilizers are the muscles and their tendons that cross the knee joint: these include the hamstrings, the iliotibial band, the pes anserine, the two heads of the gastrocnemius, the popliteus, and the extensor mechanism.
    - These muscles provide stability through compression of the joint when they are activated.
    - The hamstrings are composed of the biceps femoris, which crosses the posterolateral aspect of the knee to insert onto the head of the fibula, and the semimembranosus, which inserts onto the posteromedial aspect of the tibial plateau.
    - The semitendinosus, also a hamstring muscle, crosses the medial aspect of the knee to insert onto the anteromedial

proximal tibia along with gracilis and sartorius to form the pes anserine.
    - The iliotibial band forms from the coalescence of the gluteus maximus and tensor fascia lata and crosses the knee laterally to insert onto Gerdy tubercle, a prominence found just below the joint line on the anterolateral tibia.
    - The popliteus originates from the posterior aspect of the proximal tibia and inserts on to the lateral aspect of the lateral femoral condyle.
    - The two heads of the gastrocnemius cross posteriorly and insert onto the medial and lateral aspects of the distal femur.
- The static stabilizers include the ligaments and joint capsule.
    - The medial collateral ligament (MCL) extends from the medial epicondyle of the femur to the medial aspect of the proximal tibia metaphysis and resists valgus forces across the knee.
    - The posterolateral corner (PLC) of the knee resists varus and external rotational forces at the knee: its main components are the lateral collateral ligament, which extends from the lateral epicondyle of the femur to the proximal fibular head, the popliteus muscle, and the biceps femoris tendon.
    - The anterior cruciate ligament (ACL) extends from the posteromedial aspect of the lateral femoral condyle and runs anteriorly to insert in between and in front of the tibial spines to resist anterior displacement of the tibia relative to the femur.
    - The posterior cruciate ligament (PCL) runs from the anteromedial aspect of the medial femoral condyle to the posterior tibial sulcus to resist posterior displacement of the tibia relative to the femur.
- The extensor mechanism crosses the knee joint anteriorly and inserts onto the tibial tubercle.
    - It is composed of the four muscle bellies of the quadriceps, the quadriceps tendon, the patella, the patellar ligament, and the medial and lateral patellofemoral retinaculum.
    - It is critical to normal ambulatory function.
- The superficial femoral artery courses down the femur on the medial side underneath the sartorius muscle and then passes through the adductor hiatus to run posterior to the knee in the popliteal fossa where it becomes the popliteal artery.
    - It provides the sole blood supply to the distal extremity and, if compromised, risks viability of the leg and foot.
- The main blood supply to the knee is provided from superior and inferior lateral genicular arteries, the superior and inferior medial genicular arteries, the anterior recurrent tibial artery, and the descending genicular artery.
    - These form an anastomotic ring around the patella.

- The femoral nerve crosses the knee at the medial aspect and becomes the saphenous nerve supplying sensation to the medial leg and foot.
    - It gives off the infrapatellar branch as it crosses the knee, supplying sensation to the anteroinferior skin of the knee.
    - This nerve is sacrificed frequently during anterior midline exposures.
- The sciatic nerve bifurcates just above the popliteal fossa into the tibial and common peroneal nerves.
    - The tibial nerve joins the popliteal artery and runs directly posterior to the knee into the leg.
    - The common peroneal nerve crosses laterally and runs superficially around the neck of the proximal fibula before bifurcating in the deep and superficial peroneal nerves.
- The blood supply to the skin of the knee typically arises from medial to lateral.
    - This characteristic deserves careful attention when choosing which incision to use on a knee with multiple scars.
    - Typically the most lateral incision is chosen so that the potential area of skin at risk for necrosis is minimized.

PATHOGENESIS

- Conditions that warrant bony debridement around the knee include open fractures, chronic osteomyelitis, and periprosthetic joint infections (PJI) after TKA.
- Bony debridement is frequently required to prevent or eliminate bacteria capable of forming biofilms.
- Bacteria can exist in either a planktonic or biofilm state.
    - In contrast to planktonic microorganisms that are free-floating and rapidly dividing, a biofilm is characterized by sessile microorganisms that are embedded in a matrix capable of withstanding both the host's immune system and antibiotics.
- Once bacteria colonize and adhere to the necrotic bone or implants, they can rapidly form a biofilm.
    - Surgical debridement and removal of any implants are the most efficacious method to eradicate infection.

Open Fractures

- Open fractures involving the patella are the most common with an incidence of 6 per million per year in the general population, followed by the distal femur (5.6 per million per year) and proximal tibia (3.8 per million per year).
    - Road traffic accidents are the primary mechanism.
- The Gustilo classification system for open fractures was first published in 1976, modified in 1984, and arguably remains the most commonly used system in orthopedic surgery.[1,2]
    - This system organizes open fractures in order of worsening prognosis according to the degree of soft tissue injury, need for soft tissue coverage and vascular insult.
        - Type I: usually low energy, clean, and involve an open wound less than 1 cm in size
        - Type II: intermediate-energy, moderately contaminated wounds greater than 1 cm (but less than 10 cm)
        - Type III: farm injuries or high-energy fractures with periosteal stripping and extensively contaminated open wounds greater than 10 cm:
            - IIIA wounds can be managed with local wound coverage and skin graft only.
            - IIIB requires rotational or free flap coverage.
            - IIIC is associated with arterial damage.

- The risk of infection has been shown to directly correlate with the fracture grade.
- The true extent of underlying soft tissue damage can be appreciated only after surgical exploration and debridement in the operating room, rather than in the emergency department.
- All open fractures are considered contaminated with bacteria, and antibiotics must be administered as early as possible to prevent infection.
    - Patzakis et al. found an infection rate of 4.7% compared to 7.4% when antibiotics were given within 3 hours of injury.[3]
    - The choice of the antibiotic depends on the degree of injury and level of contamination.
        - Intravenous first-generation cephalosporins, such as cefazolin, are considered first line.
        - For Gustilo type III open fractures, extending the coverage to include gram-negative bacteria by adding an aminoglycoside is commonplace.

Osteomyelitis

- Osteomyelitis can arise from hematogenous seeding, contiguous spread from adjacent tissues or joints, or direct inoculation from surgery or trauma.
    - Hematogenous spread of bacteria typically afflicts the metaphysis in skeletally immature patients but can also seed implants especially in the case of TKA.
    - Contiguous spread and direct inoculation are seen after direct contamination from open fractures or surgical procedures.
    - The duration of symptoms designates osteomyelitis as either acute or chronic and carries important implications with regard to biofilm formation and the need for surgical debridement.
- The Cierny-Mader classification system is commonly used to categorize osteomyelitis based on the extent of bony involvement and status of the host and carries prognostic value in addition to guiding therapy.
    - Type I involves only the medullary canal.
    - Type II involves a portion of the cortex.
    - Type III is an infection that permeates the cortex into the canal, but the bone is axially stable.
    - Type IV is similarly permeative but diffuse and places the bone at risk for fracture.
    - The status of the host is divided into classes A, B, and C.
        - The A host is physiologically healthy.
        - The B host has compromised physiology from systemic effects of the infection or medical comorbidities.
        - The C host is classified as one in which the morbidity of the treatment is greater than the disease.
- Sequestrum is a key pathologic feature of osteomyelitis and represents the formation of necrotic bone.
    - Bacteria persist in devascularized bone and evade host defenses and antimicrobial agents.
    - The response of the host is to generally wall of the "bony abscess" by forming sclerotic bone around the sequestrum.
        - This is known as the involucrum.

Infection After Total Knee Arthroplasty

- Periprosthetic joint infection after TKA is a devastating condition that occurs in 0.5% to 1.9% of primary TKAs and in 8% to 10% of revision TKAs.[4–6]

- The implants provide an excellent surface for bacterial adherence, biofilm formation, and facilitate the spread of the microorganisms into the surrounding bone and soft tissues.
- Infections can occur in the perioperative period or years later after a previously well functioning TKA.
- The longer the duration of symptoms, the greater chance of biofilm formation on the implants and surrounding bone.
  - Symptom duration is commonly separated into acute (3 weeks after surgery or symptom onset) and chronic (greater than 3 weeks after surgery or symptom onset).
  - Aggressive surgical debridement and implant removal are key interventions to treat infections with suspected biofilm formation.
- Conditions that warrant soft tissue debridement around the knee include open fractures, septic arthritis, and PJI after TKA.
- Soft tissue debridement is frequently required to prevent or eliminate bacteria capable of forming biofilms.

PATIENT HISTORY AND PHYSICAL FINDINGS

Open Fractures

- Any patient presenting with an open fracture may have associated injuries to the head, chest, abdomen, pelvis, spine, and extremities.
- A standard evaluation according to the Advanced Trauma Life Support guidelines should be performed to evaluate for all potentially life-threatening injuries.
- The injury mechanism and details are helpful as high- vs low-energy injuries predict the extent of bony and soft tissue injury.
  - Low-energy trauma with an open fracture may be associated with a small inconspicuous poke hole created from inside-out injury.
  - High-energy trauma usually creates a much larger soft tissue defect or frank degloving of the skin and subcutaneous tissues.
- A detailed neurovascular exam of the lower limb involved should be done with focus on evaluating the function of the peroneal and tibial nerves, as well as the dorsalis pedis and posterior tibial pulses.
- Any suspicion of vascular injury may direct appropriate testing and consultation with a vascular surgeon.
- The soft tissues must be thoroughly inspected.
  - Any fracture with a nearby skin laceration or defect should be considered open until proven otherwise by surgical evaluation or saline challenge, utilized in evaluation of traumatic arthrotomy and to determine the presence of possible external communication with the knee joint.

Osteomyelitis

- Symptoms and signs of infection should be elicited from the patient including fever, chills, pain, and swelling.
- Prior injuries and surgeries including the presence of hardware are important to identify.
- The general medical status of the patient including factors that can contribute to an immunocompromised state should be investigated.
- The involved limb should be inspected for erythema, swelling, tenderness, and any opening in the skin that might

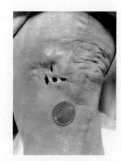

FIG 1 • Draining sinuses as a result of chronic periprosthetic knee infection.

suggest a draining sinus tract (**FIG 1**), which is indicative of chronic osteomyelitis.
- The neurovascular status of the limb should be evaluated as well as the quality of the soft tissues.
- The erythrocyte sedimentation rate (ESR) and C-reactive protein (CRP) are markers of inflammation that are typically elevated and can be useful for monitoring response to therapy.
- The white blood cell count may be normal in cases of chronic infection.

Infection After TKA

- PJIs may present acutely after surgery with persistent pain and drainage from the incision with overlying cellulitis or in a delayed fashion with pain only (**FIG 2**).
- Any pain, stiffness, or instability should warrant consideration of an infection until proven otherwise.
- Special attention should focus on the scars about the knee and neurovascular status of the limb.
- Multiple scars or poor-quality tissues may necessitate the early involvement of a plastic surgeon for soft tissue coverage at the time of the planned surgery.
- An ESR greater than 30 and CRP greater than 10 mg/L are recommended as the thresholds indicative of chronic infections.
- If there is any suspicion of PJI, the knee should be aspirated and the fluid sent for cell count, gram stain, and culture.
  - Importantly, the entry point of the needle for aspiration should not involve any skin with overlying cellulitis.
  - An aspiration that yields greater than 1700 cells/µL with a neutrophil percentage greater than 65% is highly suggestive of PJI.

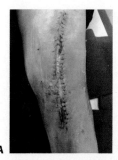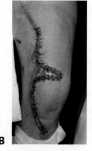

FIG 2 • **A.** Wound dehiscence postoperative day 14 in a 55-year-old woman with diabetes mellitus s/p total knee arthroplasty for osteoarthritis. **B.** Skin necrosis in a 25-year-old woman after patellofemoral arthroplasty for post-traumatic arthrosis.

IMAGING

Open Fractures

- Orthogonal radiographs of affected area including the joint above and below are important for characterizing the fracture pattern and detecting concomitant injuries, which are frequent in high-energy trauma.
  - For open extra-articular fractures involving the proximal tibia or distal femur, plain radiographs are typically all that is required for surgical planning.
  - This is true also for isolated open fractures of the patella.
- Fractures involving the tibia plateau or distal femoral condyles may be complex and require computed tomography (CT) to better visual the fracture patterns and to facilitate optimal surgical planning.
- CT angiography may be considered if there is suspicion for vascular injury.
- Magnetic resonance imaging (MRI) is not typically warranted in the acute period but may be obtained eventually if ligamentous or meniscal damage is suspected.

Osteomyelitis

- Radiographs of the involved limb should be obtained in orthogonal planes.
  - In the acute stages of osteomyelitis, the films may be unremarkable.
  - A lytic lesion may be appreciated when enough of the bone has eroded.
  - In chronic situations, the sequestrum may form and is characterized by a sclerotic focus of infected and necrotic bone that may be surrounded by a thickening of the surrounding cortex known as the involucrum with periosteal reaction.
- Computed tomography is more sensitive and better shows the bony destruction from the lesion compared to plain films.
- Magnetic resonance imaging is the most sensitive modality especially in the early stages of osteomyelitis and will show the extent of intramedullary and soft tissue involvement.
- Nuclear bone scans are a sensitive modality but nonspecific.

Infection After TKA

- Standard radiographs should be obtained and may show osteolysis with component subsidence or loosening.
- CT scans, MRI, and nuclear bone scans of little use in preoperative planning and are not typically needed.

SURGICAL MANAGEMENT

Open Fractures

- Historically, the practice in orthopedic surgery has been to perform operative debridement within 6 hours after injury to minimize the risk of infection, but there may be no advantage to performing the debridement within this time frame compared to within 24 hours after injury.
  - A thorough debridement by an experienced team during daylight hours with the appropriate ancillary staff appears to be the critical factor in preventing infection.
- All devitalized and contaminated soft and bony tissue must be identified and removed in a systematic fashion.

- Bony damage can be highly variable and demands thorough intraoperative inspection.
  - The decision of whether to retain or discard bony fragments depends on the remaining soft tissue attachments and involvement of the diaphysis, metaphysis, and articular margins.
  - Diaphyseal fragments that are stripped of their soft tissue attachments are effectively devascularized and must be removed, to prevent a nidus for infection.
  - Metaphyseal fragments, in contrast, have a greater amount of cancellous bone, which has a greater capacity to revascularize and reintegrate.
    - Thus fragments that have minimal contamination may be retained.
  - Cancellous fragments from the articular margins are also retained in order to anatomically reconstruct the articular surface.
- Repeat debridement may be necessary 24 or 48 hours later, as the zone of injury may be more extensive than initially appreciated.
- Thorough irrigation of the wound after debridement should be performed using the rationale that "the solution to pollution is dilution."
- Once the wound has been debrided back to healthy and viable soft tissue and bone, attention must be turned to achieving skeletal stabilization.
  - Stabilizing the bone is critical for creating an environment conducive not only for bone healing but soft tissue healing as well.
  - Stabilization also facilitates early mobilization of adjacent joints, preventing stiffness and further disability of the injured limb.
  - Options for stabilization will depend on the need for repeat debridement and soft tissue coverage.
  - The wound should be definitively closed within 48 to 72 hours after fracture fixation.
  - If injury is a type IIIB open fracture, then external fixation may be preferred to allow unimpeded access to the wound for soft tissue coverage followed by definitive internal fixation after the soft tissue envelope has been re-established and healed.
- High-energy injuries may result in substantial bony or soft tissue loss from the initial injury with subsequent debridement procedures creating extensive dead space.
  - Temporary antibiotic-impregnated polymethylmethacrylate (PMMA) cement beads can be placed into bony defects and used to deliver high doses of antibiotics locally.
  - Alternatively, negative pressure wound therapy may be used for similarly large soft tissue defects.

Osteomyelitis

- Once the diagnosis of osteomyelitis has been made, it requires proper staging and a multidisciplinary approach with involvement of infectious disease specialists, orthopedic surgeons, and plastic surgeons especially if the need for soft tissue coverage is anticipated.
- Though acute hematogenous osteomyelitis without associated implants may be amenable to intravenous antimicrobial therapy alone, infections that are chronic, are associated with implants, or have an identified sequestrum will require

aggressive surgical debridement if the goal is to eradicate the infection.

- All dead and nonviable bone should be removed until punctate bleeding bone is encountered.
- In the case of intramedullary infections, intramedullary reaming of the canal is an effective way to debride contaminated bone while preserving cortical stability.
- The placement of antibiotic impregnated PMMA cement into the bony and soft tissue defect to deliver high concentrations of antibiotics to the local tissue has become standard in the surgical treatment of osteomyelitis.
  - Current techniques include using an antibiotic coated intramedullary nail for situations involving the medullary canal of the tibia or femur.
  - For well-localized areas and bony defects created after the debridement, antibiotic-impregnated cement may be packed into the defect or rolled into beads and attached to suture for easy extraction and to provide a high surface area to volume ratio in order to maximize drug elution.
  - As the cement is not biodegradable and may continue to elute low levels of antibiotics for up to 5 years following implantation, a repeat procedure is typically required for removal of the cement and bone grafting of the defect to restore skeletal stability and eliminate dead space.
  - Bioabsorbable composites such as calcium sulfate have been examined as an alternative for dead space fillers and antibiotic delivery vehicles.
    - These materials have the benefits of being resorbed and possibly being replaced by bone, thus potentially eliminating the need for a second procedure.
    - McNally et al. reported an excellent eradication rate of chronic osteomyelitis treated with one stage debridement and placement of an antibiotic-impregnated bioabsorbable composite.

Infection After TKA

- The timing and duration of the infection have important implications with regard to treatment.
  - An early infection is defined as occurring within 3 weeks after undergoing the procedure or within 3 weeks after becoming symptomatic in cases of late hematogenous infection.
  - Late infections are considered all cases that present more than 3 weeks after the above.
  - The designation of 3 weeks is based on the theoretical time period that it takes for bacteria to form biofilms.
- To prevent the morbidity of explanting components, early infections are typically treated with aggressive debridement and irrigation, exchanging the polyethylene liner, and retaining the femoral and tibial components.
- Late infections are most commonly treated by a two-stage exchange arthroplasty in the United States.
  - The microorganisms by this time have likely adhered to the implants and formed biofilms, undermining the efficacy of systemic antibiotic therapy.
  - The first stage is composed of removal of all implants, cement, and infected tissue.
  - Although minimizing bone loss is a priority, the surrounding bone can contain biofilm and must be debrided back to healthy punctate bleeding bone.

- Irrigation is then performed, and an antibiotic-impregnated cement spacer is placed to provide stability, fill dead space, and deliver high concentrations of local antibiotics.
- The spacer can be dynamic or static.
  - Dynamic spacers involve the use of articulating components that allow for knee range of motion.
  - Static spacers typically involve antibiotic cement-coated humeral nails that bridge the knee after being placed in the distal femoral and proximal tibial canals.
  - Intravenous antibiotics that target the identified organism are then given for 4 to 6 weeks. Once the patient has finished the course of antibiotics and has been off therapy for 2 weeks, repeat inflammatory markers are drawn. If the ESR and CRP are normal, and the clinical exam is negative for any suspicion of persisting infection, reimplantation is then considered.
  - This entails removal of the antibiotic spacer, a thorough repeat irrigation and debridement and obtaining several intraoperative tissue specimens for cultures.
    - It is important to remove the pseudomembrane that forms between the cement and the bone in the intramedullary canal with instruments such as a ringed curette.
  - If there is no suspicion for residual infection, the distal femur, proximal tibia, and patella are prepared for reimplantation of the components, and the knee is balanced to achieve symmetric flexion and extension gaps.
  - Depending on the degree of bone loss encountered, metal augments, stems, porous cones, or sleeves may be needed to reconstruct the bony defect.

Positioning

- Supine
- Tourniquet applied to the thigh
- Bump under ipsilateral hip to internally rotate the operative leg
- Povidone-iodine (preferred) or chlorhexidine skin prep

Approach

- Medial parapatellar approach: most commonly used approach for septic arthritis of the knee and open periarticular fractures with excellent exposure to anterior structures of the knee
  - Landmarks: borders of the patella, tibial tubercle
  - Longitudinal midline or medial incision, extending proximally to 5 cm above superior pole of patella and distally to tibial tubercle depending on desired exposure
  - Develop skin flaps to expose interval between vastus medialis obliquus and quadriceps tendon proximally, medial border of patella, and medial border of patellar tendon distally
  - Medial parapatellar arthrotomy performed sharply or using cautery
  - Depending on amount of exposure needed, patella can be dislocated and flipped laterally to provide access to lateral joint structures.

■ Bone Infection Management

- The goal of bony debridement in all of these conditions is to resect all bone that is necrotic or contaminated with potential biofilm formation.
- Debridement is typically accomplished with rongeurs, curettes, and osteotomes, as well as round or pencil tipped high-speed burs.
  - The bur can be especially useful for quick debridement of the bone or removing a well-fixed implant and cement.
- The debridement should continue until punctate bleeding bone is encountered.

- To allow this, a tourniquet should not be inflated during the debridement, if possible.
- Bony resection may be extensive and can create dead space and structural instability (**TECH FIG 1A,B**).
- Antibiotic impregnated PMMA cement may be used to temporarily manage dead space and deliver antibiotics to the local tissues (**TECH FIG 1C**).
- Bone loss management is beyond the scope of this chapter but includes the following techniques: induced membrane technique, allograft reconstruction, autograft reconstruction including vascularized fibula, bone transport and distraction osteogenesis, and primary shortening of the limb.

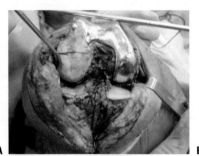
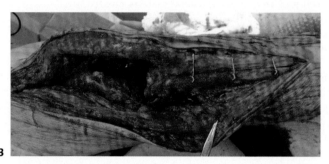
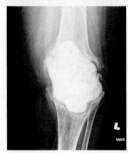

TECH FIG 1 • A. Bicompartmental knee arthroplasty being removed for chronic periprosthetic infection. **B.** Knee after extensive bony debridement and tibial tubercle osteotomy required for removal of a chronically infected total knee arthroplasty. **C.** Radiograph showing an antibiotic-impregnated polymethylmethacrylate spacer placed after removal of an infected total knee arthroplasty in the first of a planned two-stage procedure.

■ Soft Tissue Infection Management

Irrigation and Debridement

- Although there is no consensus, a high volume of low-pressure irrigant appears to be sufficient, such as with gravity irrigation using cystoscopy tubing.
  - High-pressure irrigation, though potentially beneficial for removing more bacteria and debris with less solution, may cause damage to soft tissues and the bone.
  - Pulsatile devices have also not been shown to improve outcomes compared to gravity irrigation and may actually have a decreased irrigation rate overall.
  - Bulb irrigation may not be as efficacious.
- Normal saline is the favored irrigant, with or without the use of added antibiotics in the final liter of irrigation.
  - In the setting of open fractures with a traumatic arthrotomy, the amount of irrigant used generally depends on the extent of injury. For example, employing the Gustilo classification, type I injuries can be

effectively irrigated with 3 L of saline, type II with 6 L, and type III with 9 L.
- In open fractures, debridement should involve a systematic inspection of all tissue types, including the skin, subcutaneous fat, fascia, muscle, and bone.
  - Remove all necrotic tissue until a healthy bleeding wound bed is achieved.
  - Muscle viability can be determined by color, contractility, consistency, and capacity to bleed.
  - Debridement should be performed sharply, centripetally, and radically, removing any tissue that may even appear questionably viable.
  - The cortical bone without soft tissue attachments should be removed, as it will be nonviable, though articular fragments should be retained if joint reconstruction can be achieved (**TECH FIG 2**).
  - A repeat debridement can be performed after 24 to 48 hours if tissue viability or adequacy of initial debridement is in question and at the time of definitive closure in wounds requiring a muscle flap.

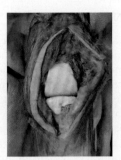

TECH FIG 2 • The knee in **FIG 1** after debridement and placement of an articulating spacer made from antibiotic-impregnated PMMA.

Adjuncts

- Hydrogen peroxide
  - May be synergistic in conjunction with chlorhexidine or povidone-iodine with regard to bactericidal activity

- Can result in wound complications, local cytotoxicity against healthy tissue, and increase risk of air embolism
- Local antibiotics
  - Antibiotic-loaded polymethylmethacrylate (PMMA, bone cement): vancomycin and aminoglycosides, such as tobramycin and gentamicin, can be effectively incorporated during mixing process and are thermostable to withstand the exothermic polymerization of the cement.
    - Can be formed into beads and placed into wound bed
    - Implants used for fracture fixation can be coated for delivery to tissues.
  - Antibiotic powder placed directly into wound
- Negative pressure wound therapy
  - Has a role in wounds left open or closed primarily
  - Reduces edema
  - Improves local microcirculation
  - Can be used to stage coverage for open wounds requiring delayed flap closure

PEARLS AND PITFALLS

Bone management	▪ Do not strip viable bone. Remove all stripped bone not attached to cartilage as these represent a nidus for future infection.
Soft tissue management	▪ Maintaining or reconstructing a viable and well-vascularized soft tissue envelope in the case of open fractures is key to preventing infection and enhancing bone healing. Maintain all viable bone. Do not pinch the skin. Use atraumatic technique.
Necrotic tissue	▪ Remove all hardware and nonviable tissue as these represent a nidus for future infection.
Cartilage	▪ Preservation of metaphyseal and periarticular fragments stripped of soft tissue is the exception as they may reintegrate in contrast to diaphyseal fragments and may be critical to reconstructing the joint line or articular surface.
Negative pressure wound dressing	▪ Do not apply over bone directly as it can desiccate the location that requires further debridement. Do not apply in active infection.
Antibiotic beads	▪ Consider for temporary management of an infected wound bed.
Well-fixed implant	▪ Cemented implants should be carefully freed from the underlying cement with a bur or saw before attempted removal to avoid fracture of key supporting structures.
Amputation	▪ If reconstruction and preservation of the limb are not feasible, amputation should be strongly considered.
Wound edges	▪ Debride rounded skin to fresh edges to facilitate healing.
Plastic surgery	▪ Consult plastic surgery early in the process of wound closure or defect management to assess primary, secondary, or flap-based closure.

POSTOPERATIVE CARE

- Open fractures
  - Antibiotics should be administered for 24 hours after definitive closure of the wound.
  - The weight-bearing status of the patient will depend on the type of fixation used and location of the injury.
  - Diaphyseal fractures treated with intramedullary nailing can typically be treated with weight bearing as tolerated, whereas periarticular fractures require several weeks of nonweight bearing to allow anatomic healing of the articular surface.
  - Early mobilization of neighboring joints is critical to prevent adjacent stiffness.

- Osteomyelitis
  - Intravenous antibiotics for at least 6 weeks is typically required with the choice depending on the sensitivities of the identified microorganism.
  - ESR and CRP levels are monitored at routine intervals.
  - Early mobilization of the patient and maintaining motion at adjacent joints is similarly critical to overall functional outcome.
- Infection after TKA
  - Intravenous antibiotics specific to the organism are continued for a minimum of 6 weeks after the initial debridement and explanation until ESR and CRP levels have resolved.

- After the patient has completed antibiotic therapy, the ESR and CRP are evaluated at least 2 weeks later.
- Reimplantation is then considered only if the ESR and CRP levels are normal.

OUTCOMES

- Open fractures
  - Successful treatment of open fractures depends on the thoroughness of the debridement, the presence of a well-vascularized soft tissue envelope, and the bony reconstruction.
  - The overall infection rate for open fractures has been shown to be around 2% to 4%, whereas Gustilo type IIIC injuries can become infected at rates as high as 20% to 40%.[7,8]
  - In open fractures treated with antibiotics at the time of admission, there is no significant difference in infection rates when debrided within or after 6 hours of injury.
- Osteomyelitis
  - Units experienced in the treatment of osteomyelitis typically achieve the best outcomes.
  - Cierny reported a cure rate of 84% at 2 years of follow-up.[9]
- Infection after TKA
  - Eradication of infection following two-stage protocol using an antibiotic spacer followed by reimplantation has reported success rates between 74% and 91%.
  - The data on articulating vs static spacers are conflicting; however, some studies have shown improved patient satisfaction, range of motion, and an easier exposure at the time of reimplantation when an articulating spacer is used.

COMPLICATIONS

- Open fractures can result in infection and osteomyelitis, nonunion, malunion, hardware failure, and amputation.
- Inadequate treatment of osteomyelitis can lead to persistent infection, sinus formation, and malignant transformation.
- Osteomyelitis may also require amputation.
- Inadequate treatment of PJI can lead to persistent infection or reinfection requiring repeat debridement and antibiotic spacer exchange, chronic suppression with antibiotics if the patient is not a surgical candidate, or amputation.

REFERENCES

1. Gustilo RB, Anderson JT. Prevention of infection in the treatment of one thousand and twenty-five open fractures of long bones: retrospective and prospective analyses. *J Bone Joint Surg Am.* 1976;58(4):453-458.
2. Gustilo RB, Mendoza RM, Williams DN. Problems in the management of type III (severe) open fractures: a new classification of type III open fractures. *J Trauma.* 1984;24(8):742-746.
3. Patzakis MJ, Wilkins J. Factors influencing infection rate in open fracture wounds. *Clin Orthop Relat Res.* 1989;(243):36-40.
4. Bozic KJ, Kurtz SM, Lau E, et al. The epidemiology of revision total knee arthroplasty in the United States. *Clin Orthop Relat Res.* 2010;468(1):45-51.
5. Kurtz SM, Lau E, Schmier J, et al. Infection burden for hip and knee arthroplasty in the United States. *J Arthroplasty.* 2008;23(7):984-991.
6. Kurtz SM, Ong KL, Lau E, et al. Prosthetic joint infection risk after TKA in the Medicare population. *Clin Orthop Relat Res.* 2010;468(1):52-56.
7. Kim PH, Leopold SS. In brief: Gustilo-Anderson classification. [corrected]. *Clin Orthop Relat Res.* 2012;470(11):3270-3274.
8. Lenarz CJ, Watson JT, Moed BR, et al. Timing of wound closure in open fractures based on cultures obtained after debridement. *J Bone Joint Surg Am.* 2010;92(10):1921-1916.
9. Cierny G. Surgical treatment of osteomyelitis. *Plast Reconstr Surg.* 2011;127(suppl 1):190S-204S.

Bone Reconstruction of the Knee

Robert J. Steffner and Raffi S. Avedian

DEFINITION

- For this chapter, we will be discussing segmental bone loss with a specific example of a metadiaphyseal hemicortical bone defect below an intact knee joint.
- Above and below the knee is a common area for segmental bone loss due to trauma, tumor, and infection.
- Bone loss in the proximal tibia with an intact joint that compromises the extensor mechanism is often best reconstructed with an intercalary fresh frozen allograft with soft tissue attachments. This facilitates extensor mechanism reconstruction.
- Joint loss is generally reconstructed with an allograft-prosthetic composite or endoprosthetic reconstruction.

ANATOMY

- Anatomy relevant to reconstruction on the medial knee includes the adductor tendon insertion on the medial distal femur and the pes anserinus tendons inserting on the proximal tibia. The surgeon will encounter the femoral artery and vein just below the medial intermuscular septum moving through the adductor hiatus to enter the popliteal fossa.
  - Pay close attention to identify and preserve the saphenous nerve branch and saphenous vein.
- The medial collateral ligament (MCL) connects the medial distal femur to the medial proximal tibia. The deep portion of the ligament inserts on the proximal tibia approximately 1 cm below the joint line. The superficial portion is broad and inserts on the proximal tibia 6 to 7 cm distal to the joint line.
  - The MCL may need to be reconstructed as part of the surgical procedure.
- On the lateral knee, the iliotibial band inserts on the proximal lateral tibia at Gerdy tubercle and the bicep femoris tendon spans the knee to insert onto the fibular head. Posterior to the bicep femoris tendon lies the common peroneal nerve. The nerve divides at the anterior fibular neck into deep and superficial branches.
- The lateral collateral ligament connects the lateral distal femur to the fibular head. Reconstruction may be required with bone defect management at the lateral knee.
- Soft tissue loss around the proximal tibia can create a precarious situation that is at increased risk of infection. The surgeon should maintain a low threshold for soft tissue coverage with a gastrocnemius flap or free tissue transfer.

PATHOGENESIS

- This technique is applicable to bone loss from bone tumor excision, bone loss from trauma such as an open fracture, and osteomyelitis requiring debridement.

NATURAL HISTORY

- Management of bone defects around the knee are a challenging problem that frequently requires multidisciplinary management between general surgery, orthopedic surgery, plastic surgery, and infectious disease.
- Before instituting the described procedure, the surgeon must obtain a clean bone defect with viable tissue that is free of infection.
- This may require multiple surgeries focusing on debridement, antibiotic cement spacer placement, bone stabilization, soft tissue coverage, and intravenous antibiotics to prepare the area for the described definitive procedure.

PATIENT HISTORY AND PHYSICAL FINDINGS

- The patient presentation and reason for the bone defect influence the treatment approach and time interval to the definitive bone grafting procedure.
- Trauma and infectious etiologies often require serial debridement and temporary stabilization with definitive stabilization and soft tissue coverage performed once a clean tissue bed is achieved.
- The surgeon should assess the neurovascular status of the involved extremity. A functional limb is a candidate for limb salvage. A severely compromised limb may be better with an early amputation.
- When pursuing limb salvage, the stability of the collateral ligaments should be tested by applying a varus and valgus stress to a slightly flexed knee.
- The patient should be asked to extend the knee against gravity to test the competency of the extensor mechanism.
- Laboratory studies depend on patient specifics and can be used to assess nutritional status, blood count recovery after chemotherapy, and inflammatory markers to assess for infection or response to antibiotics.

IMAGING

- Radiographs are used to assess defect size and provide an estimate of how much bone graft will be needed (**FIG 1A**). Further, the surgeon can plan implant needs to provide sufficient stabilization of the involved bone.

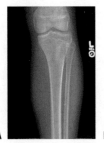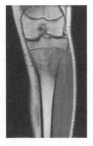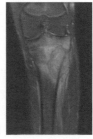

FIG 1 • **A.** AP radiograph, **(B)** coronal T1 MRI, and **(C)** coronal T2 MRI of a primary bone tumor of the lateral proximal tibia.

- Computed tomography and magnetic resonance imaging (**FIG 1B,C**) provide a detailed assessment of cortical bone and offer a volumetric assessment of the defect.

SURGICAL MANAGEMENT

- In the setting of a large bone defect (≥6 cm), surgery is generally necessary to improve function and facilitate weight bearing. The described technique has been utilized for defects up to 2.5 cm.[1]
- The treatment goal is to create a clean and viable tissue bed that is then filled with a cement spacer to maintain the defect space and induce formation of a biologically active, vascularized membrane (**FIG 2**).
  - After 4 to 6 weeks, the cement spacer is removed, and the defect is optimized for placement of autogenous bone grafting to facilitate reconstitution of the defect.[2]
- The cement spacer provides structural support to the bone, offloads the implant bridging the defect, maintains the bone void, facilitates formation of the induced membrane, and can be a conduit for local antibiotic elution.
- Bone graft is obtained using a reamer-irrigator-aspirator (RIA) system (Synthes, Paoli, PA).
  - This is a single-pass, negative pressure reaming system for obtaining intramedullary nonstructural autogenous bone graft.
- Compared to the traditional iliac crest bone used for the harvest of autogenous bone graft, RIA obtains more graft volume (on average 60 cc from the femur and 40 cc from the tibia)[3,4], and the graft appears to have equivalent osteoconductivity and better osteogenicity and osteoinductivity.[5-7] Studies also suggest a greater concentration of stem cells. Harvest of bone graft with RIA is also less invasive and associated with less donor site morbidity.[8]
- Use of RIA to obtain autogenous bone graft is indicated in skeletally mature patients with normal femur anatomy.

Relative contraindications include metabolic bone disease, presence of metastatic bone cancer in the donor bone, active osteomyelitis in the donor bone, known bleeding disorder, and osteoporotic patients with thin cortices.[5]

- Bone graft volume can be extended with cancellous allograft and demineralized bone matrix. Extension is common, and when used, we add fresh bone marrow aspirate to provide osteogenic mesenchymal stem cells to the structural allograft.[6]
- The induced membrane is a vascularized soft tissue layer that forms around the cement spacer. It is composed of an outer layer of fibroblasts and collagen and a synovium-like inner layer. It is rich in growth factors and osteoinductive elements that include BMP-2. Upon placement of autogenous bone graft, the membrane prevents graft resorption and facilitates the formation of new cortical bone.[8]

Preoperative Planning

- Bone reconstruction is a two-stage process.
- Bone defects from infection or trauma may require serial debridement with placement of a temporary cement spacer and temporary stabilization of the bone with an external fixator or long plate. The cement spacer is often loaded with antibiotics to provide a local elution.
- A clean defect can be judged by negative cultures, bleeding tissues, and maintained continuity of the defect with the intramedullary canals.
  - Once clean, the patient is eligible for stage 1 of this procedure.
- For infection, intravenous antibiotics are generally given for the 4 to 6 weeks that the cement spacer is implanted. These antibiotics are an adjuvant and do not make up for an inadequate debridement.[9]
- Patients are followed with serial inflammatory markers such as C-reactive protein (CRP) and erythrocyte sedimentation rate (ESR) to judge eradication of the infection.
  - At this point, the patient has a clean bone defect that is free of infection.
- The patient should be counseled on the risks of surgery, which include fracture of the donor bone, infection of the recipient site, and possible need for blood transfusion(s).
- Patients should know that there may be a need to surgically stabilize the donor femur due to bone perforation by the reamer head or perceived postoperative fracture risk based on the assessment of cortical thickness after RIA use.
- Patient should be aware of the donor site location and possible weight-bearing restrictions after surgery. In general, we try to use a donor bone on the ipsilateral side of the bone

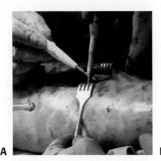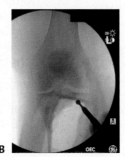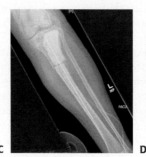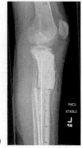

FIG 2 • **A.** Intraoperative preparation of the bone defect. **B.** Fluoroscopic view of debridement with high-speed bur. **C,D.** Placement of an antibiotic spacer into a proximal tibia bone defect.

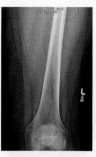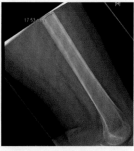

FIG 3 • **A,B.** Preoperative radiographs of the donor femur. The inner diameter of the isthmus is used to determine the reamer head size needed for bone graft harvest.

defect in order to maintain one good lower extremity to aid postoperative rehabilitation.

- Preoperative radiographs are done of the donor femur (**FIG 3**). The surgeon assesses cortical thickness, inner cortical diameter at the isthmus, and length of the femur. This facilitates decision-making on appropriate indications for RIA use, estimation of reamer head size, and determination of the appropriate length of the RIA drive shaft (360 or 520 mm).
- The size of the reamer head is determined by measuring the isthmus of the donor long bone on both AP and lateral radiographs. A head size 1 to 1.5 mm larger than the smallest measured inner cortical diameter at the isthmus should be used. If this measurement is done intraoperatively with fluoroscopy, the surgeon should factor in the distance of the ruler from the actual bone. The real canal is larger than the measurement. In general, the canal is 1 mm larger when the ruler is 2.5 cm away from bone and 2 mm larger when the ruler is 5 cm away.
- To use RIA, a power driver with 3.5 to 4.5 Nm of torque and 700 to 900 rpm should be used. Drills with torque greater than 6 Nm are too powerful and should not be used.

- In the operating room, the surgeon will need a radiolucent table, large fluoroscopy machine, 3-L bags of normal saline, a separate Mayo stand to hold the RIA, and a source of negative pressure suction.
- A tourniquet may be used at the bone defect site if brisk bleeding is present during preparation of the area. Attempts are made to avoid tourniquet use as it can compromise the assessment of tissue viability.
- The patient may benefit from a preoperative discussion with the anesthesia team regarding use of regional or neuraxial anesthesia. This can provide optimal intraoperative and postoperative pain control.

Positioning

- Patient position and draping frequently requires coordination between orthopedic surgery and plastic surgery.
- Position should facilitate debridement of the bone defect, harvest of bone graft, and any soft tissue coverage procedures. It may be necessary to change the patient's position during the surgery; a repeat sterile prep and drape is then performed.
- For bone defects about the knee, a supine position with a bump under the gluteus is often sufficient.
- A large C-arm should be placed opposite the side where bone graft will be harvested. The monitor is positioned at the end of the operating room table.

Approach

- RIA bone graft harvest from the femur is generally obtained through an antegrade approach through a greater trochanter start side. This requires an approximately 3- to 4-cm incision, approximately one hand breath above the top of the greater trochanter and 2 to 3 cm posterior to the midline axis of the greater trochanter.
- Medial and lateral/anterolateral approaches to the distal femur and proximal tibia for the bone defect are well described in surgical approach textbooks.

■ Induced Membrane With Intramedullary Autogenous Bone Grafting With Bone Marrow Aspiration and Intramedullary Nailing

■ Stage 1

Cement Spacer Placement and Internal Fixation

- For tumors, the patient starts stage 1 at the time of surgical excision of the malignancy.
- Stage 1 simply consists of placing a block of cement into a clean bone defect. The cement is hand mixed in a bowel and allowed to reach a doughy consistency. The goal is to maintain the defect space while avoiding the interdigitation of cement into the bone, which would make removal difficult (**TECH FIG 1**).
- It is important to overlap the bone ends with cement to induce a pseudomembrane longer than the defect itself.
- In the absence of infection, definitive internal fixation can be placed at this time. When possible, we prefer a titanium intramedullary nail to maintain the canal, facilitate

early weight bearing, and prevent future central necrosis of the autogenous bone graft.

- Intramedullary implants can be placed antegrade or retrograde in the femur and antegrade in the tibia. New implants allow for fixation in short bone segments.
- In defects close to the joint, a strong 4.5-mm periarticular plate with fixed-angle locking screws into the short segment is most often used.

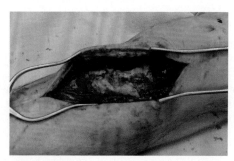

TECH FIG 1 • Placement of cement spacer into defect to generate an induced membrane.

- In the setting of infection, it is best to avoid metal implants altogether and rely on splints. Sometimes it is necessary to place antibiotic intramedullary nails or bridge plates coated in antibiotic cement for adequate bone stabilization.

Soft Tissue Coverage and Monitoring

- If soft tissue coverage is needed, it is done after placement of the cement block spacer. Defects in the proximal tibia are often augmented with a medial gastrocnemius flap (**TECH FIG 2**).
- If soft tissue coverage is not an urgent concern, muscle flap coverage can also be done at the time of definitive bone grafting.
- The patient is monitored for the next 4 to 6 weeks.
  - Weight bearing on the affected lower extremity is dictated by the strength of the cement/implant construct. At a minimum, the construct must provide enough stability to allow knee range of motion.
- Patients with infection have periodic checks of inflammatory markers.
  - At the end of intravenous antibiotics, these patients are followed for an additional 2 to 3 weeks off antibiotics to monitor for any signs of recurrent infection before proceeding with stage 2 of this procedure.

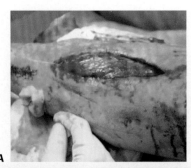

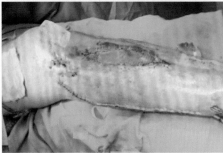

TECH FIG 2 • **A,B.** Medial gastrocnemius rotational flap of a proximal tibia bone defect.

■ Stage 2

Spacer Removal and Bone Preparation

- The second stage begins by accessing the bone defect through the prior surgical incision.
  - Patient positioning should allow access to the bone defect and the hip selected for RIA bone graft harvest.
- When exposing the bone defect site, it is very important to carefully incise the induced membrane longitudinally and use a Cobb or periosteal elevator to isolate the membrane off of the cement spacer.
- The spacer often needs to be fractured with an osteotome and removed piecemeal.
- Bone ends are gently debrided of any fibrous tissue, and if no intramedullary implant, the intramedullary canals are accessed with a flexible reamer or high-speed bur to assure continuity.
- With infection, the surgeon should maintain a high level of suspicion for persistent infection.
  - Intraoperative frozen section for high-powered fields can be done for an objective measure of continued infection.
  - In general, a finding of more than 5 to 10 WBC/HPF warrants consideration for irrigation and debridement with another 6-week cycle of cement spacer and intravenous antibiotics.
- When the bone defect site is clean with a nice induced membrane (**TECH FIG 3**), attention is turned to the intramedullary harvest of autogenous bone graft using RIA.

Inserting the Guidewire

- A large C-arm fluoroscopy positioned on the opposite side of the patient is used to localize the top of the greater trochanter.

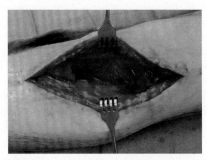

TECH FIG 3 • Clean bone defect after removal of the cement spacer. The defect is contained by the induced membrane.

- A 3- to 4-cm incision is made approximately 5 cm proximal and 2 cm posterior to the midline of the greater trochanter.
- A 3.2-mm guide pin is positioned at the tip of the greater trochanter on AP fluoroscopy and in the midline of the greater trochanter on the lateral view. The guide pin should aim for the center of the intramedullary canal at the level of the lesser trochanter (**TECH FIG 4**).
- Once the guide pin is driven 5 to 6 cm into the bone and the position confirmed on fluoroscopy, the skin and deep fascia are incised with a scalpel around the guide pin to cannulate the guide pin with a soft tissue protector.
- A 12-mm cannulated reamer is used through a soft tissue protector to drill 3 to 4 cm into the greater trochanter to create a start site.
  - The power source should be set to "drill," and the surgeon should allow the drill to spin at full speed before contacting greater trochanter bone. This will create a clean entry site.
  - Limited entry into the bone will allow more bone to be harvested.

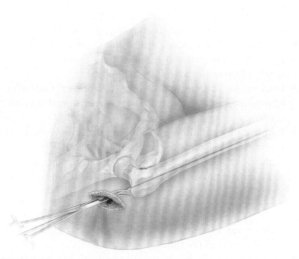

TECH FIG 4 • Illustration of the antegrade start site for RIA bone graft harvest. The guide pin is placed in-line with the center of the femoral canal.

- A 2.5 mm diameter, 950 mm in length, ball-tipped guide-wire is placed through the greater trochanter start site and inserted down the intramedullary canal of the femur to roughly 2 to 3 cm above the physeal scar of the distal femur.
  - AP and lateral fluoroscopy is undertaken to assure the guidewire is within the intramedullary canal.
  - A T-chuck handle may be placed onto the guidewire and gently tapped with a mallet to aid the guidewire passing through the metaphyseal bone of the proximal femur.
- A slight bend is often required in the distal aspect of the guidewire to direct the guidewire into a center-center position in the distal femur.
  - This helps avoid eccentric reaming and minimizes the risk of cortical perforation by the sharp reamer head.
- Measure the length of the guidewire within the femur to select the proper length of the RIA drive shaft. Length options are 360 and 520 mm.

Preparing the RIA

- The RIA system comes with a ruler that overlay the patient's skin (**TECH FIG 5A**).
  - With intraoperative fluoroscopy, the inner isthmic diameter of the femur in both AP and lateral planes can be measured to determine the size of the reamer head needed to obtain the necessary volume of bone graft.

- The intramedullary canal is often elliptical, and one measure will be smaller than the other.
  - A reamer head that is 1 to 1.5 mm larger than the smallest isthmic diameter is recommended.
  - Reamer heads are available in 12 to 19 mm diameters.
- As noted earlier, measurement of the isthmus at the skin level by intraoperative fluoroscopy requires a correction for magnification. The actual size of the isthmus is larger than the measurement. This is important when selecting the size of the reamer head.
- On a separate Mayo stand, the RIA device is assembled according to manufacturer specifications (**TECH FIG 5B**).
  - The reamer head is front-end cutting and sharp. The surgeon should assure several things: that the reamer head is mated correctly with the drive shaft, that the rubber seal is placed over the proximal drive shaft before it is connected to the power source, and that the plastic casing protecting the rotating connection between the power source and the drive shaft is locked into place.
  - Connect irrigation to RIA, it is the most proximal, smaller port labeled "I."
  - Connect suction to RIA. It is the most distal, larger port labeled "A."
  - Attach the 100-cc filter to the suction ("A" port). This has a particulate filter of 500 μm to capture the viscous autogenous bone graft.
  - Place the power source on the "drill" setting during reaming to allow for high speed and low torque.
- A 3-L bag of normal saline should be placed 3 ft. or higher above the RIA device to allow adequate gravity flow. The suction tubing should be attached to a closed, continuous suction canister with a large reservoir.

Reaming the Graft Material

- Test the RIA device on the Mayo stand outside of the patient by starting the irrigation and suction. Activate the power source to assure the reamer tip is properly revolving.
- The RIA system is single pass and continuously irrigates and suctions within the intramedullary canal. This decreases intramedullary temperatures and decreases viscosity of the graft.
- Place the RIA system over the guidewire. Before entering the patient, verify flow of irrigation. Insert the device through the soft tissue protection sleeve and turn on suction when the reamer head is set into the insertion site at the greater trochanter.

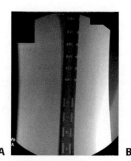
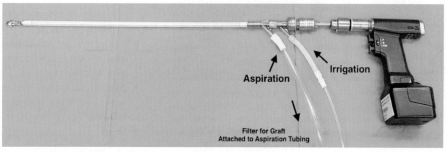

TECH FIG 5 • **A.** Intraoperative measurement of the femur isthmus using fluoroscopy. **B.** The reamer-irrigator-aspirator (RIA) device. The ports for fluid inflow and outflow are labeled. The aspiration port connects to a filter that captures the intramedullary bone graft.

- Before starting, warn anesthesia about possible blood loss due to the negative pressure suction.
- The power source should be fully activated.
- RIA is propagated through an advance-withdraw technique every 2 to 3 cm to avoid clogging of the aspiration tubing by particulate graft (**TECH FIG 6A**).
  - The surgeon should move slowly through the isthmus to allow time for appropriate emulsification of the graft (**TECH FIG 6B**). It is important not to forcibly push through resistance as incarceration of the reamer head or clogging of the aspiration tubing may occur.
- Fluoroscopy should be used liberally during active reaming to monitor the position of the reamer head.
  - The surgeon should continually assess for eccentric reaming, which most commonly takes place in the medial proximal femur and distal anterior femur.
  - It bears repeating that the surgeon must take great care to avoid incarceration of the reamer head at the isthmus and perforation of the anterior cortex as well as the knee joint distally.
- When reaming distally in the femur, a lateral fluoroscopic view is recommended to assess for perforation of the anterior femoral cortex.
- Aspiration tubing should be periodically checked to assure flow of bone graft and to assure the line is not clogged.
- When actively reaming, both irrigation and suction should be turned on. When reaming is paused, both lines should be stopped to avoid excessive blood loss.
- To obtain more graft volume, the surgeon can rotate the guidewire to capture the metaphyseal bone in the medial and lateral aspects of the distal femur.
- The RIA system should continue to be fully activated while withdrawing the drive shaft from the femur. If this is difficult, the surgeon can reverse the direction of the reamer head to facilitate removal.

Completion of Reaming

- When the reamer tip is back at the top of the greater trochanter, turn off suction and irrigation. The device is removed.
- Pack the proximal femur skin incision with gauze or a hemostatic agent.

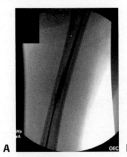 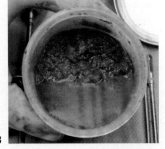

TECH FIG 6 • A. Use of intraoperative fluoroscopy to follow the reamer head during RIA bone graft harvest. It is important to assure that the sharp reamer head remains central in the intramedullary canal. **B.** Appearance of RIA autogenous bone graft after harvest.

- View the collection canister, which has markings on the outside to estimate the volume of graft obtained.
- If more graft is needed, upsize the reamer head by 0.5 to 1 mm and perform another pass down the femur. Generally, one to two passes are sufficient.
- Once graft volume is adequate, disconnect the collection canister, and move it over the sterile operating room table.
- Remove the lid, and use a plunger to compress the graft.
- Invert the filter with the plunger in place to remove the inner filter. Turn the inner filter vertical, and use the plunger to remove the graft into a sterile basin.

Harvesting Bone Marrow

- Fresh bone marrow is then obtained by palpating the medius pillar of the ilium.
- Thumb pressure can be used to push soft tissues toward the abdomen to feel the thickness of the pillar.
- A small skin puncture with a no. 11 blade scalpel is made over the medius pillar.
- A disposable 14-gauge T-handle bone marrow biopsy needle is introduced. Tactile feel is used to center over the medius pillar bone (**TECH FIG 7**).
- Gentle, sustained pressure is applied with a back and forth rotation to puncture the bone and gain access to the marrow space between the inner and outer shelves of the ilium. The needle is generally inserted around 3 cm.
- The top of the T-handle is rotated 90 degrees to remove the stylet. A 12- or 20-mL syringe is engaged to the Luerlock to aspirate bone marrow. The amount of bone marrow needed is proportional to the size of the defect. The goal is to saturate the final volume of bone graft.
- The syringe of bone marrow aspirate is disconnected, and the needle is withdrawn. Pressure is applied to the puncture site for 5 to 10 minutes, and a Steri-Strip is placed over the puncture site.

Graft Placement

- The autogenous intramedullary bone graft and bone marrow aspirate are mixed together in a sterile basin.
- The graft is extended with 1- to 4-mm cancellous allograft and demineralized bone matrix to create an appropriate graft consistency and to achieve adequate volume. The goal consistency is equivalent to gritty toothpaste.
- The recipient bone defect undergoes a final low-pressure irrigation.
- The bone graft mixture is packed into the defect with thumb pressure. Avoid dense packing of the graft with instruments such as a bone tamp.
  - Highly compacted graft does not incorporate as well (**TECH FIG 8A–D**).
- Suture the induced membrane closed (Video 1). This should completely cover the graft as it prevents resorption and promotes the formation of the cortical bone.
- All surgical sites should be closed in layers. Suture for skin closure is at the discretion of the surgeon (**TECH FIG 8E**).
- Sterile dressings are applied.

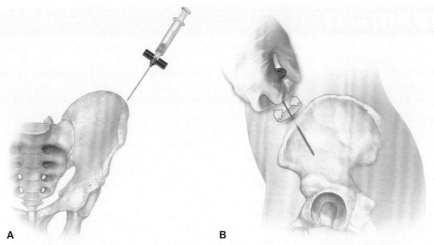

TECH FIG 7 • A. Bone marrow biopsy needle insertion site in the medius pillar of the pelvis. **B.** The needle is gently twisted back and forth as it is inserted.

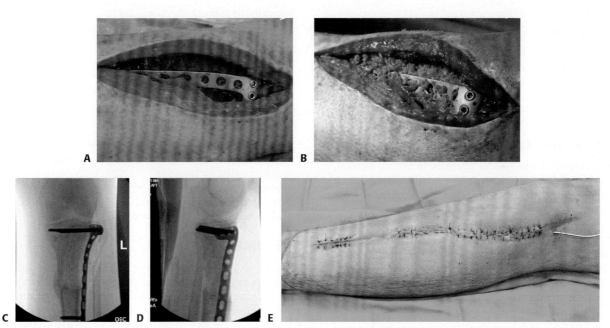

TECH FIG 8 • A,B. The bone defect is filled with bone graft with fresh bone marrow aspirate. The graft completely fills the defect, but impaction of the graft is avoided. In a different patient, **(C)** intraoperative AP and **(D)** lateral fluoroscopic views of the proximal tibia filled with autogenous bone graft and stabilized with a lateral plate. **E.** Skin closure after RIA bone grafting and stabilization into a defect with an induced membrane.

PEARLS AND PITFALLS

Bone graft harvest	▪ Try to harvest RIA from the femur ipsilateral to the bone defect. This maintains an unaffected lower extremity to facilitate postoperative rehabilitation.
	▪ While using RIA, keep the filter for the bone graft in a vertical position to avoid over washing and loss of growth factors.
	▪ When finished with RIA, disconnect the irrigation and aspiration tubing to avoid unsterile tubing coming up to the sterile field and causing contamination.
Union	▪ Central graft often remains avascular; the use of a nail or resorbable mesh to maintain the native intramedullary canal helps limit graft volume and improves the formation of cortical bone[8].
	▪ Bone stabilization with an intramedullary implant is preferred as this preserves the native medullary canal and helps to prevent the lack of incorporation seen in central graft in larger bone defects[8]. This is not always possible, however, and plate fixation may be necessary based on the defect itself (**FIG 4**).
Fracture	▪ Consider restricted weight bearing or placement of a prophylactic intramedullary nail after RIA use. Especially if the donor bone has narrow cortices or the patient is osteopenic or osteoporotic.[3]
	▪ Consider use of iliac crest bone grafting in osteoporotic patients.
	▪ Fluoroscopy in orthogonal planes is useful to assure a proper start site for RIA harvest and to assess cortical thickness of the femur after RIA use.
	▪ A greater trochanter start site for RIA harvest minimizes the reamer entry angle and decreases the risk of postoperative femoral neck fracture.
	▪ Reaming ≥ 2 mm of the inner diameter of the femoral isthmus decreases the torsional strength of the femur.
	▪ It is important to place the guidewire for RIA bone graft harvest in the center of the intramedullary canal to avoid eccentric reaming of the femoral cortex.
Blood loss	▪ RIA suction can lead to rapid blood loss. It is important to communicate this to anesthesia.
	▪ Patients should be typed and crossed before starting the procedure.
	▪ Stop RIA suction when not actively reaming.[5]
	▪ Pack the hip incision at the conclusion of RIA use to avoid a gluteal hematoma.
RIA irrigation water	▪ Filtrate water contains viable cells including mesenchymal stem cells.[10]
	▪ Adding filtrate to the harvested bone graft may improve incorporation and corticalization.

POSTOPERATIVE CARE

▪ Weight-bearing restrictions for the bone defect are advised. The length of time depends on the size of the bone defect, implant use, graft harvest technique, and patient bone stock. Implementation is at the discretion of the surgeon and is determined on a case-by-case basis.

▪ Restrictions for the bone graft harvest site are generally advised if multiple RIA passes are performed or thin femoral cortices are noted at the end of the procedure.

▪ A knee immobilizer is often used for 2 weeks to facilitate soft tissue healing. Physical therapy is then started to work on knee joint range of motion.

▪ First radiographs are done 6 weeks from surgery (**FIG 5**). Serial radiographs are used to assess the incorporation of bone graft.

▪ Bone defects stabilized with an intramedullary implant can often start partial progressive weight bearing at 3 to 4 months after surgery.

▪ Computed tomography can be used to further investigate bone graft incorporation and determine the necessity of additional bone grafting procedures.

OUTCOMES

▪ Union of a bone defect after autogenous bone grafting appears to be independent of defect length.[11] Defects up to 25 cm have been addressed with this technique (Norris).

▪ Radiographic healing is often seen by 4 months.

▪ Approximately 70% of defects heal by 6 months and 80% heal by 1 year.[1]

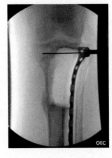

FIG 4 • Fluoroscopic image showing stabilization of a proximal femur bone defect with a 4.5-mm periarticular plate. The small amount of residual bone at the joint level did not allow for an intramedullary implant.

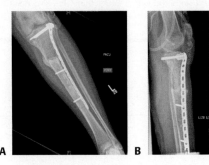

FIG 5 • **A.** AP and **(B)** lateral radiographs of the bone defect after definitive bone grafting with autogenous, intramedullary bone graft with graft extension and fresh bone marrow aspirate.

- Approximately 50% of patients heal with just one bone grafting procedure, 35% heal with more than one bone grafting procedure (McCall).
- Long-term donor site morbidity is less with RIA harvest compared to iliac crest bone graft harvest.[4,12]

COMPLICATIONS

- The complication rate with RIA harvest is 1.96% to 6.2%.[3,4]
- Iatrogenic fracture of the femur from RIA harvest is the most common complication, and it is related to technical aspects of the procedure including poor start site, eccentric reaming, and over-reaming.
- After RIA harvest, the femur is weakest in torsion.
- Femoral shaft fracture, femoral neck fracture, and anterior cortical perforation of the femur are described complications with RIA harvest.
- Heterotopic ossification of the abductors can be seen at the RIA start site and is generally asymptomatic.
- Problems encountered at the bone defect site include deep infection, nonunion, and implant loosening/failure.
- Nonunion rate is approximately 15%; causative factors include inadequate graft volume, suboptimal graft placement, and infection.[8]

REFERENCES

1. Stafford PR, Norris BL. Reamer-irrigator-aspirator bone graft and bi Masquelet technique for segmental bone defect nonunions: a review of 25 cases. *Injury.* 2010;S2:S72-S77.
2. Pelissier P, Masquelet A, Lepreux S, et al. Behavior of cancellous bong graft placed in induced membranes. *Br J Plast Surg.* 2002;55:598-600.
3. Lowe JA, Della Rocca GJ, Murtha Y, et al. Complications associated with negative pressure reaming for harvesting autologous bone graft: a case series. *J Orthop Trauma.* 2010;24:46-52.
4. Qvick LM, Ritter CA, Mutty CE, et al. Donor site morbidity with reamer-irrigator-aspirator (RIA) use for autogenous bone graft harvesting in single centre 204 case series. *Injury.* 2013;44:1263-1269.
5. Giannoudis PV, Tzioupis C, Green J. Surgical techniques: how I do it? The reamer/irrigator/aspirator (RIA) system. *Injury.* 2009;40:1231-1236.
6. Nauth A, Lane J, Watson JT, et al. Bone graft substitution and augmentation. *J Orthop Trauma.* 2015;29:S34-S38.
7. Schmidmaier G, Herrmann S, Green J, et al. Quantitative assessment of growth factors in reaming aspirate, iliac crest, and platelet preparation. *Bone.* 2006;38:1156-1163.
8. McCall T, Brokaw D, Jelen B, et al. Treatment of large segmental bone defects with reamer-irrigator-aspirator bone graft: technique and case series. *Orthop Clin North Am.* 2010;41:63-73.
9. Apard T, Bigorre N, Cronier P, et al. Two-stage reconstruction of post-traumatic segmental tibia bone loss with nailing. *Orthop Traumatol Surg Res.* 2010;96:549-553.
10. Cox G, Jones E, McGonagle D, et al. Reamer-irrigator-aspirator Indications and Clinical Results: a systematic review. *Int Orthop.* 2011;35:951-956.
11. Myeroff C, Archdeacon M. Current concepts review. Autogenous bone graft: donor sites and techniques. *J Bone Joint Surg Am.* 2011;93:2227-2236.
12. Belthur M, Conway J, Jindal G, et al. Bone graft harvest using a new intramedullary system. *Clin Orthop Relat Res.* 2008;466:2973-2980.

32 CHAPTER

Soft Tissue Coverage of the Knee: Gastrocnemius Muscle Flap

Hani Sbitany

DEFINITION

- Soft tissue defects around the knee, or the anterior third of the tibia, often cannot be treated with local fasciocutaneous flaps; instead, the most reliable local/regional coverage option is the rotational gastrocnemius muscle flap.[1]
- This is taken as a pure muscle flap, and in defects that include skin loss, the muscle is immediately skin grafted.
- This rotational muscle flap is well perfused, given its axial blood supply, and provides excellent soft tissue coverage and reliable reconstruction of defects involving the underlying bone, tendon, or exposed surgical hardware.[2]

ANATOMY

- The gastrocnemius is a bipennate muscle, located in the superficial posterior compartment of the lower extremity.
  - Other muscles in this compartment include the soleus muscle and plantaris muscle.
  - These muscles come together, via their common insertion in the posterior surface of the calcaneus, to create the Achilles tendon.
  - These muscles act to cause flexion of the ankle, when the knee is extended.
- The gastrocnemius muscle is the most superficial of these muscles, situated just deep to the posterior calf skin and subcutaneous tissue, and consists of a medial and lateral muscle head.
- The blood supply to these gastrocnemius muscles comes from the sural artery and vein, which are direct branches from the popliteal vessels; the motor nerve innervation derives from the tibial nerve.
- The medial and lateral heads of the gastrocnemius muscles can be separated from each other at their midline confluence, and each muscle belly can be isolated on its medial or lateral sural vessel pedicle, respectively.
- The medial head of the gastrocnemius muscle is usually longer and wider than the lateral head and thus has a greater arc of rotation and reach as a rotational flap; for this reason, the medial head is most commonly harvested for proximal lower extremity reconstruction.[3]
- Because the Achilles tendon is made up of contribution from all four muscles in the superficial posterior compartment, the ankle can still safely flex following harvest of one belly of the gastrocnemius muscle.

PATHOGENESIS

- As stated, the gastrocnemius rotational muscle flap is most commonly used for soft tissue reconstruction of defects situation around the knee or the proximal third of the tibia.

- There are many possible causes of defects in this region:
  - Traumatic wounds
  - Oncologic resection wounds
  - Soft tissue infection/necrotizing fasciitis
  - Burn, or burn contracture release, wounds
  - Breakdown of surgical wound after total knee arthroplasty
    - These wounds often contain exposed surgical hardware.
  - Breakdown of wound following patella or patellar tendon repair

PATIENT HISTORY AND PHYSICAL FINDINGS

- The cause and chronicity of the soft tissue wound in this area must be carefully defined.
- The patient must be questioned for a history of prior lower extremity surgery or injury along the entire limb that may have altered soft tissue anatomy or neurovascular supply.
- The specific wound location and size must be recorded and examined carefully to ensure that a rotational gastrocnemius muscle flap will adequately reach this wound with minimal tension.[4]
  - With the patient contracting the calf muscles, and flexing the ankle, the distal portion of the gastrocnemius muscle belly can be visualized or palpated, and this is the point that should be used in assessing muscle flap reach.
  - If this is not the case, then free tissue transfer must be considered.
- Physical examination of the knee and ankle must be performed, with range of motion being carefully assessed.
  - Range of motion at the knee (normal 135 degrees) must be defined, along with confirmation of normal flexion in all positions.
  - Range of motion at the ankle (normal 70 degrees) must be defined, along with normal flexion with the knee extended.
- If exam reveals normal findings, then rotational medial or lateral gastrocnemius muscle flap is safe.

IMAGING

- Routine imaging of the lower extremity is not necessary prior to gastrocnemius rotational muscle flap.
- If the patient has a history of peripheral vascular disease, a preoperative angiogram or CT angiogram can be obtained, to assess patency of popliteal and sural arteries.
- If the patient has a history of deep vein thrombosis, or venous insufficiency, then lower extremity venogram can be performed.

SURGICAL MANAGEMENT
Preoperative Planning

- Once the gastrocnemius muscle flap has been chosen as the reconstructive option, the surgeon must determine location of the muscle flap donor incision.
  - In most cases, for knee defects (anterior, lateral, or medial knee), the muscle harvest incision is separate from the wound being reconstructed, and the muscle is tunneled underneath the intervening skin bridge.
  - For wounds over the proximal third of the anterior tibia, it is common to extend the harvest incision from the defect, so that they are in continuity.

Positioning

- The patient is most commonly placed in a supine position on the operative table.
  - In some cases, based on wound location and dimensions, it is easier to harvest with the patient in a lateral decubitus position, and this is also acceptable.
  - When the patient is supine, the entire lower extremity should be circumferentially prepped into the operative field, such that the leg can be moved and manipulated during surgery.
  - This allows for placement of the leg in a "frog-leg" position, with the knee flexed and turned out, and the foot brought in such that its plantar surface is against the contralateral lower extremity.
  - This allows for easier harvest of the medial gastrocnemius muscle.

- It is also advisable to again check the arc of rotation and the reach of the gastrocnemius muscle, relative to the wound, to ensure successful soft tissue coverage, once the patient is positioned on the table.

Approach

- The incision is planned as a longitudinal incision of 10 to 15 cm length.
  - For the medial or lateral gastrocnemius muscle flap, the anterior border of the muscle is palpated through the skin and marked along its entire length.
  - The incision can be planned along this same longitudinal direction, usually one or two finger breadths posterior to this point, such that the muscle will be directly underneath the entire length of the incision, but it is still anterior enough that the harvest can easily proceed with the patient supine, and the legs in the "frog-leg" orientation.
- This incision location and length are adequate for the following necessary sites of surgical exposure:
  - Proximal exposure of the popliteal region and the sural vessel pedicle
  - Posterior exposure of the confluence between the medial and lateral gastrocnemius muscles
  - Distal exposure of the Achilles tendon
- The entire incision is made for muscle flap harvest, and dissection proceeds down through the skin, subcutaneous tissue, and superficial fascia, to enter the superficial posterior compartment of the leg.
- During this portion of dissection, when harvesting the medial gastrocnemius muscle, the saphenous vein should be identified and preserved.

■ Elevation of the Gastrocnemius Muscle Flap

- The entire incision is made for muscle flap harvest, and dissection proceeds down through the skin, subcutaneous tissue, and superficial fascia, to enter the superficial posterior compartment of the leg.
- During this portion of dissection, when harvesting the medial gastrocnemius muscle, the saphenous vein should be identified and preserved. Once the posterior compartment is entered, the gastrocnemius muscle is immediately encountered along its posterior/superficial surface.
- The entire muscle belly should then be free from the entire deep surface of the posterior fascia overlying it (**TECH FIG 1A**).
  - This should be a relatively hemostatic dissection that can be done sharply or bluntly, as this plane between gastrocnemius muscle and overlying fascia is largely avascular loose areolar tissue.
- Once this has been done, the free border of the muscle, either medial or lateral, should then be identified along its entire length and used as the access point to dissect the deep surface of the muscle belly (**TECH FIG 1B**).
  - This space is entered, and the gastrocnemius muscle is dissected free from the underlying, deeper soleus muscle.
  - In this plane, the plantaris muscle and tendon (long and thin) will be encountered and should also be preserved (if present).

- This deep dissection can be performed along the entire longitudinal length of the muscle, distally to the point of the Achilles tendon.
  - This dissection can stop at the point of confluence of the medial and lateral gastrocnemius muscles, along their deep surface, as only the half of the muscle being dissected will be elevated as a flap.
- At this point, surgical dissection should have fully freed up the deep and superficial/posterior surfaces of the gastrocnemius muscle belly (**TECH FIG 1C**).
- Next, the muscle will be elevated in a distal to proximal direction, moving up the leg.
- First, the muscle belly to be elevated is horizontally detached above the start of the Achilles tendon.
  - It is critical that the Achilles tendon not be disturbed and the entire fascial contribution of the gastrocnemius muscle within the Achilles tendon remains intact.
  - Thus, the muscle is transected one fingerbreadth above the point where the tendons of all the muscles in this compartment join to form the Achilles.
  - At this point, the gastrocnemius muscle will contain some tendon, and this can be used for suture anchoring on inset of the muscle flap in the defect.
- Next, the half of the gastrocnemius muscle being elevated then is lifted in a distal to proximal direction, by separating the medial and lateral gastrocnemius muscles from each other (the last remaining point of attachment).

T E C H N I Q U E S

- This area must be carefully identified along its entire length based on changing directionality of muscle fibers (**TECH FIG 1D**).
- Often times, this point between the medial and lateral heads of the gastrocnemius muscles is not a distinct plane, and thus, separation should be performed with electrocautery to minimize bleeding.
- Numerous minor perforators exist between the medial and lateral heads of the muscle, and these must be ligated.

- This elevation of the muscle in the proximal direction, by separating the two halves of the gastrocnemius, should be performed just beyond the point at which the freed muscle can rotate into the defect with no tension or stretch (**TECH FIG 1E**).
  - Often times, the dissection can stop well before the point where the sural vessels enter the deep surface of the muscle, as elevation to this point is not necessary for adequate rotation.[5]
  - In such cases, the sural vessels are never directly visualized, and this will reduce risk of vascular pedicle injury.
  - However, if necessary for adequate muscle rotation, dissection can proceed to this point, and the sural vessels can be identified, dissected free, and preserved.
  - In some cases, due to the need for excessive rotation, the muscle origin on the femoral condyle can be identified and transected.

- This will result in a significant increase in muscle rotation and length of transposition.
- Without the stability of the muscle insertion to prevent excess stretch on the sural vessels, they must be carefully watched during rotation and inset, to avoid excess tension and possible vascular traction injury or avulsion.

- Once the muscle has been fully dissected and elevated, it can then be rotated into the soft tissue defect (**TECH FIG 1F**).
  - If the muscle is tunneled underneath a planned skin bridge, it must be ensured that the skin bridge is not excessively tight or compressive on the underlying muscle flap.
- The muscle is usually inset with the previous posterior/ superficial surface of the muscle belly externalized in the wound, as this portion of the muscle does not contain aponeurosis or fascia and thus accepts a skin graft well.
- The muscle is then inset into the soft tissue defects and secured circumferentially to the lower extremity skin and subcutaneous tissue with sutures (**TECH FIG 1G**).
  - The proximal portion of the muscle, in the area of the sural vessels, should then be again examined after inset, to ensure no tension or stretch on this area.
- Finally, a skin graft can be placed on the superficial surface of the muscle flap at this point.
- The donor site can then be closed primarily over a drain, at the fascia and skin level.

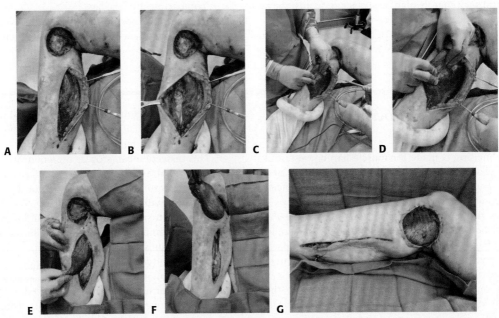

TECH FIG 1 • A. Patient with a medial knee soft tissue wound, adequately debrided, and ready for soft tissue reconstruction. Planned medial gastrocnemius muscle flap is exposed through longitudinal incision shown. Posterior leg skin, subcutaneous tissue, and fascia have been elevated off the superficial surface of the muscle flap. **B.** Dissection of the deep surface of the gastrocnemius muscle flap from the underlying soleus muscle. The aponeurosis of the soleus muscle is visible deep to the gastrocnemius muscle. The plantaris tendon is visible distally in the donor site and runs along the border of the gastrocnemius muscle. **C.** Both the deep and superficial surfaces of the medial head of the gastrocnemius muscle have been fully dissected, and the muscle has more freedom of movement. **D.** The longitudinal midline border between the medial and lateral heads of the gastrocnemius muscle is visible, by its overlying streak of fat. This will be the point of separation of the two muscle bellies. **E.** Following transection of the medial gastrocnemius muscle proximal to the Achilles tendon, and separation of the medial and lateral bellies of the muscle in the midline, the medial gastrocnemius muscle flap has now been elevated. The vascularized soft tissue bulk (width and thickness) afforded by this flap is clearly visualized. **F.** The muscle flap passed under the skin bridge and into the soft tissue wound. The size and reach of the muscle provide adequate coverage for the wound. **G.** The medial gastrocnemius muscle flap, following complete inset into the wound. The muscle is well perfused, with no pressure or tension. At this point, the muscle belly can be skin grafted, and the donor site can be fully closed in primary fashion.

PEARLS AND PITFALLS

Muscle flap elevation	▪ The muscle flap only needs to be dissected proximally to the point where it can safely be rotated and inset into the wound, without tension; often times, complete elevation proximally to the sural vessel level is unnecessary and to avoid risk of vascular disruption.
Tunneling	▪ The tunnel or skin bridge that the muscle flap passes under must be relaxed and without underlying tightness, to avoid muscle flap congestion and flap loss; if necessary, the fascia on the underside of the tunnel skin can be incised to increase the size of the tunnel.
Long muscle transposition length	▪ In cases where the muscle flap must be advanced a long distance, it can be detached from the femoral condyle, to allow for a significant increase in reach; in these cases, the sural vessels must be continuously examined for a relaxed state without stretch, as they are no longer stabilized by the proximal muscle insertion.
Hemostasis	▪ Hemostasis is critical, in both the muscle donor site, and in the wound being reconstructed, as tension from a hematoma can occlude the venous outflow and result in muscle flap loss.

POSTOPERATIVE CARE

- Postoperatively, the lower extremity is placed in a stabilizing knee immobilizer.
    - This reduces muscle stretch or tension in the acute healing phase and reduces muscle flap edema.
    - During this period, the patient may be kept nonweight bearing if deemed necessary or may be placed on limited foot pressure on the effected extremity while ambulating with crutches.
    - Immobilization is usually kept on for 2 weeks, at which point the patient can begin knee flexion and normal ambulation (**FIG 1**).
- The skin graft can be covered for 5 to 7 days with either negative pressure therapy or with a bolster dressing.

COMPLICATIONS

- Hematoma

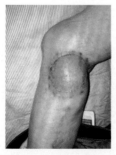

FIG 1 • Healed medial gastrocnemius muscle flap and overlying split thickness skin graft, 3 months after coverage operation in **TECH FIG 1**. Patient has stable soft tissue coverage and is ambulating without difficulty.

- Bleeding in either the donor site or the wound bed underneath the muscle flap must be treated immediately with hematoma evacuation, to avoid pressure on vascular pedicle and resultant muscle flap loss.
- Infection
    - Proper wound bed debridement and removal of all nonviable tissue prior to muscle flap coverage will reduce this risk.
    - When infection occurs, re-elevation of the muscle flap and aggressive washout should be performed.
- Flap loss
    - With complete flap loss, a secondary free flap often must be performed for wound coverage.
- Venous congestion
    - The entire flap must be elevated, and if congestion resolves, this usually indicates pressure or kinking on vascular pedicle, which must be resolved.
    - The tunnel must be checked for excessive tightness, and if this is the case, it can be opened with an incision and the muscle externalized in this area.

REFERENCES

1. McCraw JB, Fishman JH, Sharzer LA. The versatile gastrocnemius myocutaneous flap. *Plast Reconstr Surg.* 1978;62:15-23.
2. Arnold PG, Mixter RC. Making the most of the gastrocnemius muscles. *Plast Reconstr Surg.* 1983;72:38-48.
3. Hersh CK, Schenck RC, Williams RP. The versatility of the gastrocnemius muscle flap. *Am J Orthop.* 1995;24:218-222.
4. Verber M, Vaz G, Braye F, et al. Anatomical study of the medial gastrocnemius muscle flap: a quantitative assessment of the arc of rotation. *Plast Reconstr Surg.* 2011;128:181-187.
5. Daigeler A, Drücke D, Tatar K, et al. The pedicled gastrocnemius muscle flap: a review of 218 cases. *Plast Reconstr Surg.* 2009;123: 250-257.

33
CHAPTER

Soft Tissue Coverage of the Knee: Free Flaps

Goo-Hyun Mun and So Young Kim

DEFINITION

- Although most soft tissue and bony defects around the knee are usually covered with locoregional tissues, free flaps should be considered when the desired donor territory is damaged or unsuitable or if the defect is extensive or complex. Free flaps offer benefits such as shortened recovery time, plentiful availability of donor tissue, and greater flexibility in flap design.[1]
- Soft tissue defects of the knee can significantly influence gait; therefore, reconstruction should be done with proper planning and technique at an early onset.[2]
- Restoration of the thin and pliable skin for satisfactory appearance and function of the knee is an important reconstruction goal.

ANATOMY

- Popliteal vessels and vessels from the anterior knee can be recipients of microvascular free flap transfer for soft tissue coverage of knee defects.
- Recipient vessels for free flap.
  - Popliteal vessel and its branches (**FIG 1A**). The popliteal artery ranges from a proximal portion starting at the opening of the adductor canal to the distal portion lying behind the upper part of the tibia and fibula. The popliteal vessel and branches, including the superior medial

and lateral genicular vessels (**FIG 1B**), medial and lateral sural vessels (**FIG 1C**), middle genicular vessels, and inferior genicular vessels, are considered the choice of recipient vessels for a free flap in the knee region. However, the approach to the popliteal vessels can be difficult when the anterior surface of the knee is reconstructed, and sural vessels are difficult to use in a free tissue flap to the region proximal to the knee.[3] Furthermore, there is a risk of increased complications caused by compression and twisting of the flap blood vessels, depending upon the postsurgical position of the patient.

- Anterior knee (**FIG 2A**):
  - Three vessels, including the descending genicular vessel and its branches (**FIG 2B,C**), and the descending branches of the lateral circumflex femoral vessels (**FIG 2D**) and anterior tibial vessels are considered the choice of recipient vessels for a free tissue transfer for the anterior knee region.
  - These recipient candidates have several benefits with supine positioning and easy accessibility to the recipient vessel. However, these branches may be very small vessels and, if so, may be of limited value and less reliable.[3]
- The perforators along the intermuscular septum of the upper leg and lower thigh can be used as recipient vessels for free flap reconstruction of the knee, but also note that these vessels may be small.[4]

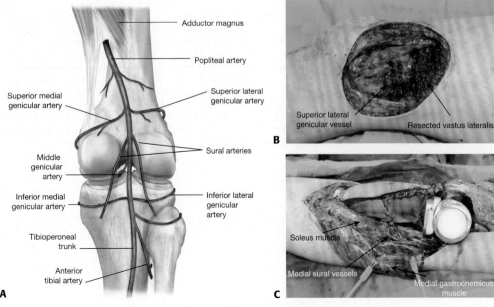

FIG 1 • A. Muscular boundaries and branches of the popliteal artery and deep neurovascular structures in the posterior knee. **B.** Superior lateral genicular vessel for recipient vessel. **C.** Medial sural vessel for recipient vessel.

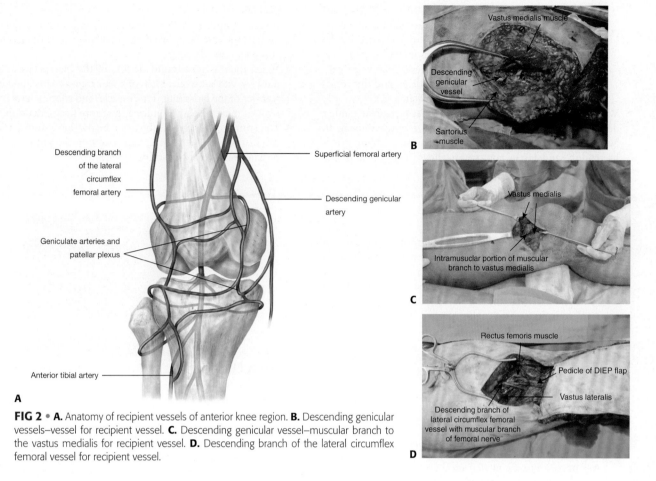

FIG 2 • A. Anatomy of recipient vessels of anterior knee region. **B.** Descending genicular vessels–vessel for recipient vessel. **C.** Descending genicular vessel–muscular branch to the vastus medialis for recipient vessel. **D.** Descending branch of the lateral circumflex femoral vessel for recipient vessel.

PATHOGENESIS

- Multiple prior operations and revision arthroplasties with atrophy/scarring of soft tissues
- Prior coverage of a total knee prosthesis and wound dehiscence due to infection
- Large post-traumatic defects
- Extensive soft tissue tumor excision
- Soft tissue necrosis and chronic infection after extremity radiation
- Necrotizing fasciitis and septic arthritis
- Burn scar contracture and post-traumatic stiff knee

PATIENT HISTORY AND PHYSICAL FINDINGS

- The patient history should focus on the exact mechanism and etiology of the defect.
- It is important to assess the medical history including vascular disease, systemic disease, and hypercoagulable state, which can influence the outcome of a microsurgical procedure.
- The preoperative evaluation for patients with a knee defect includes a detailed assessment of function limitations. The range of motion is a widely used measure of the knee joint, with a normal range of flexion of 45 to 105 degrees during routine activities and full extension to 0 degree.[5]

IMAGING

- The authors routinely perform preoperative computed tomography (CT) angiography of the lower extremity unless contraindicated to evaluate the regional vascular anatomy.
- Magnetic resonance imaging (MRI) can also be performed for evaluation of complex defects of soft tissue.

SURGICAL MANAGEMENT

- The proper selection of recipient vessels is essential for the success of a free flap and is arguably the most important factor that can affect the outcome.[4,6] Major considerations regarding the choice of appropriate recipient site for revascularizing the flap include performing the microanastomosis outside the zone of injury and avoiding the need for vein grafts.[7]
- Extending the incision from the defect is used when there is a suitable adjacent recipient; however, a separate incision with subcutaneous tunneling can be effective for a distant recipient vessel approach.
- Options of free flap:
  - Commonly chosen flaps for soft tissue reconstruction of knee defects are an anterolateral thigh (ALT) flap, rectus abdominis muscle flap, deep inferior epigastric artery perforator (DIEP) flap, tensor fascia lata flap, superficial

circumflex iliac artery perforator (SCIP) flap, latissimus dorsi musculocutaneous flap, and thoracodorsal artery perforator (TDAP) flap. The TDAP flap is favored by the authors because of several advantages including generous dimensions of the back, tissue thinness, relatively well-hidden donor scar, a long vascular pedicle, and the versatility offered by composite tissue transfer.

- When complex knee trauma accompanies a patellar tendon defect, the patellar tendon is traditionally restored using an autogenous graft, such as the semitendinosus tendon, gracilis tendon, and fascia lata, or an allograft. Because of the problem of delayed healing, fascia lata failure, and infection, a composite ALT myocutaneous flap with vascularized fascia lata can be utilized for one-stage reconstruction of complex knee defects.[8]

- When there is post-traumatic loss of the quadriceps femoris muscles with subsequent loss of knee extension, free functional transfer of the latissimus dorsi muscle[9] and contralateral rectus femoris muscle[10] can be utilized to restore knee extension.

- For stump coverage in above or below knee amputations, the distal placement of a flap to cover the entire weight-bearing surface of the stump is required.[11]

■ Wound Preparation

- The first goal of wound preparation is to debride all contaminated soft tissue or excise pathologic or necrotic lesions and to evaluate the extent of soft tissue defects in terms of size and components, including the bone, tendon, muscle, fascia, and skin (**TECH FIG 1**).
- A tourniquet is usually applied on the thigh during wound preparation.

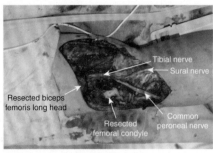

TECH FIG 1 • Wound preparation of posterior knee defect after tumor extirpation.

■ Recipient Vessel Preparation

- Approach to the medial sural artery
  - The procedure can be performed with the patient in prone or semilateral decubitus position, with the recipient extremity down and the opposite leg crossed anteriorly, with simultaneous access to the contralateral back as a donor site (**TECH FIG 2A**).
  - Arising from the posterior aspect of the popliteal vessel, the medial sural vessel enters the deep surface of the medial gastrocnemius muscle. Between the muscular head of the medial and lateral gastrocnemius, the medial sural vessel is easily approached[12] (**TECH FIG 2B**). A branch of the tibial nerve usually accompanies the dominant vascular pedicle to the gastrocnemius muscle and should be preserved.[7]
- Approach to the descending genicular artery and its branches
  - The procedure is performed with the patient in the supine position, with the knee flexed and the thigh rotated externally.
  - The descending genicular vessel is divided into three equal branches:
    - A muscular branch to the vastus medialis muscle
    - A terminal articular branch supplying the periosteum of the medial condyle
    - A saphenous (superficial) branch
  - After medial retraction of the sartorius muscle, the descending genicular vessel can be identified immediately posterior to the vastus medialis muscle[4] (see **FIG 2B**). The intramuscular portion of muscular

branch to the vastus medialis can be a candidate recipient vessel and is exposed through retrograde intramuscular dissection of a perforator overlying the vastus medialis[4] (see **FIG 2C**).

- Approach to the descending branch of the lateral circumflex femoral artery (LCFA)

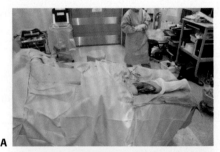

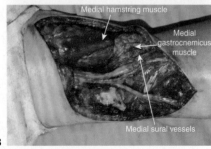

TECH FIG 2 • **A.** Lateral decubitus position with the recipient extremity down and the opposite leg scissored anteriorly for the approach to the medial sural artery. **B.** The medial sural vessel is prepared for the recipient vessel.

- The procedure can be performed in the supine position.
- The descending branch of the LCFA with adequate size as a recipient vessel can be found in an area 10 to 15 cm above the upper margin of the patella; therefore, a donor flap must have a long enough pedicle.[2] After separating the rectus femoris medially from the intermuscular septum between the vastus lateralis and the rectus femoris, the descending branch of the LCFA is exposed. It travels with the muscular branch of the femoral nerve along the anterior border of the vastus lateralis toward the knee joint (see **FIG 2D**).
- Approach to the superior medial and lateral genicular artery
  - The superior genicular vessels arise on either side of the popliteal fossa and wind around the femur immediately above its condyles to the front of the knee joint.[4]
  - In cases of a defect in the posterior knee, the superior medial genicular vessel is exposed after gentle retraction of the semimembranosus muscle at the level of the upper edge of the femoral condyle when the popliteal artery is in sight.[3]
  - The superior lateral genicular vessel is identified above the lateral condyle of the femur as it courses laterally beneath the short head of the biceps femoris and the vastus lateralis[13] (see **FIG 1B**).
- Selection of recipient vein
  - Because the use of an accompanying concomitant vein as the recipient has the benefit of straightforward insetting of the flap, the deep vein system is usually considered the first choice of a recipient vein for a free flap in the lower extremity.
  - However, in this anatomical area of the knee, a superficial vein such as the great saphenous vein passing medial to the medial femoral condyle is sometimes in a more convenient position and is a better size match for anastomosis than the deep vein system.[14]

Assessment of the Defect

- Because the knee is a large diarthrodial (synovial) joint with an extensive range of motion, free flaps in this region should provide ample skin coverage to allow unrestricted joint mobility in flexion and extension and to facilitate ambulation.[1,15]
- Final defect size and shape are exactly measured by making a transparent plastic or paper template that will be used for flap design. With the consideration both of minimizing restricted mobility of joint and avoiding redundancy of reconstructed flap, the measurement of anterior defect is usually conducted in slightly flexed knee status, and measurement of posterior defect is done in position of knee extension status.
- Dead space to be filled is also measured and accounted for in flap design/harvest.

Flap Harvest

- Outlines of the relevant muscle and other landmarks are drawn (**TECH FIG 3A**).
- Perforators are located using a handheld pencil Doppler, and the flap is designed using a template of the final defect.
- The targeted perforator(s) are identified by suprafascial dissection through a limited incision because the design of skin paddle could be potentially adjusted to capture the perforator securely within the flap, and then the whole skin paddle is elevated.
- Meticulous intramuscular dissection of the pedicle under loupe magnification with bipolar forceps is performed.
- A muscle chimeric perforator flap can be harvested as needed to fill dead space or to cover the artificial implant (**TECH FIG 3B**).
- Motor nerve branches to the muscle are maximally preserved during a perforator flap harvest, and the pedicle is divided when sufficient length is obtained.
- A closed suction drain is placed and the donor wound is primarily closed in layers (**TECH FIG 3C**).

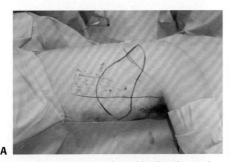
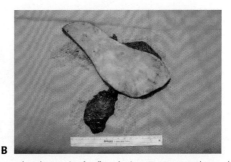

A   B

TECH FIG 3 • A. Outline of the relevant muscle and landmarks are drawn on the donor site for flap design. **B.** Harvested muscle chimeric TDAP flap.

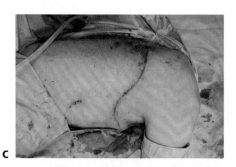

C

TECH FIG 3 (Continued) • **C.** Donor site that was primarily closed after flap harvest.

■ Microanastomosis with Temporary Inset

- Temporary inset of the flap is performed with a skin stapler.
- The vascular pedicle is comfortably laid to reach the recipient vessel without kinking, twisting, or tension. This is best accomplished by prudent preoperative planning and harvesting sufficient pedicle length.
- Wide exposure of the operative field and creation of a comfortable milieu are critical for successful microvascular anastomosis.

- Either end-to-end or end-to-side microanastomoses are performed and may depend on the size of the vessels.
- Vascular clamps are removed after completion of anastomoses. Warm saline is applied to the vessels and covered with moist gauzes for several minutes.
- After checking for patent arterial inflow and venous outflow, then perform careful hemostasis to evaluate for any bleeding points from the vascular pedicle or recipient vessels.

■ Final Inset

- Insetting of the flap is straightforward because it should have been harvested based on an exact template of the defect.
- The muscle component of a chimeric flap is placed to fill in dead space or to cover the prosthesis (**TECH FIG 4**).
- If the flap is too bulky, it may be thinned by carefully removing tissue from the deep fat layer and part of the superficial fat layer, except for a few centimeters of a cuff of subcutaneous tissue around the entry point of

the perforator(s). The use of loupe magnification or even the microscope may be advised to avoid damaging small blood vessels traveling through the fat.
- The wound is closed with placement of closed suction drains under the flap to prevent fluid collection (**TECH FIG 5**).
- A leg splint is applied for immobilization, and an elastic bandage is loosely applied so as to avoid compression over the vascular pedicle.
- Part of the flap is left open for postoperative monitoring of flap perfusion.

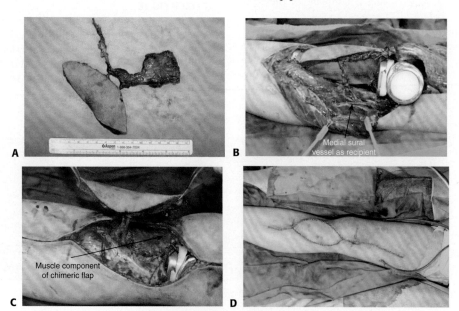

TECH FIG 4 • **A.** Harvested muscle chimeric perforator flap. **B.** After end-to-end microanastomoses to the corresponding vessels of the chosen free flap, exposed artificial bone and knee joint are seen in anterior knee. **C.** Muscle component of chimeric flap is arranged to cover the artificial implant. **D.** Transferred muscle chimeric TDAP flap in anterior knee after final inset, using the medial sural vessel as recipient.

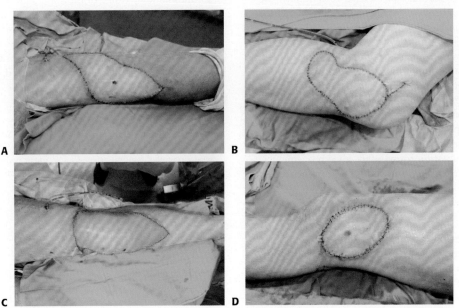

TECH FIG 5 • **A.** Transferred muscle chimeric TDAP flap in posterior knee after final inset, using the medial sural vessel as recipient. **B.** Transferred TDAP flap in medial knee after final inset, using muscular branch of the descending genicular vessel as recipient. **C.** Transferred DIEP flap in anterior knee after final inset, using muscular branch of the descending genicular vessel as recipient. **D.** Transferred TDAP flap in lateral knee after final inset, using the superolateral genicular vessel as recipient.

PEARLS AND PITFALLS

Planning	▪ Meticulous preoperative planning for recipient vessels, donor site, flap composition, and positioning of the patient is crucial for successful reconstruction. ▪ A multidisciplinary approach with comprehensive communication between oncologic and/or orthopedic surgeons will enable better treatment outcomes.
Selection of recipient vessel	▪ The recipient vessel option includes the descending genicular vessel and its branches, descending branch of lateral circumflex femoral vessel and anterior tibial vessel in the anterior knee, and superior medial and lateral genicular vessel, medial and lateral sural vessel, middle genicular vessel, and inferior genicular vessel in the popliteal area. Surgeons may choose a recipient vessel based on the proximity to the defect, concomitant injuries, vessel availability, and vessel size match. ▪ The deep vein system is usually considered as the first choice of recipient vein for a free flap in the lower extremity. However, in this anatomical area of the knee, a superficial vein such as the great saphenous vein is sometimes in a more convenient position and is a better size match for anastomosis than the deep vein system.
Assessment of the defects	▪ Free flaps in this region should provide ample skin coverage to allow unrestricted joint mobility in flexion and extension and to facilitate ambulation. ▪ Defect size and shape are exactly measured by making a template for subsequent flap design.
Microanastomosis and flap inset	▪ It is important to avoid twisting and kinking of the pedicle. ▪ Tension on the pedicle should be avoided and sufficient acquisition of pedicle length is a safe strategy. ▪ Defatting of the perforator flap at the time of inset is an effective technique to obtain aesthetic contour but must be performed carefully to avoid compromising blood supply.

POSTOPERATIVE CARE

▪ Most surgeons who perform free flaps in the lower extremity rely upon clinical observations including subjective visual inspection, capillary refill, turgor, and temperature of the flap, in combination with a handheld pencil Doppler for monitoring the flap.[16] The protocol varies according to surgeon, but the authors perform clinical assessment of flap status, combined with a handheld Doppler examination, every 3 hours for the first 48 hours and then every 6 hours for the next 48 hours after surgery.

▪ Although preferences regarding anticoagulation regimens vary widely among microvascular surgeons, medication for perioperative anticoagulation can be used to minimize the risk of postoperative thrombosis. The major classes include antiplatelet, heparin-based anticoagulant, and plasma expander drugs.

- Postoperatively, lower extremity edema and overly aggressive mobilization can compromise the free flap, especially causing venous congestion.[17] Although the duration of immobilization time varies based on the orthopedic injuries, generally progressive weight bearing and ambulation are achieved when the patient is tolerating dangling at least 30 minutes, six times per day.[17]

- Postoperative rehabilitation to maintain knee movement is an essential part of treatment and should be commenced in the early postoperative period.[15]

OUTCOMES

- Published success rates for free tissue transfers to the knee vary according to the etiology of the defect, but a microvascular free flap in this region is a safe procedure, with a success rate ranging from 97% to 100%.[1,15,18]

- A microvascular free flap is a reliable reconstructive option for defects of various sizes in various locations in the knee. The type of perforator flap, whether cutaneous or muscle chimeric (**FIG 3**), is selected according to tissue requirement.

COMPLICATIONS

- Vascular complications such as venous and arterial thrombosis
  - Prompt emergent exploration is demanded when these conditions are suspected.
- Hematoma
  - Early diagnosis of a hematoma under the flap is critical so that it can be evacuated promptly to prevent compression of the anastomotic site due to an expanding hematoma. Any time a postoperative hematoma is noted, the surgeon must suspect venous obstruction.
- Infection
  - When the defect accompanies an infected prosthesis and chronic infection of the bone or joint, a late infection or recurrence of infection after free tissue transfer can develop.[18,19] Therefore, it is critical that the wound be sufficiently debrided of necrotic, infected, or pathologic tissue before definitive flap reconstruction.

- Suboptimal knee range of motion
  - Suboptimal knee range of motion may result from increased periods of restricted knee extension followed by allowance of very limited knee range of motion during free flap maturation.[1] Therefore, early range of motion is advised once flap viability is established.

REFERENCES

1. Louer CR, Garcia RM, Earle SA, et al. Free flap reconstruction of the knee: an outcome study of 34 cases. *Ann Plast Surg.* 2015;74:57-63.
2. Kim JS, Lee HS, Jang PY, et al. Use of the descending branch of lateral circumflex femoral artery as a recipient pedicle for coverage of a knee defect with free flap: anatomical and clinical study. *Microsurgery.* 2010;30:32-36.
3. Park S, Eom JS. Selection of the recipient vessel in the free flap around the knee: the superior medial genicular vessels and the descending genicular vessels. *Plast Reconstr Surg.* 2001;107:1177-1182.
4. Fang T, Zhang EW, Lineaweaver WC, Zhang F. Recipient vessels in the free flap reconstruction around the knee. *Ann Plast Surg.* 2013;71:429-433.
5. Laubenthal KN, Smidt GL, Kettelkamp DB. A quantitative analysis of knee motion during activities of daily living. *Phys Ther.* 1972;52:34-43.
6. Basheer MH, Wilson SM, Lewis H, Herbert K. Microvascular free tissue transfer in reconstruction of the lower limb. *J Plast Reconstr Aesthet Surg.* 2008;61:525-528.
7. Hallock GG. The medial approach to the sural vessels to facilitate microanastomosis about the knee. *Ann Plast Surg.* 1994;32:388-393.
8. Yagi Y, Ueda K, Shirakabe M, et al. Reconstruction of knee ligaments with a free tensor fascia lata myocutaneous flap transfer. *Br J Plast Surg.* 2002;55:155-157.
9. Hallock GG. Restoration of quadriceps femoris function with a dynamic microsurgical free latissimus dorsi muscle transfer. *Ann Plast Surg.* 2004;52:89-92.
10. Wechselberger G, Ninkovic M, Pulzl P, Schoeller T. Free functional rectus femoris muscle transfer for restoration of knee extension and defect coverage after trauma. *J Plast Reconstr Aesthet Surg.* 2006;59:994-998.
11. Higgins JP. Descending geniculate artery: the ideal recipient vessel for free tissue transfer coverage of below-the-knee amputation wounds. *J Reconstr Microsurg.* 2011;27:525-529.
12. Beumer JD, Karoo R, Caplash Y, et al. The medial sural artery as recipient vessel and the impact on the medial gastrocnemius. *Ann Plast Surg.* 2011;67:382-386.
13. Wiedner M, Koch H, Scharnagl E. The superior lateral genicular artery flap for soft-tissue reconstruction around the knee: clinical experience and review of the literature. *Ann Plast Surg.* 2011;66:388-392.
14. Lorenzo AR, Lin CH, Lin CH, et al. Selection of the recipient vein in microvascular flap reconstruction of the lower extremity: analysis of 362 free-tissue transfers. *J Plast Reconstr Aesthet Surg.* 2011;64:649-655.
15. Ulusal AE, Ulusal BG, Lin YT, Lin CH. The advantages of free tissue transfer in the treatment of posttraumatic stiff knee. *Plast Reconstr Surg.* 2007;119:203-210.
16. Xipoleas G, Levine E, Silver L, et al. A survey of microvascular protocols for lower extremity free tissue transfer II: postoperative care. *Ann Plast Surg.* 2008;61:280-284.
17. Rohde C, Howell BW, Buncke GM, et al. A recommended protocol for the immediate postoperative care of lower extremity free-flap reconstructions. *J Reconstr Microsurg.* 2009;25:15-19.
18. Cetrulo CL Jr, Shiba T, Friel MT, et al. Management of exposed total knee prostheses with microvascular tissue transfer. *Microsurgery.* 2008;28:617-622.
19. Hierner R, Reynders-Frederix P, Bellemans J, et al. Free myocutaneous latissimus dorsi flap transfer in total knee arthroplasty. *J Plast Reconstr Aesthet Surg.* 2009;62:1692-1700.

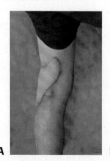 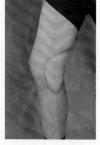

A   **B**

FIG 3 • **A,B.** Satisfactory result of muscle-chimeric free flap to the posterior knee defect.

Repair of Patella Tendon

Patrick Horrigan, Michael Bellino, and Julius Bishop

DEFINITION

- Rupture of the patellar tendon is a disruption of the knee extensor mechanism between the patella and the tibial tubercle.
- Complete ruptures cause significant disability, pain, hemarthrosis, and an inability to extend the knee.
- Prompt treatment nearly always involves surgery and early motion during rehabilitation.
- Missed or delayed diagnosis and treatment can result in significant pain and dysfunction.[1]

ANATOMY

- The patellar tendon is a continuation of the quadriceps tendon, a confluence of the vastus medialis, intermedius, and lateralis tendons and the rectus femoris tendon. It is derived primarily from extending fibers of rectus femoris traversing the anterior surface of the patella.
- The tendon itself consists of 90% type I collagen. Its fibers are arranged longitudinally relative to the axis of the lower extremity.
  - It measures approximately 32 mm in width and narrows by several millimeters near its insertion on the tibial tubercle.
  - Its thickness in normal knees is approximately 6 mm at its proximal extent and 6 mm distally.[2,3]
- The blood supply of the patellar tendon is derived from the inferior genicular arteries proximally and from the anterior tibial recurrent artery distally. It shares a portion of its blood supply posteriorly with the infrapatellar fat pad.[3,4]

PATHOGENESIS

- Because degenerative changes are present in most cases, tendinopathy is increasingly given the primary pathogenic role in rupture.[5]
- Rupture can also occur in the setting of direct trauma, recent corticosteroid injections for tendonitis, and systemic disease (patients with chronic acidosis or nephropathy requiring hemodialysis, systemic lupus erythematosus).[6]
- A classic described mechanism is forceful contraction of the quadriceps musculature with the knee in greater than 45 degrees of flexion.[7]

PATIENT HISTORY AND PHYSICAL FINDINGS

- Patients will typically describe an acute popping or tearing sensation during a brief period of forceful quadriceps contraction. This is often followed by acute-onset knee pain, swelling, and inability to bear weight.

- A palpable infrapatellar defect around a swollen joint can sometimes be appreciated on the symptomatic knee.

IMAGING

- Plain anteroposterior and lateral radiographs of the knee are usually sufficient for diagnosis of patella tendon rupture (**FIG 1**).[7]
- In cases of uncertain physical examination, MRI or ultrasonography may be useful for confirmation of diagnosis.

DIFFERENTIAL DIAGNOSIS

- Quadriceps tendon rupture
- Patella fracture
- Medial/lateral collateral ligament rupture
- Anterior cruciate ligament rupture
- Meniscus tear
- Patellar dislocation/subluxation event

NONOPERATIVE MANAGEMENT

- Management of patellar tendon ruptures in medically stable adults is surgical. Nonoperative treatment predictably results in tendon retraction and loss of active knee extension strength and extensor lag.[7]

SURGICAL MANAGEMENT

- Surgical goals include restoration of the knee extensor mechanism with strength to allow for early postoperative rehabilitation.
- Secondary goals include avoidance of overcorrection resulting in patella baja and altered knee kinematics.

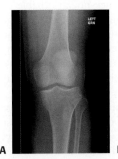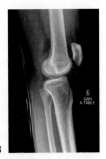

FIG 1 • A,B. Anteroposterior and lateral radiographs of a 32-year-old man with a sudden popping sensation and left knee pain after landing from a jump while playing basketball. Radiographs show a knee effusion, absence of fracture and patella alta best seen on the lateral projection.

- The most commonly described technique to date consists of an augmented primary repair using transosseous patellar tunnels and nonabsorbable suture fixation.[8]

Preoperative Planning

- AP and lateral radiographs of the affected and contralateral knee can be reviewed for comparison and to look for other concurrent abnormalities such as calcific tendonitis, abnormal patellar morphologies, or previous surgeries.

Positioning

- The patient is positioned supine on a radiolucent table with arms abducted. A bump is placed under the ipsilateral buttock and low back to facilitate internal rotation of the operative knee to neutral.
- A nonsterile tourniquet is applied.
- Hair over the operative site and anticipated dressing placement is trimmed with clippers.
- C-arm fluoroscopy may be available for confirmation of tunnel placement or for delineation of any occult fracture fragments not noted on initial radiography.

Approach

- An anterior approach to the patellar tendon provides the most direct and extensile access to the site of injury and planned repair.

T E C H N I Q U E S

■ Transosseous Suture Technique

Anterior Approach to the Patellar Tendon and Extensor Retinaculum

- Landmarks: patella, tibial tubercle, and patellofemoral joint line.
- Exsanguinate the leg and inflate a tourniquet as needed for hemostasis
- Make a midline incision longitudinally from the superior pole of the patella to the proximal aspect of the tibial tubercle.
- Elevate thick skin flaps to the prepatellar bursa. Hematoma is often encountered at this point.
- Identify patellar paratenon for later repair if not traumatically disrupted.
- Identify the area of patellar tendon rupture and the extent of retinacular involvement.
- Evacuate intra-articular hematoma.

Preparation of Tendon

- Identify the area of the tear; most patellar tendon ruptures are from the distal patellar pole, leaving a long distal limb for suture anchoring.
- Debride the tendon and infrapatellar pole of any nonviable strands or areas of degeneration and thickening. Excise any free bony fragments that originated from the inferior patellar pole that cannot be incorporated into the repair construct.
- Using two separate thick nonabsorbable braided suture (no. 5 FiberWire) and starting at the most proximal aspect of the distal segment, pass the Krackow sutures on either side of the tendon, traversing for approximately four or five passes before creating a second row per suture and ultimately creating four total suture strands exiting near the suture's entry point (**TECH FIG 1**).
- Separate the four strands into three groups: one medial, two central, and one lateral. Cut the central strands to two different lengths that can still pass through the length of the patella and be tied down. This will differentiate them during suture fixation.

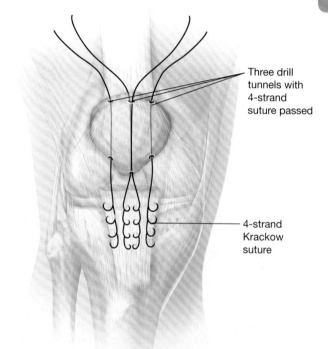

Three drill tunnels with 4-strand suture passed

4-strand Krackow suture

A

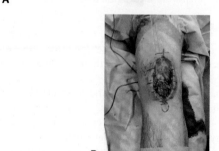

B

TECH FIG 1 • A. Diagram of Krackow suture repair of torn patellar tendon. **B.** Left knee patellar tendon repair with four-strand Krackow sutures placed.

Creation of Bone Tunnels

- Identify the medial and lateral borders of the patella. Divide this total width into fourths, taking into account areas of thin cortical bone, particularly at the lateral facet.
- Using a long 2.5-mm drill, create three retrograde drill holes at the central divisions of each of the zones described in step one (**TECH FIG 2**). Mark the entry point of each drill pass with electrocautery. Consider using multiple drill bits or saved fluoroscopic views to ensure the drill paths do not cross.

Suture Passage and Knot Tying

- Flex the knee to approximately 20 degrees with a small bump behind the knee. This is to ensure suture passage anterior to the quadriceps tendon to permit knot tying as close to the patella as possible.
- Use a 2.4-mm Beath pin with eyelet to pass each of the four suture strands through the three drill holes using the designation created earlier. All strands will then be superior to the patella (**TECH FIG 3A–C**).
- Pass the central limbs through the quadriceps tendon to their corresponding medial and lateral limbs using a free needle. This avoids soft tissue bridging and possible loosening (**TECH FIG 3D,E**).
- Hand tie at least five surgical knots, using a slip knot or needle driver to hold the initial knot tight. Leave 4-mm tails of suture.

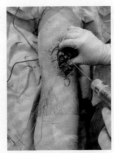

TECH FIG 2 • Drill holes placed retrograde with long 2.5-mm drill.

Completion and Assessment of Repair

- Repair any ruptured retinaculum with large absorbable braided suture.
- Move the knee through passive motion under direct visualization of repair.
  - Note any gapping or opening of the repair. This will be the limit of range of motion in the early postoperative period.
- Deflate tourniquet, irrigate, obtain hemostasis, and close in layers with paratenon closure if possible.
- Apply a soft dressing and a hinged knee brace locked in extension.

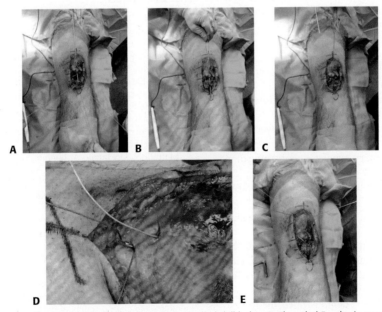

TECH FIG 3 • **A.** Beath pin passed retrograde through each of three marked drill holes. **B.** Threaded Beath pin passing through central drill hole with two suture strands. **C.** Central thread strands now passed through drill hole and quadriceps tendon with knee slightly flexed. **D.** Free needle used to pass central suture strands closer to their respective medial and lateral strands so as to avoid soft tissue bridging. **E.** All four suture strands ready for creation of two hand-tied knots.

PEARLS AND PITFALLS

Indications	▪ Confirm diagnosis with examination under anesthesia to rule out the more proximally oriented quadriceps tendon rupture.
Tendon preparation	▪ Ensure at least three passes of each row of Krackow suture to limit the possibility of suture pullout and subsidence of fixation.
Creation of bone tunnels	▪ Avoid intra-articular penetration of drill, using fluoroscopic guidance or via proprioceptive feedback with the patella held between the thumb and index finger. ▪ Oscillate when drilling tunnels so as not to bind suture in drill bit. ▪ Mark bone tunnel placement in surrounding soft tissues with electrocautery for accuracy of Beath pin passage. ▪ Avoid crossing of bone tunnels, which can create suture entanglement and prevent secure tightening of repair knots.
Suture passage and knot tying	▪ Use a free needle to pass suture close to its accompanying strand and avoid soft tissue bridging. ▪ Avoid over- or undertensioning of suture and subsequent alteration of patellofemoral mechanics.

POSTOPERATIVE CARE

▪ In isolated tendon injuries, the patient may be discharged to home with hinged knee brace locked in extension for 2 weeks. No active knee extension is permitted for 6 to 8 weeks.

▪ At the initial 2-week postoperative follow-up visit, the brace is unlocked for range of motion exercises up to the limit noted at the time of operation.

▪ Thirty-degree increases may be made every 2 weeks, and then knee brace is unlocked and weaned entirely for the remainder of rehabilitative therapy.

▪ Stretching and strengthening are permitted at 8 weeks, with return to full activity as tolerated at 12 to 16 weeks.

OUTCOMES

▪ Gilmore et al. analyzed the different techniques of acute and chronic patellar tendon repair in a recent review.[9]
  ▪ In searching techniques of primary repair, they noted 383 patellar tendon ruptures repaired primarily.
    • Seventy-seven percent of the primary repairs were with nonabsorbable suture.
    • Sixty-six percent of primary repairs underwent some form of augmentation.
    • The most common suture method was the Krackow technique.
  ▪ Five different outcome scoring systems were used to grade the success of repair.
    • While no comparisons in functional outcome could be made between specific techniques, primary repairs with augmentation demonstrated the best mean knee range of motion of 0 to 129 degrees.
  ▪ Augmented primary repair also demonstrated the lowest failure rate at 2%.

COMPLICATIONS

▪ In Gilmore et al.'s review,[9] augmented primary repair demonstrated the lowest failure rate at 2%.

▪ Described complications of patellar tendon repair include[1]:
  ▪ Improper tendon tensioning leading to patella alta or baja
  ▪ Failure of repair/ rerupture
  ▪ Infection
  ▪ Knee stiffness
  ▪ Prominent suture knots requiring removal
  ▪ Deep vein thrombosis

REFERENCES

1. Volk WR, Gautam PY, Uribe JW. Complications in brief: quadriceps and patellar tendon tears. *Clin Orthop Relat Res.* 2013;472(3):1050-1057.
2. Andrikoula S, Tokis A, Vasiliadis HS, Georgoulis A. The extensor mechanism of the knee joint: an anatomical study. *Knee Surg Sports Traumatol Arthrosc.* 2006;14:214-220.
3. Pang J, Shen S, Pan WR, et al. The arterial supply of the patellar tendon: anatomical study with clinical implications for knee surgery. *Clin Anat.* 2009;22(3):371-376.
4. Nemschak G, Pretterklieber ML. The patellar arterial supply via the infrapatellar fat pad (of Hoffa): a combined anatomical and angiographical analysis. *Anat Res Int.* 2012;(3):1-10.
5. Maffulli N, Del Buono A, Loppini M, Denaro V. Ipsilateral hamstring tendon graft reconstruction for chronic patellar tendon ruptures. *J Bone Joint Surg Am.* 2013;95:e1231-e1236.
6. Rose PS, Frassica FJ. Atraumatic bilateral patellar tendon rupture: a case report and review of the literature. *J Bone Joint Surg Am.* 2001;83A:1382-1386.
7. Matava MJ. Patellar tendon ruptures. *J Am Acad Orthop Surg.* 1996;4:287-296.
8. Black JC, Ricci WM, Gardner MJ, et al. Novel augmentation technique for patellar tendon repair improves strength and decreases gap formation: a cadaveric study. *Clin Orthop Relat Res.* 2016;474:2611-2618.
9. Gilmore JH, Clayton-Smith ZJ, Aguilar M, et al. Reconstruction techniques and clinical results of patellar tendon ruptures: evidence today. *Knee.* 2015;22:148-155.

Excision of Soft Tissue Tumors of the Thigh

Raffi S. Avedian

DEFINITION

- Soft tissue sarcomas are malignant tumors that arise from mesenchymal cells and are classified according to their cell of origin such as the muscle, tendon, or fat.
- Peripheral nerve sheath tumors arise from neural crest cells but are typically grouped with sarcomas because of similarities in location, natural history, and treatment.
- The World Health Organization groups soft tissue sarcomas into ten categories based on the tissue of origin.
- Most sarcomas occur in a deep location meaning below the muscle fascia, whereas one-third of sarcomas occur in a subcutaneous location.
- Patients with soft tissue sarcomas and patients with benign tumors often present with the same chief complaint of having a soft tissue mass.
- Rendering an accurate diagnosis prior to surgery is important because the treatment plan may vary based on the nature of the diagnosis. For example, a benign tumor may be monitored or removed with a simple excision, whereas in the case of a sarcoma, the goal of surgery is to remove the tumor with a wide margin.
- With appropriate planning, radiotherapy and/or chemotherapy is often incorporated into the treatment plan either before or after definitive surgery.[1]

ANATOMY

- The critical anatomic structures that should be preserved when performing an excision of tumor in the thigh are the femoral artery, sciatic nerve, and femoral nerve.
- The common femoral artery enters the thigh under the inguinal ligament. As it travels distally, it gives several branches, the largest of which is the profundal femoral artery (PFA). This branch travels on top of the adductor brevis until the muscle inserts onto the linea aspera at which point the distal half of the PFA continues just posterior to the femur.
- Several perforator branches from the PFA pierce the lateral intermuscular septum and go into the anterior compartment. In most patients, limb salvage can be performed even if the PFA is ligated near its takeoff from the common femoral artery.
- The superficial femoral artery (SFA) is the most important blood vessel when considering tumor excision. It must be preserved or reconstructed if excised to maintain viable limb perfusion. As the SFA travels distally, it is located on the anterior surface of the psoas, adductor longus, and then adductor magnus until it courses through the adductor canal into the popliteal fossa. The sartorius muscle acts as a cover to the superficial femoral vessels throughout the middle of the thigh.
- There are three muscle compartments of the thigh: anterior, medial, and posterior.
- The sciatic nerve travels in the posterior compartment. It branches into the common peroneal nerve, which can reliably dissected and found just medial and anterior to the biceps femoris in the popliteal fossa. The tibial nerve portion of the sciatic nerve stays midline with the popliteal vessels.
- The femoral nerve divides into several branches that spread out and innervate the anterior compartment muscles soon after passing under the inguinal ligament. Unlike the sciatic nerve, which can be isolated throughout the thigh, the femoral nerve is rarely identified during tumor removal because it branches so proximally.

PATHOGENESIS

- The mechanism for sarcoma formation is not known.
- Risk factors for sarcoma development include radiation exposure, radiotherapy, pesticide exposure, and hereditary conditions including Li-Fraumeni syndrome and neurofibromatosis.

NATURAL HISTORY

- All sarcomas have the potential for local recurrence and metastasis.
- Tumor variables that are associated with increased risk of metastasis include high grade and large size (greater than 5 cm).[2]
- Lungs are the most common location of metastasis.

PATIENT HISTORY AND PHYSICAL FINDINGS

- Determining when the mass was first noticed and how rapidly it is growing can help the clinician differentiate between benign and malignant tumors.
- The presence of pain is often associated with a benign tumor such as a schwannoma or vascular malformation and may not be present with sarcomas until late in the disease course.

- Determining the size of the tumor, manual muscle strength testing, and sensory examination are useful to determine if there is neurological compromise. Limb edema assessment and pulse examination can help determine if the tumor is causing vascular or lymphatic compromise.
- Range of motion testing and gait assessment are helpful in assessing a patient's mobility and functional status to guide a perioperative and postoperative counseling.

IMAGING

- Magnetic resonance imaging is the modality of choice for soft tissue tumor evaluation.[3]
- Fat-sensitive images such as T1-weighted sequences are best for identifying critical anatomic structures such as nerves and vessels (**FIG 1**).
- Fluid-sensitive images including T2-weighted and STIR sequences highlight pathology very well.
- Contrast-enhanced sequences are used to differentiated cystic from solid areas in tumors and identify reactive peritumoral edema, which will be high signal on fluid sequences but not enhance with contrast.
- Some benign tumors such as lipoma and schwannoma may be diagnosed on MRI; however, most soft tissue tumors require a biopsy for diagnosis.

DIFFERENTIAL DIAGNOSIS

- Benign tumors
- Sarcoma
- Lymphoma of soft tissue
- Infection/abscess

SURGICAL MANAGEMENT

- The appropriate treatment for any musculoskeletal tumor is based on its diagnosis and natural history.
- Performing a surgery without consideration of the diagnosis and the appropriate margin may cause harm to patients.[4]
- In cases where MR imaging is not diagnostic, a biopsy should be performed.

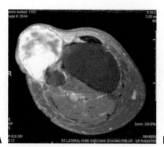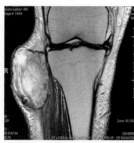

FIG 2 • **A.** Axial MRI of the thigh demonstrating a subcutaneous sarcoma. **B.** Coronal MRI of the thigh showing a subcutaneous sarcoma.

- Treatment strategy including the use of preoperative radiation and specific surgical plan should be formulated by a multidisciplinary team specializing in sarcoma care.

Preoperative Planning

- A patient is considered ready for surgery after completion of staging and multidisciplinary review of pertinent imaging, pathology, and treatment strategy.
- The surgical plan is created by thorough study of the preoperative MR scan. A plane of surgical dissection is planned to remove the tumor in its entirety while maintaining a clean margin around it (**FIG 2**).
- If the tumor encases important vascular structures, a plan for vascular reconstruction is made with a vascular surgeon.
- Anticipated soft tissue coverage needs are assessed such as skin graft, local rotation flap, or free tissue transfer.

Positioning

- The patient is placed in the supine position when the tumor is in the anterior or medial compartment (**FIG 3**).
- The patient is placed in the prone position when the tumor is in the posterior compartment.
- The site of a flap harvest must be completely isolated from the tumor site to avoid contamination and tumor spread. A separate back table and clean instruments should be used.

Approach

- The surgical approach varies based on the location of the tumor.
- Previous biopsy and surgical scars are considered contaminated and must be excised en bloc with the tumor.

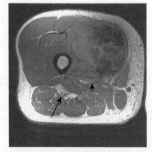

FIG 1 • Axial T1-weighted image demonstrating compartments of the thigh and relevant anatomy of the thigh. The *arrow* points at the sciatic nerve and the *arrowhead* at the femoral vessels, and there is a sarcoma in the vastus medialis.

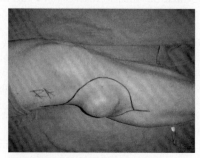

FIG 3 • Intraoperative photograph demonstrating patient positioning.

■ Wide Resection of Subcutaneous Sarcoma

- Subcutaneous sarcomas are located in the adipose tissue above the muscle fascia. There is no anatomic barrier to longitudinal tumor spread in this location; however, the deep fascia can act as a natural barrier to deep penetration of the tumor. Careful review of preoperative MR imaging and physical palpation are important when determining tumor extent and the location of the surgical incision.
- A surgical incision is planned 2 cm to 3 cm peripheral to the edge of the tumor as determined by palpation and MRI. Typically, a large paddle of the skin is removed along with the tumor (**TECH FIG 1**).

- The dissection is carried through the subcutaneous fat angling away from the tumor.
- The deep fascia is identified and cut circumferentially around the tumor.
- The fascia and subcutaneous tissue containing the tumor are kept in continuity, and a small cuff of muscle is removed with the fascia to ensure a clean deep margin.
- The tumor and surrounding fat, fascia, and muscle are removed in their entirety.
- Take care not to shear off the fat from the fascia during dissection.
- Avoid retractors on the tumor side of the dissection.
- Most surgeries require a skin graft or muscle flap for closure. Do not sacrifice margin to save tissue for a primary closure.

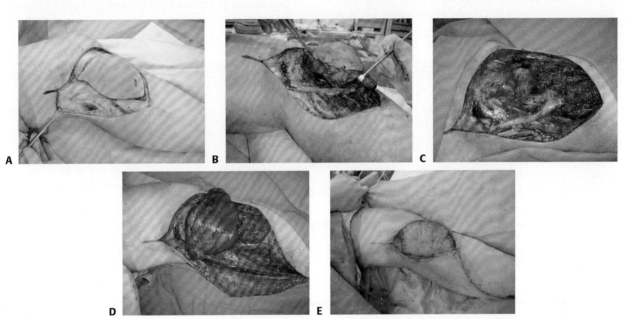

TECH FIG 1 • Operative technique for resecting a subcutaneous sarcoma. **A.** Dissection of the skin and subcutaneous tissue around the tumor, notice the large paddle of skin that extends approximately 2 cm beyond the palpable tumor to ensure adequate resection margin. **B.** Dissection through the deep plane leaving the fascia and small, approximately 1-cm, cuff of underlying muscle on the tumor that serves as the deep margin. **C,D.** The skin was then reapproximated, and preparation for skin grafting was completed. **E.** A split-thickness skin graft was obtained from the contralateral thigh using completely separate instruments, back table, and clean gowns and gloves to avoid seeding the harvest site with tumor.

■ Wide Resection of a Deep Sarcoma

- Because fascia acts as a natural anatomic barrier, tumors tend to grow longest in a longitudinal dimension; as a result, larger margins in the longitudinal plane com-

pared to the mediolateral/anteroposterior planes are recommended.
- Tumors often abut major nerves and blood vessels in which case the epineurium around the nerve and adventitia surrounding the vessel can be used as margins[5] (**TECH FIG 2**).

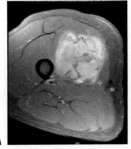
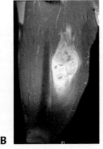
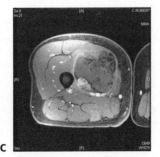

TECH FIG 2 • **A.** Axial T1 fat-suppressed contrast MRI showing a high-grade sarcoma within the vastus medialis and abutting the femoral artery and vein. **B.** Coronal T1 fat-suppressed contrast MRI. **C.** Axial T1 fat-suppressed contrast MRI after completion of preoperative radiation showing decreased enhancement suggesting tumor necrosis.

■ Incision and Dissection

- A longitudinal incision is made over the tumor by incorporating the previous biopsy site.
- Subcutaneous skin flaps are raised circumferentially around the tumor making sure to the keep the deep fascia intact as a margin around the tumor.
- Begin the deep dissection by palpating the tumor and incising the deep fascia several centimeters further out from the tumor. If the tumor abuts the fascia, then leave the fascia intact, trace it back to its insertion on the bone, and remove it in its entirety as a margin around the tumor thus avoiding inadvertent tumor penetration or exposure (**TECH FIG 3**).
- It is recommended that several centimeters of muscle be removed from cranial and caudal to the tumor. The deci-

sion on how much muscle to remove is based on preoperative evaluation of the MRI, palpation of the tumor, and visual inspection of the muscle to ensure the plane of dissection is outside of the tumor and any associated abnormal tissue such as a pseudocapsule.

- If the tumor abuts the bone but there is no evidence of bone penetration, use a periosteal elevator to lift the periosteum off the bone with the tumor on top. The periosteum acts as the deep margin.
- If there is bone penetration, then depending on the extent of bone involvement, either a hemicortical or complete resection should be performed and reconstructed with either allograft, vascularized fibula, or endoprosthesis.
- If the tumor encases the major blood vessels of the limb, they should be removed en bloc with the tumor followed by vascular reconstruction.

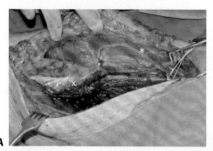 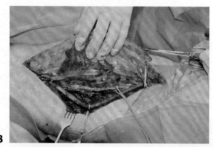 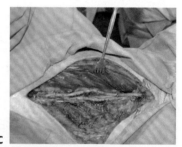

A   **B**   **C**

TECH FIG 3 • Operative technique for resection of a deep sarcoma of the thigh. **A.** Photograph showing deep dissection of tumor, * indicates proximal end of sartorius, *X* indicates cut distal end of adductor magnus. The adventitia of the vessels are dissected and left with the tumor. **B.** Photograph showing complete mobilization of the vessels, the medial intermuscular septum and vessel adventitia "*" serve as the deep margin. **C.** Photograph after the remaining muscles around the tumor are cut and the tumor is removed with a clean margin. The wound is closed in layers with multiple suction drains.

■ Completion

- After tumor removal, irrigate the wound thoroughly and assess the dead space. An attempt to myodese (muscle-to-muscle approximation with sutures) surrounding

muscles to eliminate as much dead space as possible is recommended.
- Other strategies to manage dead space are local or free muscle transfer, closing over multiple drains, and rarely delayed closure using a negative pressure dressing.

PEARLS AND PITFALLS

Hematoma	■ Dead space after tumor removal should be managed with drains, muscle flap, free tissue transfer, or a combination of these techniques. ■ Seroma drainage in the clinic may be necessary.
Wound breakdown	■ Incisional negative pressure dressings, aggressive dead space management, and maximizing patients' nutrition may reduce wound problems. ■ Patients should be counseled about potential need for reoperation for wound management.
Positive margins	■ Appropriate preoperative planning is important to minimize risk of unplanned positive margins. ■ Planned positive margins around critical structures such as nerves and vessels may be appropriate in certain settings.

POSTOPERATIVE CARE

- Mobilization and weight bearing depend on the extent of surgery.
- Extremity elevation is recommended while patient is in bed.
- Range of motion and therapy may begin after wound healing is sufficient.
- Postoperative radiotherapy may take place 4 to 6 weeks after surgery.

OUTCOMES

- Oncological outcomes include local recurrence and metastasis. Surveillance for recurrence should be managed by a multidisciplinary sarcoma team.
- Functional outcomes depend on the extent of tissue resection, patient overall health status, and late effects of radiation. Aggressive wound care and physical therapy may help maximize patient function.[6,7]

COMPLICATIONS

- Wound healing problems that require operative intervention can occur in up to 33% of patients who undergo preoperative radiotherapy and 17% of patients who undergo postoperative radiotherapy.[1]

- Local recurrence occurs in a minority of patients and is more common in patients with positive margins. Radiotherapy decreases the risk of local recurrence.

REFERENCES

1. O'Sullivan B, Davis AM, Turcotte R, et al. Preoperative versus postoperative radiotherapy in soft-tissue sarcoma of the limbs: a randomised trial. *Lancet.* 2002;359(9325):2235-2241.
2. van Praag VM, Rueten-Budde AJ, Jeys LM, et al. A prediction model for treatment decisions in high-grade extremity soft-tissue sarcomas: Personalised sarcoma care (PERSARC). *Eur J Cancer.* 2017;83:313-323.
3. Demas BE, Heelan RT, Lane J, et al. Soft-tissue sarcomas of the extremities: comparison of MR and CT in determining the extent of disease. *AJR Am J Roentgenol.* 1988;150(3):615.
4. Pretell-Mazzini J, Barton MD Jr, Conway SA, Temple HT. Unplanned excision of soft-tissue sarcomas: current concepts for management and prognosis. *J Bone Joint Surg Am.* 2015;97(7):597-603.
5. O'Donnell PW, Griffin AM, Eward WC, et al. The effect of the setting of a positive surgical margin in soft tissue sarcoma. *Cancer.* 2014;120(18):2866-2875.
6. Davidge KM, Wunder J, Tomlinson G, et al. Function and health status outcomes following soft tissue reconstruction for limb preservation in extremity soft tissue sarcoma. *Ann Surg Oncol.* 2010;17(4):1052-1062.
7. Davis AM, O'Sullivan B, Bell RS, et al. Function and health status outcomes in a randomized trial comparing preoperative and postoperative radiotherapy in extremity soft tissue sarcoma. *J Clin Oncol.* 2002;20(22):4472-4477.

36 CHAPTER

Excision of Bone Tumors of the Femur

Raffi S. Avedian

DEFINITION

- Bone tumors of the femur may be benign or malignant (bone sarcoma) and exhibit a variable natural history ranging from latent to rapid growth. Aggressive benign tumors and malignant tumors typically cause pain, dysfunction, and fracture.

ANATOMY

- The femoral artery, sciatic nerve, and femoral nerve are important structures that need to be accounted for during surgery of the femur.
- The common femoral artery enters the thigh under the inguinal ligament. As it travels distally, it gives several branches, the largest of which is the profundal femoral artery (PFA), which travels on top of the adductor brevis until the muscle inserts onto the linea aspera at which point the distal half of the PFA continues just posterior to the femur.
- Several perforator branches from the PFA pierce the lateral intermuscular septum and go into the anterior compartment. The PFA is located near the linea aspera and is often ligated when resecting segments of the femur.
- The superficial femoral artery (SFA) is the most important blood vessel when considering tumor excision. It must be preserved or reconstructed if excised, to maintain viable limb perfusion. As the SFA travels distally, it is located on the anterior surface of the psoas, adductor longus, and then adductor magnus until it courses through the adductor canal into the popliteal fossa. The sartorius muscle acts as a cover to the superficial femoral vessels throughout the middle of the thigh.
- The sciatic nerve travels in the posterior compartment. It branches into the common peroneal nerve, which can reliably be dissected and found just medial and anterior to the biceps femoris in the popliteal fossa. The tibial nerve portion of the sciatic nerve stays midline with the popliteal vessels.

PATHOGENESIS

- The mechanism for bone tumor formation is not known.
- Risk factors for sarcoma development include radiation exposure, radiotherapy, pesticide exposure, and hereditary conditions including Li-Fraumeni syndrome and retinoblastoma gene mutation.

NATURAL HISTORY

- Active benign tumors, such as giant cell tumor of the bone, chondroblastoma, and aneurysmal bone cyst, will progress over time and may recur after excision but are not lethal.

- All bone sarcomas have the potential for local recurrence and metastasis.
- Some bone sarcomas such as low-grade chondrosarcoma exhibit a slow rate of growth and low risk of metastasis, whereas aggressive tumors like high-grade osteosarcoma and dedifferentiated chondrosarcoma grow rapidly and have a relatively high risk of metastasis.
- Tumor variables that are associated with increased risk of metastasis include high grade and large size (greater than 8 cm).
- Lungs and other osseous sites are the most and second most common location of metastasis, respectively.

PATIENT HISTORY AND PHYSICAL FINDINGS

- Pain is a common presenting symptom for aggressive bone tumors.
- A thorough history and examination are important to assess duration of symptoms, comorbidities, physical dysfunction, organ involvement, overall health, and patient expectations to best tailor treatment strategy for the individual patient.
- Neurovascular examination is mandatory for any extremity tumor.

IMAGING

- Plain radiographs are used to formulate a differential diagnosis and a preoperative plan (**FIG 1A**).
- Magnetic resonance imaging is routinely used to determine the extent of intramedullary tumor involvement, presence of soft tissue extension, status of the neurovascular structures, and preoperative planning (**FIG 1B**).

DIFFERENTIAL DIAGNOSIS

- The differential diagnosis for a bone tumor includes benign tumors, sarcomas, lymphoma of the bone, infection, and metabolic lesions (eg, hyperparathyroidism).
- The most common bone sarcomas are osteosarcoma, chondrosarcoma, and Ewing sarcoma.

SURGICAL MANAGEMENT

- The appropriate treatment for any musculoskeletal tumor is based on its diagnosis and natural history.
- Biopsy incisions are considered contaminated and must be resected at the time of definitive surgery. Care should be taken to place the biopsy in a location that does not interfere with the final surgical plan.

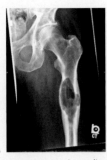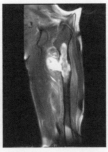

FIG 1 • **A.** Anteroposterior radiograph of a 67-year-old man with high-grade chondrosarcoma of the proximal femur seen as a large lucent lesion. **B.** Coronal T2-weighted MRI of the same patient demonstrating extensive soft tissue component and intramedullary involvement by chondrosarcoma.

- Intralesional curettage is the preferred treatment for benign tumors. Radical resection with a clean margin is required for bone sarcomas.
- Reconstruction depends on the extent of bone excision and may include simple bone grafting, endoprosthetic implants, bulk allografts, osteoarticular implants, or vascularized fibula.
- The goal of surgery is to remove the tumor adequately to minimize recurrence and restore the mechanical integrity of the bone and joints so that the patient may have sufficient function to perform activities of daily living with minimal pain.[1,2]

Preoperative Planning

- A patient is considered ready for surgery after completion of staging and multidisciplinary review of pertinent imaging, pathology, and treatment strategy.

- The surgical plan is created by a thorough study of the preoperative radiographs and MR scan.
- Bone cuts are planned by examining preoperative imaging and measuring the distance from an intraoperatively identifiable landmark (eg, femoral condyle, greater trochanter) to the desired osteotomy site.
- The soft tissue margin depends on the size and location of a soft tissue component to the tumor. For example, an anterior soft tissue mass along the distal femur can be safely resected by incorporating a portion of the vastus intermedius as the margin.
- When tumor abuts but does not encase blood vessels or nerves, they can be dissected free by leaving adventitia and epineurium on the tumor as the margin.

Positioning

- Patient positioning is based on the surgeon's assessment of the critical anatomy of the surgery and how best to visualize it during surgery.
- Distal femur resections are typically performed in the supine position. Proximal femur tumors are often performed in the lateral position.
- If a flap is to be used, the harvest must be performed using a separate back table and instruments and the surgical sites completely isolated to avoid contamination.

Approach

- The surgical approach varies based on the location of the tumor.
- Previous biopsy and surgical scars are considered contaminated and must be excised en bloc with the tumor.

■ Femur Resection and Allograft Reconstruction

- Tourniquet is used at discretion of the surgeon using gravity exsanguination rather than Esmarch to avoid tumor dissemination.
- A longitudinally oriented incision is created that includes a fusiform skin excision of the biopsy site. Skin flaps are created as needed to ensure adequate visualization of the tumor and critical anatomy.
- Dual incisions may be useful for hemicortical resection, but otherwise are rarely used.
- Soft tissue dissection around the tumor is performed with the following principles:
  - Adequate visualization must be achieved.
  - Margin of healthy tissue is kept on the tumor.
  - Nerves are dissected free. The epineurium may be used as margin if tumor abuts the nerve. Sciatic nerve branches to hamstring muscles may be cut as needed to adequately mobilize nerve away from tumor.
  - Vessels are mobilized and the adventitia may be used as margin if tumor abuts the vessels.

- Bone cuts are performed based on preoperative planning and measurements to ensure complete tumor removal. Easily identifiable anatomic landmarks such as the femoral condyles, epicondyles, greater trochanter, and vastus ridge serve as reference points for measurements that can be transferred from preoperative plans to intraoperative execution.
- Fluoroscopy may be used at the discretion of the surgeon.
- Hemicortical resection is an option if the tumor does not involve the entire diameter of the bone.
- Reconstruction is performed to restore mechanical stability of the extremity.
  - Endoprosthetic implants, if used, may be cemented or press fit into the native bone.
  - Allografts are fashioned to fit the defect and secured in place with internal fixation (**TECH FIG 1**).
- The deep fascia, if available, is closed over drains, followed by a subcutaneous fascia and dermal layer. Deep drains are used to avoid hematoma and minimize pressure on the skin repair.

TECHNIQUES

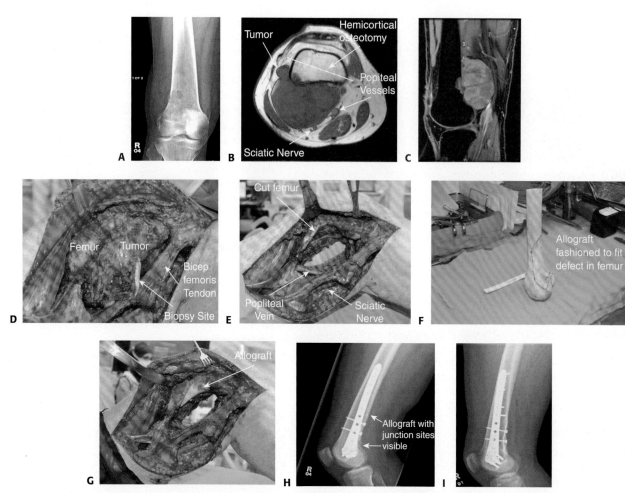

TECH FIG 1 • A. Anteroposterior radiograph of a 74-year-old man demonstrating bone sarcoma with soft tissue mass. **B.** Axial T1-weighted MRI showing tumor eroding into femur and abutting sciatic nerve and popliteal vessels. **C.** Sagittal MRI showing craniocaudal extent of tumor. **D.** Intraoperative photograph demonstrating soft tissue dissection to expose tumor, mobilize popliteal vessels and sciatic nerve, and expose femur in preparation of osteotomy. **E.** Intraoperative photograph showing the femur after tumor resection. **F.** Allograft femur with ink lines outlining how the graft will be fashioned to fit the defect. **G.** Intraoperative photograph after allograft has been secured into the native femur. **H.** Lateral radiograph of the distal femur 3 weeks after surgery. **I.** Lateral radiograph of the distal femur 36 months after surgery. The allograft has incorporated into the patient's femur.

PEARLS AND PITFALLS

Hematoma	■ Dead space after tumor removal should be managed with drains, muscle flap, free tissue transfer, or a combination of these techniques. ■ Seroma drainage in the clinic may be necessary.
Wound breakdown	■ Incisional negative pressure dressings, aggressive dead space management, and maximizing patients' nutrition may reduce wound problems. ■ Patients should be counseled about potential need for reoperation for wound management.
Positive margins	■ Appropriate preoperative planning is important to minimize risk of unplanned positive margins. ■ Planned positive margins around critical structures such as nerves and vessels may be appropriate in certain settings.
Allograft nonunion/fracture	■ Common complications may be minimized by good cortical apposition of graft to the native bone. ■ Restrict weight bearing until evidence of bone healing is observed. ■ Counsel patients that reoperation for nonunion is possible.

POSTOPERATIVE CARE

- Mobilization and weight bearing depend on the extent of surgery.
- Extremity elevation is recommended while patient is in bed.
- Range of motion and therapy may begin after wound healing is sufficient.
- May administer antibiotics in the perioperative period.

OUTCOMES

- Oncological outcomes include local recurrence and metastasis. Surveillance for recurrence should be managed by a multidisciplinary sarcoma team. Local recurrence is greater when margins are positive.
- Functional outcomes depend on the extent of tissue resection and patient overall health status. Most patients will experience some form of disability that is proportional to the volume of muscle and bone resected.[3,4]

COMPLICATIONS

- Allograft nonunion and fracture are relatively common and require additional surgery to achieve a limb salvage.[5]

- Local recurrence occurs in a minority of patients and is more common in patients with positive margins.
- Deep infection can occur at any time after surgery and requires aggressive therapy including surgical debridement and antibiotic therapy to achieve limb salvage. Removal of implants may be necessary to eradicate infection.

REFERENCES

1. Bacci G, Forni C, Longhi A, et al. Local recurrence and local control of non-metastatic osteosarcoma of the extremities: a 27-year experience in a single institution. *J Surg Oncol*. 2007;96(2):118.
2. Grimer RJ, Taminiau AM, Cannon SR; Surgical Subcommittee of the European Osteosarcoma Intergroup. Surgical outcomes in osteosarcoma. *J Bone Joint Surg Br*. 2002;84(3):395.
3. Nagarajan R, Neglia JP, Clohisy DR, Robison LL. Limb salvage and amputation in survivors of pediatric lower-extremity bone tumors: what are the long-term implications? *J Clin Oncol*. 2002;20(22):4493.
4. Renard AJ, Veth RP, Schreuder HW, et al. Function and complications after ablative and limb-salvage therapy in lower extremity sarcoma of bone. *J Surg Oncol*. 2000;73(4):198.
5. Hornicek FJ, Gebhardt MC, Tomford WW, et al. Factors affecting nonunion of the allograft-host junction. *Clin Orthop Relat Res*. 2001;(382):87-98.

37
CHAPTER

Femoral Bone Debridement

Robert J. Steffner, David W. Lowenberg, and Sahitya K. Denduluri

DEFINITION

- Femoral bone debridement is generally needed for osteomyelitis (acute or chronic), symptomatic nonunion, and open fracture.

ANATOMY

- The femur contributes to the hip and knee joints and withstands significant stress in motion.
- Vital structures around the femur include the sciatic and femoral nerves, the superficial and deep femoral artery and vein, and the extensor mechanism for knee extension.

PATHOGENESIS

- Open fracture leads to gross contamination, soft tissue stripping, and avascular bone. Direct inoculation occurs, which will lead to infection in the absence of prompt surgical care.
- Hematogenous spread of bacteria to the bone can create osteomyelitis. Acute infection tends to produce rapid symptoms and the accumulation of purulent fluid. Chronic infection is more indolent and produces waxing and waning symptoms. After a week or two of infection, bacteria form a protective avascular matrix called biofilm. Antibiotics cannot penetrate this layer.
- Nonunion is a fractured bone that will not heal. Hypertrophic nonunion comes from too much fracture site motion. Atrophic nonunion is from poor blood supply and inadequate substrate for bone healing. Infection can also lead to nonhealing bone and sometimes creates a false joint known as a pseudarthrosis.
- In all of these instances, surgical debridement is required to promote bone recovery and healing.

NATURAL HISTORY

- Neglected open fractures and osteomyelitis can lead to systemic infection and sepsis, which is life threatening.
- Chronic infection can produce a nonhealing wound with drainage. This limits quality of life and can also lead to squamous cell carcinoma at areas of long-standing skin ulceration.[1]

- Nonunion in the femur limits weight bearing and mobilization. Pain is often present with activity. Quality of life is significantly diminished.

PATIENT HISTORY AND PHYSICAL FINDINGS

- Ask about prior trauma, surgical procedures, and any complications or wound healing problems.
- Specifically ask about cellulitis and draining sinus tracts.
- Assume infection until proven otherwise.
- Assess impact on the patient's quality of life.
- Inquire about recent antibiotic use.
- Determine host factors such as nutrition, nicotine use, medical comorbidities, use of immunosuppressive and anti-inflammatory medications, and any prior radiation exposure to the area of interest.
- Visually inspect the patient's thigh. Look for deformity, leg length discrepancy, and rotational change from the contralateral side.
- Lab work including WBC, ESR, and CRP can help determine the presence of infection.

IMAGING

- Plain radiographs can demonstrate nonhealing bone, erosive cortical changes seen in acute infection, and sclerotic thickening seen in chronic infection (**FIG 1**).

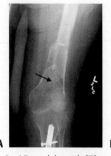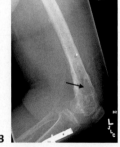

A   **B**

FIG 1 • **A.** AP and lateral **(B)** radiographs of a distal femur chronic osteomyelitis in the setting of prior internal fixation for an open distal femur fracture. Original hardware removed with exception of a broken screw. Radiolucent changes (**arrows**) seen in the metaphysis of a patient with clinical evidence of a draining sinus tract.

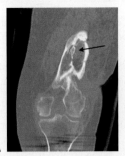
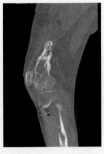

FIG 2 • **A.** Coronal and sagittal **(B)** CT scan of the distal femur with chronic osteomyelitis demonstrating sclerotic rim of the bone (involucrum) surrounding a spicule of the bone (sequestrum, **arrow**).

- Full-length, weight-bearing radiographs of the lower extremities show deformity and leg length discrepancy.
- CT scan is best for bony detail. It is the modality of choice to identify a nidus of dead bone (sequestrum) and surrounding sclerotic bone (involucrum) seen in chronic osteomyelitis (**FIG 2**).
- MRI imaging assesses the level of intramedullary bone and soft tissue involvement with bone infections. This is crucial in determining the extent of surgical debridement.

NONOPERATIVE MANAGEMENT

- Nonhealing bone and bone infection in the femur are almost always operative given the structural importance for weight bearing and ambulation.
- Exceptions include low-demand patients with minimal symptoms, patients who adapt well with assist devices, and patients at high surgical risk due to medical comorbidities.
- Nonunion patients without infection can try bracing and bone stimulation devices before surgery.

SURGICAL MANAGEMENT

- It is important to set patient expectations. Several debridement procedures may be needed to create a favorable bone and soft tissue bed for reconstructing and healing. Persistent or recurrent nonunion or infection may happen despite aggressive surgical management.

Preoperative Planning

- Address modifiable host factors including smoking cessation, nutrition, glycemic control, and medication use (anti-inflammatories, corticosteroids, etc.).
- In the lower extremity, quantify the degree of limb shortening, malalignment, and malrotation. Shortening greater than 2 cm and deformity greater than 10 degrees tend to limit a patient's quality of life.
- Anticipate the extent of debridement and appropriately plan for bony stabilization, dead space management, and soft tissue coverage.

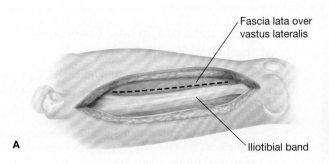
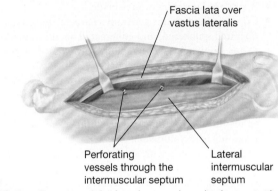

FIG 3 • Illustration of the lateral approach to the femur. **A.** The iliotibial band is divided in-line with the skin incision, and the vastus lateralis is raised off the intermuscular septum with clips placed on perforating branches of the profunda femoris artery and vein **(B)**.

- A reamer-irrigator-aspirator device can assist with intramedullary debridement in long bone osteomyelitis.[2]
- Hold antibiotics for culture. Multiple cultures should be obtained and sent for aerobic, anaerobic, fungal, and yeast assessment. Cultures will guide postoperative medical therapy.
- Send soft tissue and bone for surgical pathology. This will help determine the presence and chronicity of infection, especially if cultures are negative.

Positioning

- Both lateral decubitus with an axillary roll and supine position with hip bumps and a leg ramp are acceptable for a lateral approach to the femur.
- Lateral position is best for the upper half of the femur, and supine position with leg ramp is best for the distal half of the femur.
- Use a radiolucent table to allow intraoperative fluoroscopy.

Approach

- Planned access to the femur is generally through a lateral approach (**FIG 3**). Traumatic wounds and prior incisions can sometimes lead to alternative approaches.

TECHNIQUES

■ Debridement of Chronic Osteomyelitis of the Distal Femur

- Patient is positioned supine with an ipsilateral hip bump on a radiolucent table. A small leg ramp can be added to facilitate intraoperative imaging.
- Antibiotics are held for culture and then given.
- Open wounds are prepped with Betadine scrub and paint.
- Before incision, the involved anatomic location is identified with intraoperative fluoroscopy.
- A straight lateral incision is made.
- Compromised skin is generally characterized as multiply operated, puckered, and adherent. This skin, in addition to any sinus tracts, should be sharply excised. Remaining skin should have bleeding edges.
- The iliotibial band is split in-line with the skin incision, and the vastus lateralis muscle is raised off the lateral intermuscular septum. The muscle is retracted upward to identify perforating vascular branches from the deep profunda artery and vein.
- Ligating branches with surgical clips preserves branches for possible microsurgical anastomosis.
- Using a combination of a microsaw, osteotomes, and high-speed bur, a long cortical window is created in the lateral femoral cortex. The high-speed bur is then used from inside-out to widen the elongated ellipse to improve access to the intramedullary canal (**TECH FIG 1A**). Irrigating during use of the bur can limit heat necrosis of the bone.
- Multiple cultures are obtained from the soft tissue and bone. The bone is sent for surgical pathology.
- Aggressive debridement involves excision of all nonviable soft tissue and bone (**TECH FIG 1B**), including seques-

tra (**TECH FIG 1C**). Surgical tools for debridement include curettes, rongeurs, osteotomes, high-speed bur, and fresh surgical blades.
- Wound irrigation is performed with low-flow cystoscopic tubing. Many liters of normal saline with antibiotics are advised.
- An adequately debrided field demonstrates bleeding tissues with normal color and properties such as contractility.
- Polymethyl methacrylate (PMMA) is mixed with medications to create filler for the defect created from the debridement. The medications used, which may include antibiotics, antifungals, and antiparasitics, should be discussed before surgery with infectious disease and pharmacy colleagues.
- Appropriate drug concentrations with PMMA should also be discussed with a pharmacist.
- PMMA beads can be made either by hand or with a mold. A line of beads is placed along a thick monofilament suture. It is important to document the number of beads being implanted.
- Pack the dead space with antibiotic beads (**TECH FIG 1D**).
- Surgical stabilization should bridge the defect. Options include external fixation, an antibiotic-impregnated cement intramedullary nail, or a locking plate coated in antibiotic cement (**TECH FIG 1E,F**).
- Final fluoroscopic or radiographic images should be taken to document implants.
- Deep drains are utilized to help with dead space management.
- Remaining soft tissues should be healthy and bleeding. Attempt to isolate deep fascial layers for a tiered closure. Primary closure should not have a lot of tension. The surgeon should maintain a low threshold for rotational or free tissue coverage.

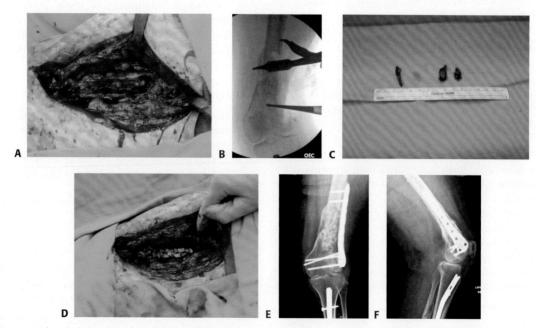

TECH FIG 1 • A. Clinical photograph of an exposed distal femur with the creation of a long cortical window with evidence of infected soft tissue within the intramedullary canal. **B.** Fluoroscopic image showing debridement of the femur intramedullary canal with a curette. **C.** Photograph of sequestra removed during debridement of the distal femur. **D.** Photograph of cement antibiotic beads placed into the bone defect after debridement of chronic osteomyelitis. **E.** Postoperative AP and lateral **(F)** radiographs of the distal femur after debridement, placement of antibiotic beads, and stabilization of the defect.

PEARLS AND PITFALLS

Hip and knee	■ In the setting of infection, consider aspirating adjacent joints to ensure there is no associated septic arthritis. ■ Surgical stabilization should be robust enough to allow joint passive range of motion during recovery.
Debridement	■ Retained hardware likely has a bacterial biofilm. Efforts should be made to remove all foreign bodies during the debridement.
Tumor	■ Bone tumors can look like bone infection. If there is any uncertainty, a biopsy should be performed before debridement.
Bacteria	■ Some microbiology labs can run polymerase chain reaction (PCR) to identify microbial DNA.
Antibiotic nail	■ Bone defects can be supported with an antibiotic intramedullary nail. Inject a chest tube with cement mixed with antibiotics and let dry with a guide wire inserted into the cement. A small injection nozzle is often needed. Once dry, bend the guide wire at the top to facilitate removal of the nail. Bone must be reamed to a diameter 1.5 mm larger than the diameter of the chest tube.

POSTOPERATIVE CARE

■ Dressings can be removed in 48 hours and the patient may shower with soap and water.

■ Encourage early range of motion of surrounding joints to avoid stiffness.

■ Intravenous medications are tailored to operative cultures and are determined in consultation with infectious disease specialists. Cultures may not grow because many patients receive antibiotic therapy before debridement and some bacteria require special media.

■ Patients with infection are monitored clinically and with serial lab studies (ESR and CRP). After antibiotics are complete, the patient is observed for a few weeks for signs of recurrent infection. If there are no concerns, management of the bone defect can ensue. Many physicians will perform intraoperative frozen section studies assessing the number of neutrophils per high-powered field at any subsequent surgeries. It is wise to maintain suspicion of infection.

■ Persistent or recurrent infection starts the process over again.

OUTCOMES

■ Coagulase-negative *Staphylococcus* and *Staphylococcus aureus* are the most common causes of bacterial osteomyelitis.[3]

■ Age (60 years and older) and diabetes are risk factors for osteomyelitis.[4]

■ The most common cause of persistent infection is inadequate debridement.[5] Often times, the site of inadequate debridement is the intramedullary canal.

COMPLICATIONS

■ The bone that does not heal after debridement, stabilization, and possible antibiotic therapy should trigger additional workup to examine host factors, poor vascularity of tissues, presence of unidentified metabolic conditions, and possible persistent or new infection.

■ Nonhealing bone should also consider the need for more stability (hypertrophic nonunion) or more biology (atrophic nonunion).

REFERENCES

1. Kerr-Valentic MA, Samimi K, Rohlen BH, et al. Marjolin's ulcer: modern analysis of an ancient problem. *Plast Reconstr Surg.* 2009;123:184-191.

2. Tosounidis TH, Calori GM, Giannoudis PV. The use of reamer-irrigator-aspirator in the management of long bone osteomyelitis: an update. *Eur J Trauma Emerg Surg.* 2016;42:417-423.

3. Lew DP, Waldvogel FA. Osteomyelitis. *Lancet.* 2004;364:369-379.

4. Kremers HM, Nwojo ME, Ransom JE. Trends in the epidemiology of osteomyelitis: a population-based study, 1969–2009. *J Bone Joint Surg Am.* 2015;97:837-845.

5. Wagner JM, Zöllner H, Wallner C. Surgical debridement is superior to sole antibiotic therapy in a novel murine posttraumatic osteomyelitis model. *PLoS One.* 2016;11:1-13.

38

CHAPTER

Reconstruction of Femur

Vishwanath R. Chegireddy, Michael J. A. Klebuc, and Anthony Echo

DEFINITION

- Femoral shaft bone defects usually result from tumor resection, traumatic loss, chronic osteomyelitis, congenital skeletal defects, failed allografts, or infected nonunions.[1,2]
- Extensive resection of long bone can lead to large intercalary osseous defects necessitating reconstruction, which was traditionally achieved with allografts or allograft prosthetic composites. These allografts were associated with high rates of complications, including joint instability, fracture of the allograft, and infection of the allograft.[3]
- Vascularized bone flaps are essential for successful bone reconstruction due to their ability to incorporate into the recipient site and provide early bone consolidation while maintaining stability of the appendicular skeletal structure. Owing to its independent blood supply, such a flap is well incorporated into the recipient bone despite compromised surrounding tissue from previous surgery or radiation therapy.
- The advantage of vascularized bone flap over nonvascularized bone grafts is the intrinsic ability to integrate into the recipient bone similar to standard fracture healing instead of creeping substitution.
- The fibula is an ideal vascularized bone flap for femur reconstruction due to its ease of access for harvest while preserving the stability of the proximal and distal tibial-fibular syndesmosis despite segmental resection. It has a negligible influence on knee and ankle joint stability without compromising weight-bearing ability or function of the lower extremity.
- The vascularized fibular flap undergoes hypertrophy overtime in response to continuous pressure load, which translates to remarkable long-term durability.[4-6]

ANATOMY

- The femur is the longest and strongest bone in the body and is subject to large amounts of axial loading as well as significant rotational angular stresses.
- The fibula is a long and thin cortical bone with a small medullary component. In adults, the width of the fibula is 1.5 to 2 cm with a length of 35 cm of which approximately 25 cm of the fibular diaphysis can be harvested for free tissue transfer.
- Vascular supply to the diaphysis of the fibula is via a dominant nutrient endosteal artery and minor musculoperiosteal branches from the peroneal artery and veins. These vessels

run parallel to the fibula and course between the flexor hallucis longus (FHL) and tibialis posterior muscle group.

- The dominant nutrient artery branches 6 to 14 cm from the peroneal artery bifurcation and enters the fibula posterior to the interosseous membrane. It then courses into the nutrient foramen located in the middle third of the diaphysis and further divides into an ascending and descending branch.
- Musculoperiosteal vessels are derived from the peroneal artery and travel within the posterolateral septum, through the FHL and tibialis posterior muscle, giving segmental rise to four to eight branches that supply the muscles in the anterior compartment, soleus muscle, and lateral leg skin territory. The majority of the periosteal branches are located in the middle third of the fibula (**FIG 1**).
- Soft tissue defect coverage is achieved with a skin paddle supplied by perforators traversing through the posterior crural septum with the majority concentrating at the proximal and distal ends of the fibula. These fasciocutaneous perforators supply a skin paddle up to 10 × 20 cm in size.[7]

PATIENT HISTORY AND PHYSICAL FINDINGS

- Detailed preoperative evaluation is required for patients undergoing extensive long bone resection and intercalary bone defect reconstruction.
- A thorough medical history should be obtained to evaluate the peroneal artery for free fibula graft. Pertinent history includes trauma, deep venous thrombosis, peripheral vascular disease, lymphedema, or venous insufficiency. Patients with peripheral vascular disease may not be a candidate for surgery.
- Physical exam should include an evaluation of knee and ankle joints for range of motion and laxity, and a foot Allen test with a Doppler probe to access dorsalis pedis and posterior tibial arteries.
- Peronea arteria magna is a congenital variant of the arterial inflow to the foot, which affects about 1% to 8% of the population, where both the anterior and posterior tibial arteries are hypoplastic or absent with the peroneal artery serving as the single arterial supply below the knee.
- Patients with an abnormal vascular exam or a history of trauma to the affected extremity will need additional preoperative imaging such as an arteriogram, computed tomography angiogram (CTA), duplex ultrasound, or magnetic resonance angiography (MRA) to identify atherosclerotic occlusive disease or congenital anomalies.

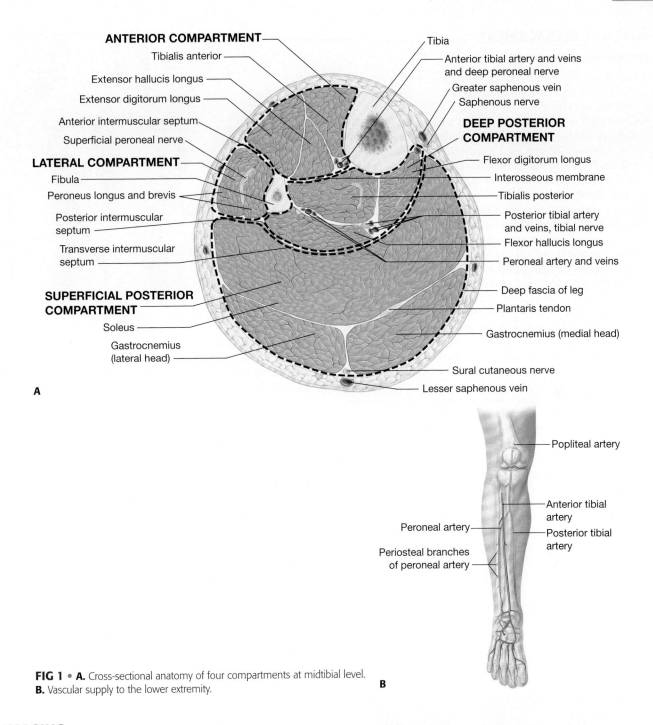

FIG 1 • **A.** Cross-sectional anatomy of four compartments at midtibial level. **B.** Vascular supply to the lower extremity.

IMAGING

- Preoperative imaging of both the recipient and donor sites should include an evaluation of:
- Recipient site:
  - The extent of bone resection, length and diameter of the intercalary defect, and potential soft tissue defect (**FIG 2**). This allows the surgeon to determine the extent of the tumor burden, traumatic bone loss, or chronic osteomyelitis and plan for reconstructive options.
- Donor site:
  - Evaluate vascular supply with Doppler ultrasound (anterior tibial, posterior tibial, and dorsalis pedis arteries), and exclude any fibular deformities.
  - Angiogram to look for vessel patency and flow to the foot.

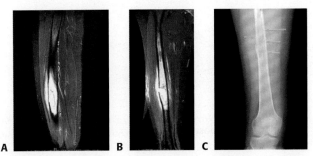

FIG 2 • **A.** Anterior and lateral **(B)** preoperative MRIs showing a right midfemur chondroblastoma. **C.** Plain radiograph of the right femur showing chondroblastoma.

SURGICAL MANAGEMENT

Preoperative Planning

- Free fibula bone graft can be transferred with a generous skin paddle and adjacent muscles such as soleus, peroneal muscles, or FHL.
- Either right or left leg can be used as a donor for fibula flap. The left side is preferable in most patients because it is the less dominant leg and used less frequently while driving a vehicle. However, thoughtful planning of vessel orientation in the recipient site should be considered, when deciding upon laterality.
- Prior to incision, anatomical landmarks including the head of the fibula, lateral malleolus, and anterior and posterior border of the fibula are marked. The posterior border of the fibula correlates with the posterior intermuscular septum encasing the vascular supply to the skin paddle (**FIG 3**).
- Intraoperative Doppler probe is used to identify perforator vessels to design the skin paddle centered over the posterior crural septum. Sometimes, the perforators pass through the FHL and/or soleus muscles and lie posterior to the septum.
- Area of fibula bone resection is marked with superior margin 4 cm below the head of the fibula and inferiorly 6 cm above the lateral malleolus. By preserving the proximal fibula, the stability of the knee is maintained without disrupting the attachment of the tibia to the fibula, fibular collateral ligament to the head of the fibula, and biceps femoris muscle. Also, the common peroneal nerve courses inferior to the head of the fibula, and identifying this location can prevent injury during dissection.

Positioning

- Positioning can allow two surgical teams to work simultaneously, if the contralateral fibula flap is used (**FIG 4**):
  - The patient is placed in the supine position on the operative table with the donor side knee flexed 90 degrees. A roll is placed under the ipsilateral hip to internally rotate the pelvic girdle and keep the hip and knee flexed.
  - A heel stop can be placed on the operative room table to help knee at 90 degrees, when harvesting in the supine position.
- The patient can also be placed in lateral decubitus position if donor and recipient site is in the same limb:

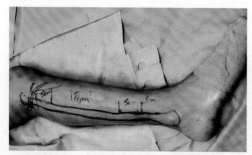

FIG 3 • Intraoperative marking of anatomical landmarks for an ipsilateral fibula harvest in the lateral decubitus position: head of the fibula, lateral malleolus, and anteroposterior fibular border.

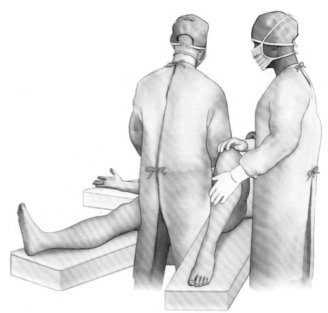

FIG 4 • If the contralateral fibula flap is desired, the patient can be placed in a supine position, which allows two teams to work simultaneously for recipient preparation and donor site harvest.

- A bean bag can help keep the patient in the lateral position.
- All pressure points should be carefully padded and protected.

Approach

- Plastic surgeons and orthopedic surgical team will need to work together to coordinate resection of the affected femur segment and reconstruction of the subsequent intercalary defect. Preservation of potential recipient vessels is of the upmost importance.
- Reconstruction of long femoral intercalary defects with vascularized fibula alone is not sufficient due to inadequate stability and fragility of the bone to tolerate early weight bearing. The Capanna method is ideal in this scenario, using a femoral allograft as a peripheral shell and telescoping the free fibula graft through the allograft segment.[7]
- Reconstruction of smaller intercalary defects up to 13 cm can be achieved with double-barreled fibular flap, keeping the arterial blood supply intact while performing an osteotomy in the fibula flap.
- Initial exposure by the plastic surgeon serves to protect the recipient vessels for microvascular anastomosis at a later point. Although any artery or vein of adequate caliber can be utilized as the recipient vessel, the descending branch of the lateral femoral circumflex artery and vein is the preferred vessel because of its location.
- If extensive soft tissue defect is anticipated due to trauma or tumor/chronic osteomyelitis resection, then a skin paddle can be harvested with the fibular flap by sharing the same vascular pedicle, which helps with early detection of flap compromise and provides tension-free skin closure of recipient site.

■ Free Fibula Flap

- After the bone tumor or chronic osteomyelitis resection by the orthopedic surgical team, the dimensions of the intercalary bone defect are measured (**TECH FIG 1A**).

- Prior to flap harvest, a sterile tourniquet is placed on the midthigh while avoiding compression over the fibular head and common peroneal nerve.
- By tracing the anatomical landmarks, a midlateral vertical incision is made over the fibula, and skin flaps are elevated at the level of the fascia.

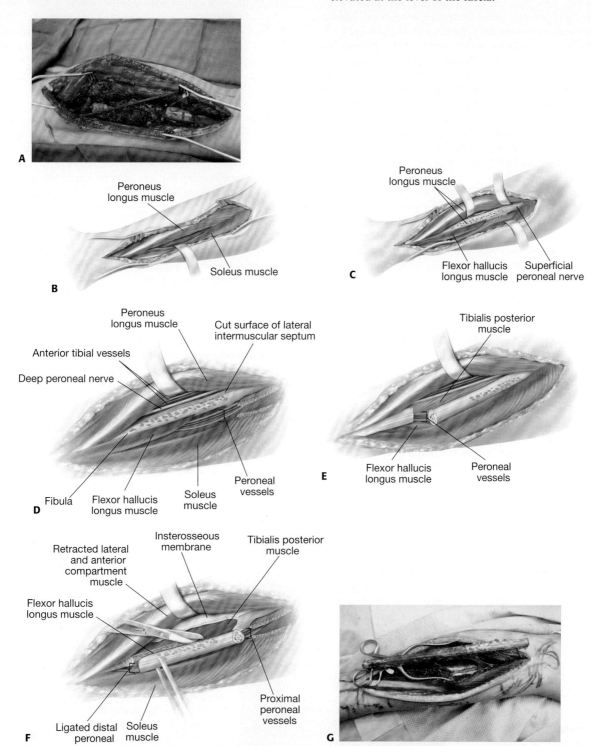

TECH FIG 1 ● A. Right femoral intercalary defect remaining after the tumor resection. **B.** Exposure of peroneus longus and soleus at the midtibial level. **C.** Dissection around the fibula and lateral muscle compartment. Dissection proceeds proximally to identify and protect the superficial peroneal nerve. **D.** Dissection anterior to the fibula through the anterior intermuscular septum and protecting the deep peroneal nerve and anterior tibial vessels. **E.** After the distal fibula osteotomy, the peroneal vessels located between FHL and tibialis posterior muscle groups should be ligated distally. **F.** Adequate fibula length is freed, and proximal osteotomy is performed carefully while protecting the pedicle vessels. **G.** Isolated fibula graft with intact peroneal vessels.

- Dissection is carried through the investing fascia of the lateral compartment, anterior to the posterior intermuscular septum (**TECH FIG 1B–D**):
  - Care should be taken to preserve fasciocutaneous perforators traveling through the posterior intermuscular septum if a skin island is needed for osteocutaneous flap.
- During proximal dissection, identify and preserve the common peroneal nerve traversing around the head of the fibula to become the superficial peroneal nerve.
- The peroneal muscles are dissected off the anterior surface of the fibula and reflected anteriorly to expose the anterior intermuscular septum. The septum is incised to gain access to the anterior compartment and reflect extensor digitorum and hallucis muscles to identify and preserve anterior tibial vessels and deep peroneal nerve.
- The interosseous membrane is incised to enter the deep posterior compartment, and the peroneal vessels are located between tibialis posterior and flexor hallucis longus (FHL) muscles.
- After adequate length of the fibula is marked for reconstruction, towel clamps are used to apply lateral traction on the proximal and distal fibula while osteotomizing with an oscillating saw or Gigli saw. If possible, a strip of periosteum overlying the osteotomy site should be included to overlap the osteotomy sites at the recipient site.

- Prior to performing osteotomy, a microvascular clamp can be applied to the peroneal artery distal to the osteotomy site to ensure adequate supply to the foot and then divided (**TECH FIG 1E**):
  - The vascular pedicle is dissected starting distally and carried proximally up to the origin of tibioperoneal trunk and ligated with approximately 2 to 6 cm of pedicle length.
- Next, the peroneal vessels are identified proximally and distally, and dissection is propagated circumferentially around the fibula while staying medial to the vessels using a large right-angle clamp. The vascular pedicle should be maintained during dissection.
- After the fibula graft is fully mobilized with the pedicle (**TECH FIG 1F,G**), the tourniquet is released. One should see robust arterial inflow and venous outflow and healthy back bleeding from both the periosteum and intramedullary canal.
- An osteomuscular flap can also be harvested in similar fashion to include soleus and FHL muscles. This can aid in filling the dead space in patients with extensive soft tissue defect.
- If the distal osteotomy is close to lateral malleolus, a screw fixation to the tibia can be utilized to prevent valgus deformity and ankle instability, which is more important in a pediatric patient.

■ Capanna Method

- The Capanna technique combines a vascularized fibula graft with massive allograft to reconstruct large defects of the femur to provide structurally competent reconstruction with vascular perfusion and osteogenic capability to achieve lower rates of infection, fracture, and nonunion.[8]
- The free fibula graft can be harvested in similar fashion mentioned earlier:

  - The allograft is cut to match the resected defect, and the medullary canal of the allograft is enlarged with a reamer to create a space for fibula graft (**TECH FIG 2A**).
  - A bur is used to create a window in the allograft to accommodate the vascular pedicle without external compression (**TECH FIG 2B**).
- The fibula is telescoped into the intramedullary canal of the allograft and delivered into the recipient site. This is anchored to the femur proximally and distally with

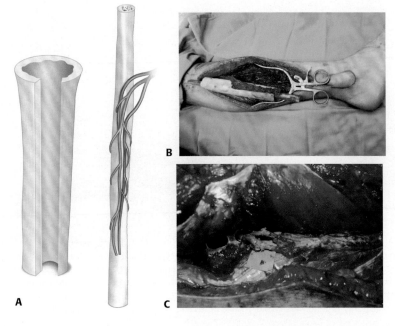

TECH FIG 2 • A. In the Capanna technique, the allograft is cut to match the femur defect size, and the fibula is telescoped into the intramedullary canal of the allograft. Care should be taken to accommodate the vascular pedicle. **B.** The Capanna technique using a femoral allograft. **C.** Microvascular anastomosis between the recipient vessels (descending branch of the lateral femoral circumflex artery and vein) and the flap vessels (peroneal artery and vein).

compression plates and screws. During this step, care is taken to prevent any damage to the nutrient vessel.

- Standard microvascular anastomosis is performed between the recipient vessels and peroneal artery and accompanying venae comitantes (**TECH FIG 2C**):

- Additionally, several fat grafts can be placed around the pedicle in an effort to prevent compression.
- A well-padded posterior leg splint is applied to keep the foot in extension to prevent an equinus deformity.

▪ Double Barrel Fibula Technique

- This technique can be useful for reconstruction of smaller femur defect without the use of an allograft:
  - Larger defects will not be able to be reconstructed with a single fibula in a double-barreled fashion; both fibulas would need to be harvested which is not usually recommended.
- The fibula graft is harvested in similar fashion as described previously. This technique provides a graft that doubles the cross-sectional area of the flap but only requires single arterial and venous anastomosis (**TECH FIG 3**).
- At the site of the proposed osteotomy, the vascular pedicle is carefully elevated off the bone flap in the subperiosteal plane with an elevator over a segment of 2 to 3 cm, which will allow a malleable retractor to be placed to protect the pedicle.
- The graft is osteotomized at the midpoint, with care taken to preserve the peroneal vessels.

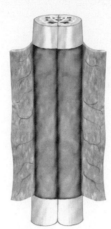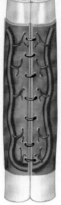

TECH FIG 3 ▪ In the double-barrelled fibula repair, free fibula is harvested with the peroneal vessels intact. The graft is then osteotomized at the midpoint and folded.

PEARLS AND PITFALLS

Flap inset	▪ The goal is to maximize bone-to-bone contact between the recipient bone ends and fibula flap. ▪ Opposition and stability can be achieved by making wedges, steps, or another method that articulates the bone ends together. Creating adequate opposition helps with bone healing while minimizing the number of screws placed into the fibula flap for fixation.
Vascular pedicle	▪ Any fixation needs to consider the vascular pedicle of the flap. The plate should not be placed over the vascular pedicle. In some cases, the screws placed within the bone flap may need to be unicortical. The plastic surgeon should be actively involved with the fixation and inset of the flap.
Vascular variations	▪ Peronea arteria magna is a congenital variant of the arterial inflow to the foot, where both the anterior and posterior tibial arteries are hypoplastic or absent with the peroneal artery serving as the single arterial supply below the knee.
Injury to common peroneal nerve	▪ The nerve courses inferior to the head of the fibula and should be identified during proximal dissection to prevent injury.
Careful dissection of skin perforators	▪ Preserve the posterior intermuscular septum, which carries perforators to the skin paddle.

POSTOPERATIVE CARE

- Monitor donor site for signs and symptoms of vascular insufficiency or compartment syndrome.
- Assess the drains daily and remove if output is less than 20 to 30 cc/day.
- Monitor the flap postoperatively with clinical exam and using Doppler probe every hour for the first 24 hours. Flap monitoring should continue until discharge to check microanastomotic patency and skin island perfusion.

- An internal implantable Doppler can be utilized to monitor a bone flap without a skin paddle.
- No ambulation for 2 weeks postoperatively. Afterward, start with partial weight bearing with crutches until full weight bearing when bone union is achieved.
- If an osteocutaneous flap used for reconstruction fails due to vessel thrombosis, the skin island can be debrided or allowed to heal secondarily. The bone graft can remain in place, and hyperbaric oxygen therapy can be utilized to increase the chance of bone revascularization.

OUTCOMES

- Limb functionality varies depending on trauma, tumor, or infectious etiology.
- Patient counseling is crucial: numerous revision procedures (8.7 per patient)[9] common for best results
- 64% of lower extremity flap complications resolve conservatively; 36% require additional bone grafting or flap revisions.[10]
- Full bone healing: 86% of patients
- Ambulation: all patients (100%) at an average 9.5[9] to 14.3 months[11]
- Joint stiffness (40%) and pain (18%) are frequent.[9]
- Return to work: 63.5% of patients with primarily salvaged limbs[12]

COMPLICATIONS

- General complications:
  - Wound infection (9.6%–23.2%)[9,11,13,14]
  - Bleeding (6.7%)[6]
  - Delayed wound healing or dehiscence (10.0%)[6]
  - Cosmetically unpleasant scar
- Recipient site:
  - Flap failure (3.8%–5.8%)[12,14] due to compromised flap perfusion (eg, anastomotic thrombosis)
  - Minor necrotic areas (11.5%)[14] due to temporary interruptions of the vascular supply
  - Bone nonunion (15.5%–31.0%)[12,13]
  - Osteomyelitis (8.6%–17.3%)[12,13]
  - Revision surgery and need bone for grafting
  - Amputation as ultima ratio (3.9%–7.3%)[12,13]
- Donor site:
  - Knee/ankle instability with secondary pseudoarthrosis (2.0%)[9]
- Prevention: sparing 6 cm at the proximal and 6 cm at the distal end of the fibula in order not to violate the connective structures:
  - Inability to flex the great toe due to extensive dissection of FLH
  - Loss of sensation of peroneal nerve (10.0%)[9]
  - Skin graft failure after donor site closure
- Because of the improvements of microsurgical training and techniques, the use of autologous tissue for lower extremity reconstructions is continuously increasing and offers lower complication rates compared to allografts.[6]

ACKNOWLEDGMENTS

Thank you to D. Zavlin, MD, and Michael J. A. Klebuc, MD, of Houston Methodist Hospital and Weill Cornell Medicine, Houston, Texas, for their help in preparing this chapter.

REFERENCES

1. Bickels J, Meller I, Henshaw RM, Malawer MM. Reconstruction of hip stability after proximal and total femur resections. *Clin Orthop Relat Res.* 2000(375):218-230.
2. Friesecke C, Plutat J, Block A. Revision arthroplasty with use of a total femur prosthesis. *J Bone Joint Surg Am.* 2005;87(12):2693-2701.
3. Getty PJ, Peabody TD. Complications and functional outcomes of reconstruction with an osteoarticular allograft after intra-articular resection of the proximal aspect of the humerus. *J Bone Joint Surg Am.* 1999;81(8):1138-1146.
4. Capanna R, Campanacci DA, Belot N, et al. A new reconstructive technique for intercalary defects of long bones: the association of massive allograft with vascularized fibular autograft. Long-term results and comparison with alternative techniques. *Orthop Clin North Am.* 2007;38(1):51-60.
5. Malizos KN, Zalavras CG, Soucacos PN, et al. Free vascularized fibular grafts for reconstruction of skeletal defects. *J Am Acad Orthop Surg.* 2004;12(5):360-369.
6. Zaretski A, Amir A, Meller I, et al. Free fibula long bone reconstruction in orthopedic oncology: a surgical algorithm for reconstructive options. *Plast Reconstr Surg.* 2004;113(7):1989-2000.
7. Chen ZW, Yan W. The study and clinical application of the osteocutaneous flap of fibula. *Microsurgery.* 1983;4(1):11-16.
8. Bakri K, Stans AA, Mardini S, Moran SL. Combined massive allograft and intramedullary vascularized fibula transfer: the capanna technique for lower-limb reconstruction. *Semin Plast Surg.* 2008;22(3):234-241.
9. Pelissier P, Boireau P, Martin D, Baudet J. Bone reconstruction of the lower extremity: complications and outcomes. *Plast Reconstr Surg.* 2003;111(7):2223-2229.
10. Innocenti M, Menichini G, Baldrighi C, et al. Are there risk factors for complications of perforator-based propeller flaps for lower-extremity reconstruction? *Clin Orthop Relat Res.* 2014;472(7):2276-2286.
11. Weichman KE, Dec W, Morris CD, et al. Lower extremity osseous oncologic reconstruction with composite microsurgical free fibula inside massive bony allograft. *Plast Reconstr Surg.* 2015;136(2):396-403.
12. Saddawi-Konefka D, Kim HM, Chung KC. A systematic review of outcomes and complications of reconstruction and amputation for type IIIB and IIIC fractures of the tibia. *Plast Reconstr Surg.* 2008; 122(6):1796-1805.
13. Harris AM, Althausen PL, Kellam J, et al. Complications following limb-threatening lower extremity trauma. *J Orthop Trauma.* 2009; 23(1):1-6.
14. Kang MJ, Chung CH, Chang YJ, Kim KH. Reconstruction of the lower extremity using free flaps. *Arch Plast Surg.* 2013;40(5):575-583.

Soft Tissue Coverage of the Thigh—Pedicled Rectus Flap

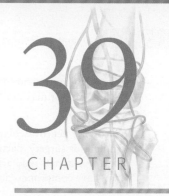

CHAPTER 39

Brock Lanier and Alex Wong

DEFINITION

- Soft tissue defects of the thigh can involve critical anatomy including the neurovascular structures of the femoral triangle (i.e. common femoral artery, common femoral vein, and femoral nerve) and/or bone.
- Prior infection, radiation, trauma, tumor resection, or other pathologies can render local or pedicled flaps from the thigh unusable for reconstruction. In such scenarios the pedicled rectus flap is a reliable workhorse for thigh defects.
- The rectus flap is very versatile. It can be used as a pedicled muscle or myocutaneous flap. The available flap dimensions can range from a small segment of muscle to a large flap incorporating an extended skin component.[1]

ANATOMY

- The rectus abdominis muscle spans the vertical length of the abdominal wall. It originates from the pubis, inserts at the fifth to seventh costal cartilage, and is situated in pairs along the paramedian axis of its anterior wall. It is a Mathes and Nahai type III muscle with two codominant vascular pedicles: the superior epigastric artery and the inferior epigastric artery (**FIG 1**).

- In order to use the pedicled rectus flap for thigh reconstruction, the superior epigastric artery is transected and the flap is rotated maintaining the blood supply from the inferior epigastric artery.
- Perforating branches from the inferior epigastric artery are concentrated around the umbilicus. As such, the periumbilical area should be incorporated into the design of any myocutaneous flap's skin paddle.
- If the periumbilical perforators to the skin are utilized, an almost infinite number of skin paddle designs are possible. Large (*size*) skin paddles can be transposed to the thigh defect if needed.[2]

PATIENT HISTORY AND PHYSICAL FINDINGS

- Most soft tissue defects involving the thigh are associated with either trauma or cancer.
- Focused examinations of the abdomen and lower extremity should be performed:
  - The abdominal examination should evaluate for previous surgical scars, the presence of abdominal wall hernias, and skin laxity if a myocutaneous flap is being considered:
    - Transverse midabdominal laparotomy scars indicate that the rectus abdominis was likely transected.

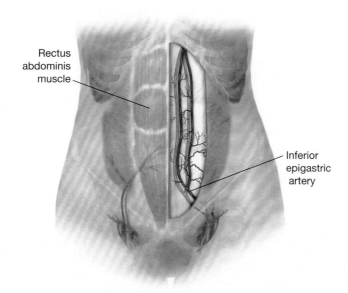

FIG 1 • VRAM clinical anatomy. The rectus abdominis muscle originates from the pubis and inserts at the fifth to seventh costal cartilage. It has codominant vascular pedicles: the superior epigastric artery and the inferior epigastric artery. The VRAM skin paddle must include periumbilical skin perforators.

Rectus abdominis muscle

Inferior epigastric artery

- Low transverse scars associated with prior cesarean sections may or may not have violated the inferior epigastric pedicle.

■ Check the neurovascular status of the lower extremities. Trauma or surgery, particularly vascular surgery, involving the external iliac artery or common femoral artery, may have compromised the inferior epigastric pedicle.

IMAGING

■ Imaging is not mandatory but can be considered if the patient's physical exam is concerning regarding the integrity of the inferior epigastric artery.

■ CT angiography can assess the pedicle and can concurrently evaluate the abdominal wall for occult hernias and other pathologies.

■ MR angiography and ultrasonography are other modalities that can also be considered.

NONOPERATIVE MANAGEMENT

■ Nonoperative treatment of soft tissue defects of the proximal thigh is limited, especially when critical structures of the femoral triangle or osseous structures of the lateral thigh are exposed.

■ Temporary coverage using vacuum-assisted wound care devices can be considered depending on the contents of the wound.

SURGICAL MANAGEMENT

■ Surgical management decisions include timing (immediate vs delayed reconstruction) and choice of the flap.

■ Flap options include local pedicled flaps of the thigh such as the anterolateral thigh flap, tensor fascia lata flap, gracilis flap, and sartorius flap.

■ Free flaps are also an option if appropriate regional options do not exist.

TECHNIQUES

■ Flap Design

■ The size and depth of the soft tissue defect should be defined following tumor resection or wound debridement.

■ Critical landmarks include the symphysis pubis and the anterior superior iliac spine (ASIS), which defines the inguinal ligament.
  ■ The origin of the inferior epigastric artery is at the halfway point of the distance between the symphysis pubis and the ASIS.

■ The paramedian location of the rectus abdominis muscle is marked.

■ If desired, a template of the defect can be constructed (e.g., using wrapping paper from sterile gloves) to facilitate creation of the design of the skin paddle. It is suggested that the length of the muscle and the size of the skin paddle be slightly larger than the defect.

■ The donor site of muscle flaps will almost always close primarily.
  ■ The donor site of skin paddle of a myocutaneous flap should be assessed during flap design. A pinch test can ensure that the donor site will be able to close primarily.

■ In pedicled flaps such as the rectus abdominis, the pivot of the flap about its vascular pedicle should be considered during flap design (**TECH FIG 1**).

■ Typically, the flap will rotate externally to reach a lateral thigh defect and internally to reach a medial thigh defect. A sterile towel or laparotomy pad can be used to simulate the arc of rotation of the flap about its pivot point to ensure adequate length of the flap during flap design.

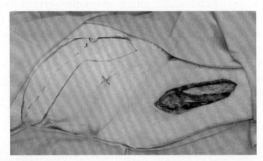

TECH FIG 1 • Lateral view of the abdomen and right thigh, demonstrating proximal anterolateral thigh full-thickness defect with exposed femur. The extended vertical rectus myocutaneous (eVRAM) flap has been marked incorporating the flap's periumbilical perforators into its design.

■ Flap Harvest

■ For a muscle flap without skin island, the approach may be via a paramedian incision directly over the muscle or a low transverse abdominoplasty incision.
  ■ Once the anterior rectus sheath is exposed, it is entered sharply in the middle of the muscle and reflected medially and laterally to expose the muscle.
  ■ For smaller defects of the thigh, a segment of the muscle can be harvested, leaving the remaining muscle supplied by the superior epigastric artery.

■ For a myocutaneous flap (**TECH FIG 2A**), the skin paddle must be in continuity with the anterior rectus sheath to incorporate perforating vessels.
  ■ At the medial and lateral surface, the fat and skin can be elevated 1 to 3 cm off of the anterior sheath to allow for the donor site to be closed directly.

■ To complete harvest, the muscle is circumferentially dissected off of the posterior rectus sheath (**TECH FIG 2B**).
  ■ Below the arcuate line, the posterior sheath is thin because it consists only of transversalis fascia.

- Neurovascular bundles associated with intercostal nerves are controlled with either suture ties or clips.
- The inferior epigastric pedicle is identified at the inferolateral aspect of the muscle approximately 4 cm cranial to the origin.
- The flap's pedicle can be dissected back to its external iliac origin to maximize the arc of rotation.

- Care should be taken not to exert excessive tension or pressure on the pedicle during the dissection.
- The cranial aspect of the muscle is transected at the costal margin, taking particular attention to identifying the superior epigastric artery.
  - The caudal aspect of the muscle can also be divided from the pubic origin for additional length.

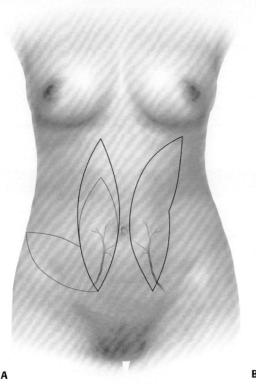
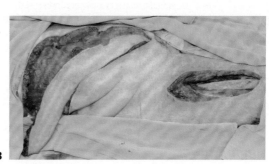

TECH FIG 2 • **A.** Examples of skin paddle designs of VRAM and extended VRAM. **B.** Dissected extended VRAM in situ at the donor site.

■ Flap Inset and Completion

- According to the location of the soft tissue defect, the flap can be rotated or tunneled to the defect (**TECH FIG 3A**).
  - With the flap in situ at the recipient site, its vascular status should be assessed before inset.
  - The pedicle can be checked to ensure there is minimal twisting and no acute turns compromising flow.
  - For myocutaneous flaps, the skin paddle's cutaneous Doppler signal sites should be examined and can be

marked with ink or small suture (e.g., 5-0 polypropylene) to facilitate postoperative monitoring.
- The flap is inset in layers using suture and/or staples. A skin graft can be applied if appropriate (**TECH FIG 3B**).
- The anterior rectus sheath donor site is repaired directly with sutures (e.g., no. 1 PDS).
  - When a skin paddle is incorporated into the flap, mesh is usually required to minimize tension on the repair.[3]

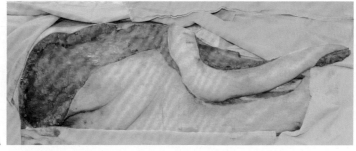

TECH FIG 3 • **A.** Rotation of VRAM flap demonstrates that it can reach past midthigh.

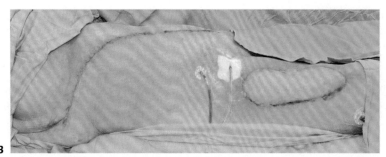

B

TECH FIG 3 (Continued) • **B.** Final intraoperative lateral view appearance of the abdomen and right thigh with the eVRAM donor site closed primarily and the flap inset after de-epithelization and tunneled through the subcutaneous space.

PEARLS AND PITFALLS

Artery preservation	■ In the setting of large soft tissue defects involving the proximal thigh, it is essential to ensure that the origin of the inferior epigastric artery has been preserved. ■ Radical resections involving the ipsilateral common femoral artery or external iliac artery will likely compromise the flap's pedicle. The need for vascular reconstruction of these vessels should alert the reconstructive surgeon.
Flap design	■ The flap can be trimmed and customized to a smaller size during inset. It cannot be enlarged once it has been dissected. ■ For this reason, a larger flap is recommended (longer rectus and/or larger skin paddle). Consider a 20% larger design than what is suggested by the initial measurements of the soft tissue defect.

POSTOPERATIVE CARE

■ The abdominal donor site can be dressed with a sterile occlusive dressing (e.g., gauze, adhesive tape, or topical liquid bonding product).

■ The dressing for the flap depends on the type of the flap (muscle with or without skin graft, skin paddle) and preference of the surgeon.

■ Pedicled flaps to the proximal thigh are at risk with early postoperative motion. A short period of immobilization, especially for flaps with overlaying skin grafts, should be considered.

■ Flap checks examining the color, turgor, temperature, and/or Doppler signal should be performed in accordance with institutional standards. Many protocols call for hourly flap checks during postoperative day 1, every 2 hours on postoperative day 2, and every 4 to 6 hours thereafter.

OUTCOMES

■ The pedicled rectus abdominis flap has a constant blood supply, making it a safe and reliable option for small to large soft tissue defects of the proximal thigh (**FIG 2**).

COMPLICATIONS

■ Obesity, smoking, uncontrolled diabetes, and prior abdominal surgery are factors that have been associated with an increased risk of complication.[4]

■ Intraoperative vascular complications related to twisting or kinking of the pedicle during inset

■ Acute venous insufficiency is rare but can occur in patients with a dominant superficial venous system. If this is encountered, then the flap can be returned to its native position, and its inset can be postponed for a few days allowing for the delay phenomenon to occur.

■ Partial flap necrosis may occur at the distal aspect of the skin island in myocutaneous flaps.[5]

■ Postoperative hematoma or seroma[5]

■ Donor site bulge or hernia (12%)[5]

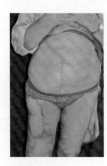

FIG 2 • Result 1 year postoperatively, demonstrating the postoperative appearance of the healed eVRAM donor site and flap.

REFERENCES

1. Gottlieb ME, Chandrasekhar B, Terz JJ, Sherman R. Clinical applications of the extended deep inferior epigastric flap. *Plast Reconstr Surg.* 1986;78(6):782-792.

2. Lee MJ, Dumanian GA. The oblique rectus abdominis musculocutaneous flap: revisited clinical applications. *Plast Reconstr Surg.* 2004;114(2):367-373.

3. Küntscher MV, Mansouri S, Noack N, Hartmann B. Versatility of vertical rectus abdominis musculocutaneous flaps. *Microsurgery.* 2006; 26(5):363-369.

4. Nelson RA, Butler CE. Surgical outcomes of VRAM versus thigh flaps for immediate reconstruction of pelvic and perineal cancer resection defects. *Plast Reconstr Surg.* 2009;123(1):175-183.

5. Parrett BM, Winograd JM, Garfein ES, et al. The vertical and extended rectus abdominis myocutaneous flap for irradiated thigh and groin defects. *Plast Reconstr Surg.* 2008;122(1):171-177.

40
CHAPTER

Soft Tissue Coverage of Thigh—Free Flaps

Ulrich Kneser and Thomas Kremer

DEFINITION

- Soft tissue defects of the thigh requiring free flap reconstruction are rare, because of a sufficient soft tissue envelope that frequently allows other reconstructive options such as split-thickness skin grafting, local random pattern, or pedicled flaps.
- Exposure of functional structures such as neurovascular bundles, tendons, or bone may require reconstruction using free microvascular tissue transfer.

ANATOMY

- Anatomy of the thigh is characterized by a sufficient number of strong muscles:
  - Anterior:
    - The quadriceps muscle (medial, lateral, and vastus intermedius muscle as well as rectus femoris muscle)
    - The sartorius muscle
  - Medial:
    - The adductor muscles (gracilis, adductor magnus, adductor longus, adductor brevis, and pectineus muscle)
  - Posterior:
    - Biceps femoris muscle
    - Semitendinosus muscle
    - Semimembranosus muscle
- Perfusion of the thigh is maintained by the femoral artery and its branches:
  - Profunda femoris artery (with medial circumflex and lateralis artery)
  - Descending genicular artery
  - Popliteal artery
  - Peripheral branches of the inferior gluteal artery for the proximal dorsum
- Major nerves of the thigh are:
  - The femoral nerve (quadriceps, sartorius, and pectineus muscle)
  - Obturator nerve (adductor muscles)
  - Sciatic nerve (posterior muscles of the thigh)
- Venous drainage of the thigh is provided by deep veins and the saphenous vein.

PATIENT HISTORY AND PHYSICAL FINDINGS

- Defects at the thigh may results from trauma, infection, or oncologic resection. Each of these entities should be evaluated and requires special focus during patient examination.
- Patients with traumatic soft tissue defects of the thigh should be asked for the mechanism of injury. This may help to identify the true extent of the defect and concomitant trauma consequences.

- Infections of the thigh should be evaluated for dynamics, systemic consequences (eg, fever, fatigue), pain, prior antibiotic treatment, as well as potential causes and infectious portals of entry.
- The major goal in patients after oncologic resection is to evaluate prognosis, prior treatment, and adjuvant treatment options, since this information strongly influences therapeutic as well as reconstructive choices.
- Additional important factors influencing reconstruction are patients' demands: patients who were ambulating normally prior treatment may require more extensive reconstructive attempts than patients who are chair- or even bed-bound.
- Inspection of the thigh in patients suffering from soft tissue loss should assess the extent and depth of the defect as well as exposed functional structures. Additionally, the surroundings of the defect should be carefully evaluated: scarring, tension, and former incisions should be noted. Prior radiation therapy may lead to wound healing disturbances and subsequent postoperative morbidity and should therefore be taken into account.
- When free flap reconstruction is required, potential donor vessels should be evaluated. The distance from these vessels to the most distant part of the defect should be measured and significantly influences flap choices. In some patient, even more invasive strategies such as arteriovenous loops or bypasses may be necessary.
- Patients should be asked for varicosity or prior venous surgery (such as venous stripping or bypass surgery).

IMAGING

- Photographs of the defect should be performed including the complete thigh as well as detailed pictures focusing on the defect.
- Conventional x-rays of the femur in two perpendicular views (anteroposterior and lateral) may show concomitant fractures or nonunions in traumatic cases, osteomyelitis after infection, or oncologic osseous lesions in oncologic patients.
- Magnetic resonance imaging and computed tomography may reveal the real extent of the defect or sequelae of infection of the bone as well as soft tissue. However, both options should not postpone onset of treatment in special patients such as cases with necrotizing infections.
- Radiologic examination of donor vessels is required in patients prior to microsurgery for thigh defects. MRI or CT angiographies are sufficient in most cases. The advantage of conventional angiographies in these patients is that endoluminal interventions are possible, if necessary.

- Doppler or duplex ultrasound is indicated to evaluate the superficial venous system and for venous mapping if vein grafts may be required.

SURGICAL MANAGEMENT

- Indications for free flap reconstruction at the thigh are relatively rare. Most cases can be managed using local random pattern or pedicled flaps as well as split-thickness skin grafting. However, extensive defects with exposure of functional structures such as bone, neurovascular bundles, or tendons may require free tissue transfer.
- Another reason for microsurgical flap transplantation is radiation therapy. Tissues from distant donor sites that are not radiated may improve the healing capacity of irradiated wound beds. This is especially important because soft tissue sarcoma of the limbs most commonly occur at the thigh.[1] Here, defect reconstruction using free flaps can even be indicated when primary wound closure would be possible with tension. In these patients, complications rates can be reduced when reconstruction with nonradiated flaps is applied.
- Any reconstructive attempt should only be started when wounds are sufficiently debrided. No signs of infection or devitalized tissue should be present.
- In some cases, vacuum-assisted closure (VAC) therapy can be performed to prepare wounds for soft tissue reconstruction.

Preoperative Planning

- Different parameters influence the choice for various reconstructive options:
  - The aim of reconstruction (eg, palliative vs curative intention, limb salvage vs major amputation; ability to walk or just to sit)
  - Structures or functions requiring reconstruction, extent of the defect (eg, soft tissue loss, bone damage, muscle function, nerve injury)
  - Perfusion of the wound bed (eg, in patients with peripheral arterial disease, after radiation therapy)
  - The patients' individual needs and compliance as well as concomitant diseases
  - Donor site morbidity
  - Adjuvant therapy options or further surgery
- Another important information is the distance from potential donor vessels to the most distant part of the defect. If this distance is too long, the risk of partial flap loss ("where

you need it most") is increased. In these cases, arteriovenous loops or vessel interpositional grafts should be considered.
- Patients with atherosclerosis should be evaluated by angiography and should be presented to vascular surgeons or interventional radiologists prior to surgery.
- If multidisciplinary approaches are required (eg, osseous internal fixation, soft tissue reconstruction and/or vascular surgical interventions), a detailed preoperative discussion is required. The sequence and extent of different surgical steps, postoperative care, and operative strategy has to be considered. Here, interdisciplinary extremity boards similar to oncologic tumor boards have been shown to be very efficient.

Positioning

- Patient positioning depends on donor vessels, flap choice, as well as additional surgical interventions (eg, osteosyntheses, vascular surgery, harvest of vein grafts).
- Supine positioning allows:
  - Common flaps: anterolateral thigh flap, gracilis flaps, rectus abdominis myocutaneous flaps, tensor fascia lata flaps, vastus lateralis flaps, lateral arm flap, forearm flaps
  - Donor vessels: femoral artery and vein in the groin and adductors canal
- Lateral decubitus position (**FIG 1**):
  - Common flaps: flaps from the subscapular system
  - Donor vessels: femoral artery and vein in adductor canal
- In some patients, it is not possible to perform the complete procedure in one position (eg, when internal osseous fixation is required). Here, intraoperative repositioning may be necessary.

Approach

- The surgical approach to defects at the thigh is defined by defect localization as well as extent and cannot be discussed here in detail.
- Recipient vessels at the thigh predominantly are the femoral vessels. These can best be approached in the groin and the adductors canal.
- In patients with unfavorable defect localization, microvascular anastomoses can be performed to arteriovenous loops (that can be performed in the same procedure or separately in prior procedures) or interpositional vein grafts.
- If different approaches to the defect, vessels, and bone have to be combined, the surgeons should carefully discuss operative incisions in advance to prevent skin malperfusion.

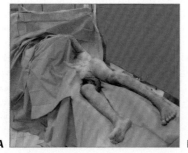 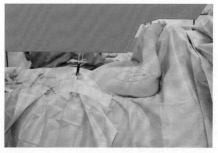

A   **B**

FIG 1 • The lateral decubitus position of patients allows exposure of the thigh and femoral vessels, if the contralateral leg is placed backward. **A.** Care has to be taken for the upper arm that has to be prevented from any compression to prevent compartment syndromes in lengthy procedures. **B.** Flaps from the subscapular system can easily be harvested.

■ Approach to the Groin

- The femoral artery and vein can easily be identified in the groin (**TECH FIG 1**). These vessels arise from the external iliac artery and course under the inguinal ligament into the thigh. Here, the artery can usually be found by palpation. The femoral vein is located medial to the artery, whereas the femoral nerve courses laterally.
- The course of the vessels across the thigh is between the vastus medialis muscle (laterally) and the adductor muscles. Distally, the sartorius muscle lies superficial to the vessels.
- Major arterial branches in the groin are the deep femoral artery, the superficial epigastric, and the circumflex iliac artery. The saphenous vein can likewise be identified in the groin.

- The skin incision is performed distal to the inguinal ligament over the vessels that were previously identified by palpation or Doppler probe. During subcutaneous preparation, the saphenous vein should be identified and preserved.
- Because the femoral vessels lie on the muscles in the groin, these structures can easily be dissected. For safety reasons, the major branches should be identified (especially the deep femoral artery) and secured using vessels loops.
- After dissection of the femoral artery and vein over several centimeters, an adventitiectomy should be performed to prepare the vessels for anastomosis that is usually performed in an end-to-side fashion.

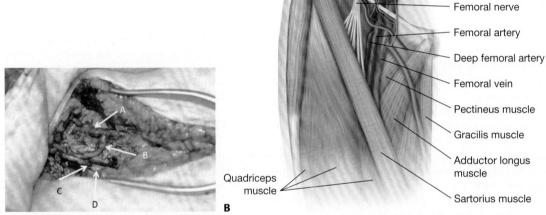

Femoral nerve

Femoral artery

Deep femoral artery

Femoral vein

Pectineus muscle

Gracilis muscle

Adductor longus muscle

Quadriceps muscle

Sartorius muscle

A   **B**

TECH FIG 1 • A. The femoral vessels can be exposed in the groin. Here, the femoral vein (*A*) is visualized caudal to the inguinal ligament. Dissection was performed to the entry of the saphenous vein. (*B*) Here, the saphenous vein is pulled cranially (left) to form an arteriovenous loop through an end-to-side anastomosis (*C*) to the femoral artery (*D*) in the groin. **B.** Illustration of the femoral vessels in the groin.

■ Approach to the Adductor Canal

- The anatomical borders of the adductor canal are:
  - Dorsally: adductor longus muscle (**TECH FIG 2A**)
  - Ventrally: vastoadductor membrane between the tendons of the vastus medialis and adductor longus muscles (see **TECH FIG 2A**)
  - Medially: adductor magnus muscle
  - Laterally: vastus medialis muscle
- The femoral vein is located under ("deep") the femoral artery.
- Additional structures in the adductor canal are the saphenous nerve and the descending genicular artery.
- The approach to the femoral artery and vein is possible in supine as well as lateral decubitus position.

- The skin incision is performed at the medial thigh (**TECH FIG 2B**). During subcutaneous dissection, the saphenous vein can be found and prepared for anastomosis.
- After incision of the fascia of the thigh, the descending genicular artery can be identified (**TECH FIG 2C**). This structure can be used as a guide into the adductor canal, and the femoral artery and vein can easily be found. Both vessels are then dissected (**TECH FIG 2D**).
- Care has to be taken to preserve the femoral vein behind (deep) to the femoral artery. Several arterial and venous branches arise from the femoral vessels in the adductor canals. Some of these generally seem to be sufficient for anastomosis. However, the authors recommend ignoring these vessels because complication rates are significantly higher when compared to direct end-to-side anastomoses to the "big" femoral vessels.

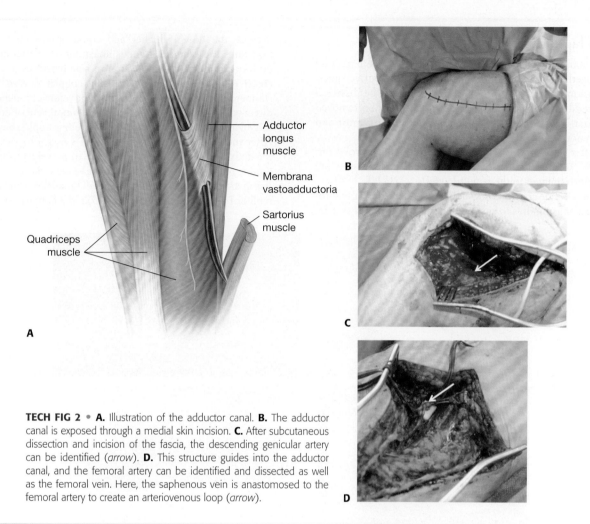

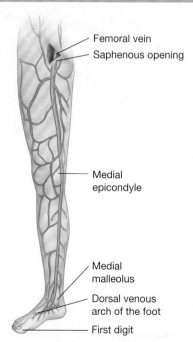

TECH FIG 2 • A. Illustration of the adductor canal. **B.** The adductor canal is exposed through a medial skin incision. **C.** After subcutaneous dissection and incision of the fascia, the descending genicular artery can be identified (*arrow*). **D.** This structure guides into the adductor canal, and the femoral artery can be identified and dissected as well as the femoral vein. Here, the saphenous vein is anastomosed to the femoral artery to create an arteriovenous loop (*arrow*).

Labels in TECH FIG 2A: Quadriceps muscle; Adductor longus muscle; Membrana vastoadductoria; Sartorius muscle

■ Dissection of the Saphenous Vein

- The saphenous vein collects the blood of the dorsum of the foot and courses superficially at the lower leg. Around the knee, it courses dorsal to the medial femoral condyle before it runs anteriorly at the thigh and penetrates the fascia in the groin where it enters the femoral vein (**TECH FIG 3**).
- The entire course of the saphenous vein is epifascially.
- During dissection, numerous branches can be identified. These should be ligated with sutures rather than vessel clips, because the latter often prove to be insufficient and postoperative bleeding occurs. This is especially important, when parts of the vein are inserted into the arterial system in arteriovenous loops, since vessel clips frequently fail to withstand arterial pressure.
- If the saphenous vein is exposed to arterial pressure, it significantly lengthens. This effect has to be considered when arteriovenous loops are performed. Here, the arterial part of the loop should be planned slightly shorter than the venous side.

Labels in TECH FIG 3: Femoral vein; Saphenous opening; Medial epicondyle; Medial malleolus; Dorsal venous arch of the foot; First digit

TECH FIG 3 • The saphenous vein collects the blood of the dorsum of the foot and courses superficially at the lower leg. Around the knee, it courses dorsal to the medial femoral condyle before it runs anteriorly at the thigh and penetrates the fascia in the groin where it enters the femoral vein.

■ Flap and Anastomosis

- If muscle flaps are performed, these should be harvested together with skin islands to allow postoperative supervision of perfusion. These skin islands can be dissected based on one perforator and can therefore be removed after 7 to 10 days just by ligation of the perforator and to not require a second procedure.
- After flap harvest (**TECH FIG 4A**), the flap is provisionally secured to the thigh, and the recipient vessels are approximated to the femoral vessels.
- End-to-side anastomoses should be preferred over end-to-end anastomoses to side branches for the arterial system, because the flow is higher and consecutive complication rates are reduced. Venous anastomosis is routinely performed in end-to-end fashion to side branches of the (**TECH FIG 4B–E**) femoral vein using coupler devices or standard suture. In cases of insufficient venous branches, direct end-to-side anastomosis to the femoral vein or end-to-end anastomosis to the saphenous vein is applicable.
- After the anastomoses are finished, it is useful to secure the anastomotic site using fibrin glue to prevent postoperative repositioning and subsequent vessel kinking.
- Adequate perfusion of the flap is either checked by capillary refill or by brisk capillary bleeding from the flap margins.

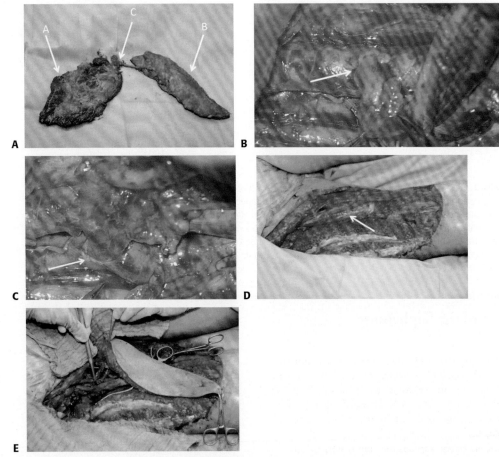

TECH FIG 4 • A. A combined latissimus (*A*) and parascapular (*B*) flap was harvested to reconstruct an extensive traumatic defect after a motor bike accident (*C*). The vascular pedicle was dissected to the subscapular artery and vein **B.** End-to-side anastomosis (*arrow*) was performed of the subscapular artery to the femoral artery. **C.** Venous anastomosis (*arrow*) was likewise done to the femoral vein. **D.** An extensive traumatic defect at the thigh with exposed femur required reconstruction using free tissue transfer because the femoral vessels were exposed (*arrow*). **E.** After anastomosis to the femoral vessels.

■ Flap Inset, Skin Grafting

- After flap reperfusion, manipulation to the anastomotic side should be avoided for some minutes. During this period, anastomotic flow is established and minor anastomotic bleeding terminates.
- Flap inset is the performed temporarily using suture clips. The anastomotic site and flap pedicle are then checked for optimal positioning before the flap is definitely sutured to the defect. Skin-to-skin closure is preferred in fasciocutaneous flaps, whereas muscle flaps are fixed under the defect margins that should be elevated. Here, running sutures using absorbable monofilament material are preferred over nonresorbable sutures.
- Muscle flaps should be covered using split-thickness skin grafts (**TECH FIG 5**). In these cases, it can be useful to provide vacuum-assisted closure therapy to the skin-grafted

area (using low pressures such as 75 mm Hg) to allow optimal wound healing.

- Split-thickness skin grafting can be performed under monitor skin islands already, if these are harvested based on perforators.

- Care has to be taken to prevent any compression to the anastomosis or flap pedicle when wound dressings are applied.

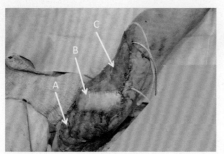
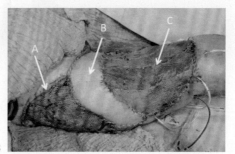

TECH FIG 5 • A,B. Flap inset was performed, and the latissimus flap as well as the proximal thigh musculature were skin grafted (*A*, proximal thigh muscles; *B*, parascapular flap; *C*, latissimus dorsi flap with split-thickness skin grafts).

PEARLS AND PITFALLS

Preoperative planning	▪ A detailed analysis of the defect is necessary prior to surgery to identify every structure that needs to be reconstructed. ▪ For flap choice, the distance from the anastomotic site to the most distant part of the defect has to be considered. ▪ The bulk of the flap has to be considered, when skin-to-skin closure is attempted.
Arterial disease	▪ If the patient suffers from peripheral arterial disease or varicosity, a vascular surgeon or interventional radiologist should be involved in the treatment team.
Patients' needs	▪ The patients' needs have to be evaluated prior to surgery. The reconstructive aim significantly varies if the patient is ambulating normally or if he is chair- or bed-bound. ▪ Palliative surgery vs curative attempts in oncologic patients.
Anastomosis	▪ End-to-side anastomoses to the femoral vessels are preferred over end-to-end anastomoses to side branches, because blood flow is greater and complication rates are reduced.
Postoperative care	▪ Flap perfusion has to be monitored on a regular base for the first postoperative days. ▪ Monitoring is possible clinically in fasciocutaneous flaps, or monitor skin islands of muscle flaps. The latter can be harvested based on a perforator to allow removal without additional surgery.

POSTOPERATIVE CARE

- Postoperative positioning of the patient can be crucial. Compression of the pedicle or flap has to be avoided. Here, postoperative positioning has to be discussed with the patient preoperatively. This increases the patients' understanding and compliance.
- External fixators can be helpful to allow adequate postoperative positioning.
- Postoperative anticoagulation is part of an ongoing debate.[2] In general, less intervention is preferred over aggressive anticoagulation. The authors only prescribe low molecular weight heparin for thromboembolic prophylaxis. Higher doses or intravenous heparin are only applied in bypass free flaps or after revision surgery. If patients develop thrombocytosis or arterial clots, acetylsalicylic acid can be useful.
- Flap perfusion has to be monitored on a regular base (hourly) to allow immediate revision surgery if arterial inflow or venous drainage is compromised.
- After 5 to 7 days, the flap should be exposed to gravity (so-called dangling procedure), and the patients should be mobilized.[3]

- Physical therapy has to be applied from the first postoperative days.
- Compression garments are usually required to avoid bulky flaps and scars as well as contractures. Scar massage is beneficial in most patients.
- Physical therapy and rehabilitation have to be planned in most patients. However, these are mostly defined as the individual defect and rarely depend on the microsurgical procedure itself (**FIG 2**).

OUTCOMES

- Outcomes after free flap surgery to thigh defects mostly depend on the underlying condition rather than on the microsurgical procedure itself.
- Outcomes in traumatic patients mainly depend on wound healing, osseous healing, and long-term function due to scarring or post-traumatic arthritis.
- Prognosis in oncologic patients depends on the tumor itself and is determinated by size, location, tumor biology, immunology, and distant metastases.

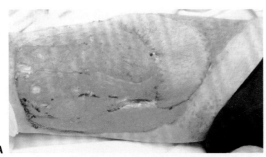 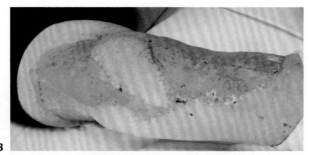

FIG 2 • Results after 2 months with uneventful wound healing (medial view **(A)**, lateral view **(B)**).

- Infectious control is of utmost importance in consecutive patients. Here, flap perfusion is as important as postoperative antibiotic treatment that can be required for long periods, when osteomyelitis is evident.

COMPLICATIONS

- Flap failure rates vary significantly depending on defect causes and localization. Failure rates between 1% and 10% are described internationally.[4]
- Other complications include wound infection, incomplete healing or ongoing infection, as well as partial flap loss. The latter can be as detrimental as a complete flap loss und should therefore be prevented if possible. Here, flap dimensions should not be extended as much as possible. If large defects have to be reconstructed, flaps should be combined, or microsurgical effort has to be increased for maximum safety (eg, inclusion of multiple perforators with in-flap anastomoses, use of arteriovenous loops, bypass free flaps, combined or chimeric flaps).

REFERENCES

1. Bains R, Magdum A, Bhat W, et al. Soft tissue sarcoma—a review of presentation, management and outcomes in 110 patients. *Surgeon.* 2016;14(3):129-135.
2. Kremer T, Bauer M, Zahn P, et al. [Perioperative management in microsurgery—consensus statement of the german speaking society for microsurgery of peripheral nerves and vessels]. *Handchir Mikrochir Plast Chir.* 2016;48(4):205-211.
3. Neubert N, Vogt PM, May M, et al. Does an early and aggressive combined wrapping and dangling procedure affect the clinical outcome of lower extremity free flaps?—A randomized controlled prospective study using microdialysis monitoring. *J Reconstr Microsurg.* 2016;32(4):262-270.
4. Xiong L, Gazyakan E, Kremer T, et al. Free flaps for reconstruction of soft tissue defects in lower extremity: a meta-analysis on microsurgical outcome and safety. *Microsurgery.* 2016;36(6):511-524. doi:10.1002/micr.30020.

Nerve Repair and Reconstruction—Sciatic Nerve and Femoral Nerve

Gabrielle B. Davis and Catherine Curtin

CHAPTER 41

SCIATIC NERVE

DEFINITION

- The sciatic nerve is the largest peripheral nerve in the body.
- Its role is critical for lower extremity protective sensation and ambulation.
- Sciatic nerve injury in the setting of lower extremity trauma was historically an indication for amputation.
- Recent advancements in microsurgical techniques have led to improved outcomes and viability of the extremity.

ANATOMY

- The origin of the sciatic nerve is from the ventral divisions of L4, L5, S1, S2, and S3.
- The confluence of nerve fibers joins in the pelvis and exits via the greater sciatic foramen and below the piriformis muscle (**FIG 1**).
- In the buttocks, the sciatic nerve is located posterior to the gluteus maximus muscle and anterior to the superior gemellus, obturator internus, inferior gemellus, and quadratus femoris.

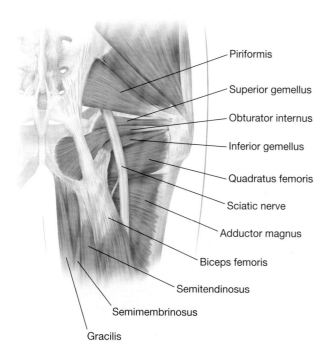

FIG 1 • Course of the sciatic nerve as it exits the pelvis below the piriformis muscle.

Labels: Piriformis; Superior gemellus; Obturator internus; Inferior gemellus; Quadratus femoris; Sciatic nerve; Adductor magnus; Biceps femoris; Semitendinosus; Semimembrinosus; Gracilis

- It courses inferiorly, midway between the greater trochanter and the ischial tuberosity.
- In the posterior thigh, it travels deep to the long head of the biceps femoris.
- There are two distinct divisions of the sciatic nerve traveling within the same sheath, the peroneal and tibial divisions.
- In the upper thigh, the tibial division gives off braches to all of the hamstring muscles (semitendinosus, semimembranosus, biceps femoris) except for the short head of the biceps femoris (**FIG 2**).
- The peroneal nerve distribution innervates the short head of the biceps femoris and the ischial portion of the adductor magnus muscle.
- The two divisions will separate completely at the level of the popliteal fossa.
- The posterior tibial nerve continues its course posteriorly to innervate the muscles in the posterior leg compartment.
- The common peroneal nerve will course laterally around the head of the fibula to innervate the muscles of the anterior and lateral compartments.
- The inferior gluteal artery provides majority of the blood supply to the sciatic nerve.

Innervation/Function

- In the upper thigh, the sciatic nerve is responsible for motor function to the hamstrings muscles, which allow for flexion at the knee.
- The common peroneal and tibial branches are responsible for all of the motor function below the knee.
- It provides cutaneous sensory innervation to the posterior thigh.
- Its terminal branches provide sensation to the lateral aspect of the knee, lateral lower leg, and the dorsal and plantar surfaces of the foot.

Mechanisms of Injury

- The sciatic nerve is at risk for entrapment as it passes through the sciatic notch, especially in the setting of pelvic fractures.
- Traumatic injuries, particularly in penetrating trauma, can occur at any level with variable grades of severity.
- Iatrogenic injuries are not uncommon and result from pelvic and hip surgery, as well as injection site injuries.
- Revisional hip surgeries and patients with developmental dysplasia are at higher risk.[1]
- Direct compression neuropathy is rare but has been described in comatose patients during prolonged anesthesia or long periods of sitting on a hard surface.[2] Piriformis syndrome is a compressive neuropathy of the sciatic nerve as it travels underneath the piriformis muscle.

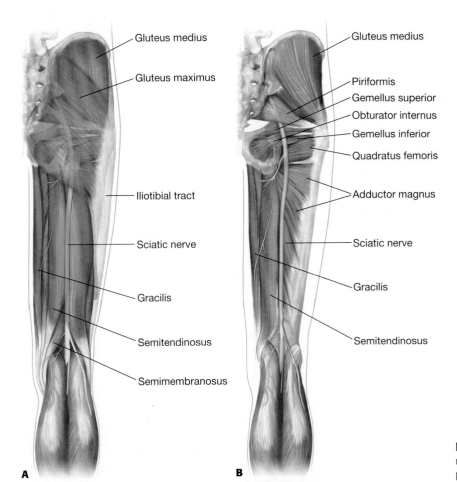

FIG 2 • A,B. The sciatic nerve path in the posterior thigh as it divides in the popliteal fossa into the peroneal and tibial divisions.

PATIENT HISTORY AND PHYSICAL EXAM

- Detailed history and physical examination must be obtained prior to the decision for operative management.
- Documentation of muscle strength using the Medical Research Council (MRC) scale and sensory deficits by two-point discrimination along the cutaneous distribution of the nerve.
- The extent of sensory deficit can also be measured by the "ten-test for sensation." The patient grades the level of sensation to touch on the injured side using a scale from 1 to 10. This number is compared to the level of sensation to similar touch on the uninjured side.
- Physical manifestations will be dependent on the level of injury, extent of each nerve division involved, and if it is a partial or complete injury.
- High injury can lead to significant morbidity, as buttock-level sciatic nerve lesions will result dysfunction of knee flexion, foot extension, flexion, inversion, eversion, and all movement of the toes.
- Sensory losses of variable degrees result in the posterior thigh and the entire foot and lower leg except for the medial aspect of the lower leg, which is supplied by the saphenous nerve.
- Injuries below the level of the hamstring can allow ambulation with an intact femoral nerve as the patient can have active flexion, extension, and locking of the knee.
- Patients with piriformis syndrome complain of buttock pain and numbness. This can also result in pain radiating down the leg and thigh "sciatica."

- Patients with piriformis syndrome may have a history of buttock trauma, and symptoms are exacerbated by prolonged sitting or activities resulting in adduction and internal rotation of the leg.
- On physical exam, the proximal sciatic is tested by asking the patient to flex the knee against resistance with the lower leg extended.
- The peroneal branch is tested by assessing foot extension, eversion, and abduction of the toes against resistance.
- The tibial branch is tested by assessing foot plantar flexion and flexion of the toes against resistance.
- To test for piriformis syndrome, the "AIF" maneuver should be performed. The AIF maneuver consists of adduction, internal rotation, and flexion of the hip.
- Pain on AIF maneuver is diagnostic for piriformis syndrome.

IMAGING

- Detailed physical exam detailing sensory and motor deficits will help delineate the level of injury.
- Nerve conduction studies can also assist with localization of the injury.
- Of note, electromyography (EMG) has limited utility in the acute setting, as muscles may not demonstrate signs of denervation for several weeks.
- For piriformis syndrome, imaging may demonstrate hypertrophy of the piriformis muscle, anomalous vessels, or bands around the muscle.

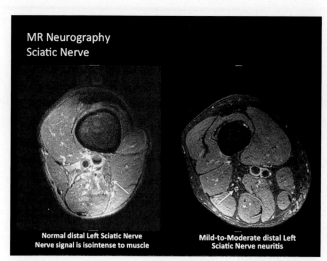

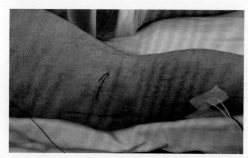

FIG 4 • Patient prepared for surgery of distal sciatic injury after knee dislocation. *Arrow* marks the area of nonadvancing Tinel. Note the needles in place for baseline motor responses during the intraoperative nerve monitoring.

FIG 3 • MRI neurogram showing bright fascicles of the sciatic nerve.

- Magnetic resonance (MR) neurogram is an emerging technique in which edema or inflammatory changes around a nerve could help identify location of injury (**FIG 3**).

NONOPERATIVE MANAGEMENT

- If the injury is closed or due to compression, a trial of conservative management should first be attempted.
- Physical therapy should be initiated early, focusing on ambulation with bracing and orthotics.
- Pain management for relief of neuropathic pain includes pharmacologic modalities and therapy for desensitization.
- If no significant return of function is noted by 3 months, then surgical exploration is warranted.
- Unrelenting pain could indicate neuroma formation and may warrant surgical exploration even if signs of spontaneous recovery are evident.
- Treatment for piriformis syndrome is typically conservative including stretching of the muscle and image-guided steroid injections.

- If conservative treatment fails, then surgical release of the piriformis can be considered.

SURGICAL MANAGEMENT

- Concern for laceration to one or both branches as demonstrated by significant motor or sensory deficits warrant early operative exploration.[3]
- Intraoperative electrophysiologic studies can serve as a guide to determine the area of injury for compression, stretch, or blunt injuries that have not spontaneously recovered (**FIG 4**).
- If nerve action potentials are detected across the injured site, external neurolysis should be performed.
- Nerve repair or reconstruction should be performed in the setting of a nerve not in continuity or intraoperative nerve testing that finds no recovery across the zone of injury.
- Primary repair should always be attempted if there is not significant tension on the repair.
- If primary repair without tension cannot be performed, reconstruction should be performed with nerve grafting.
- Neuropathic pain is a common concern. The use of antineuropathic pain medications should be part of the patient's multimodal treatment.

■ Upper Sciatic Nerve: Hip and Buttock Pathology

- The patient should be placed in the prone position.
- A bump can be placed beneath the pelvis to provide flexion at the hips.
- The contralateral lower extremity should also be prepped and draped in the event a sural nerve graft is required for repair.
- A curvilinear incision is made starting at the posterior superior iliac spine, traveling laterally to the greater trochanter, and inferiorly to the gluteal crease.
- The dissection is carried down to the level of the gluteus maximus muscle.
- The superior and lateral aspect of the gluteus maximus muscle is released from the iliotibial tract.

- A 2- to 3-cm cuff of the muscle is left to the superolateral attachment to facilitate closure.
- An avascular plane below the gluteal maximus muscle should be developed by retracting the muscle medially to expose the sciatic nerve.
- Careful hemostasis using bipolar electrocautery is critical for good visualization.
- Care must be taken not to injure the hamstring branches as they typically run superior and medial to the main sciatic trunk.
- The gluteal neurovascular structures travel along with the sciatic nerve, and care must be taken to preserve these vessels.
- In some cases, the piriformis muscle will need to be detached from the femur laterally and retracted medially for improved exposure of the nerve at the sciatic notch.

TECHNIQUES

T E C H N I Q U E S

■ Lower Sciatic Exposure: Thigh Pathology

- The patient is placed in the prone position.
- An incision is made over the suspected level of injury.
- Tourniquet may not be feasible, given proximal lesion and need for nerve monitoring; therefore, preinject suspected site prior to prepping with bupivacaine with epinephrine.
- Dissection can be carried down to the popliteal fossa for full exposure of the nerve depending on the level of injury (**TECH FIG 1A**).

- A plane is developed between the biceps femoris and the semitendinosus muscle.
- Careful hemostasis using bipolar electrocautery is critical for good visualization.
- The sciatic nerve can be exposed running deep to the biceps femoris (**TECH FIG 1B**).
- The sheath should be divided exposing the two divisions of the nerve for full inspection of injury.
- Further isolation of the nerve should be performed under an operating microscope, with adequate exposure of the nerve proximal and distal to the lesion.
- The nerve should be resected to healthy nerve fascicles.

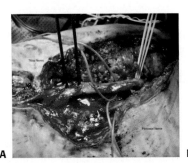
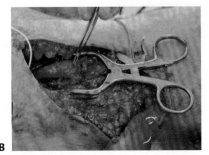

TECH FIG 1 • A. Nerve-to-nerve monitoring of the sciatic nerve to tibial nerve to assess for neuroma in continuity. The *black arrow* represents the division becoming the tibial nerve, the *blue arrow* the peroneal nerve. **B.** Lacerated sciatic nerve exposed in the posterior thigh. Note the large caliber of this nerve.

■ Primary Nerve Coaptation

- Nerve repair should be performed via end-to-end epineural coaptation with 9-0 monofilament permanent sutures.
- Fibrin sealant can also be used to reapproximate and seal nerve ends.

- A sural nerve graft can be interposed between the two ends if primary repair is not possible.
- The peroneal and tibial components should be repaired separately aligning their respective fascicles.

PEARLS AND PITFALLS

Hemostasis	■ Preinject incision with bupivacaine with epinephrine. ■ A solution of 1 amp of epinephrine diluted in 100 cc of saline can be used to moisten a gauze, which is then dabbed in the wound to help with visualization.
Technique	■ In the thigh, there are numerous branches of the sciatic nerve to the hamstring muscles, and care must be taken not to injure these branches during dissection.
Intraoperative monitoring	■ Communication between neurology and anesthesia teams is critical to ensure that patient does not receive medications that will hinder intraoperative monitoring. ■ The machines for the sequential compression device and warming blankets can cause background that interferes with intraoperative monitoring. ■ Do not use tourniquet if planning intraoperative monitoring as ischemia of the nerve can result in neuropraxia.
Diagnosis	■ Must determine sciatic nerve injury vs pelvic plexus trauma, as repair of the latter may be contraindicated.

POSTOPERATIVE CARE

- If there is concern for tension across the nerve repair, range of motion exercises should wait for at least 3 weeks.
- Physical therapy should be initiated early focusing on ambulation with the use of braces and orthotics.
- Early therapy for desensitization and scar management are useful to minimize postoperative pain.
- If pain is severe, a multidisciplinary approach with pain management, psychology, and therapy should be initiated.

OUTCOMES

- Factors associated with worse outcomes include delay in repair of more than 4 months, length of nerve defect, and division of nerve involved.[4]
- One of the largest series evaluating outcomes of civilian sciatic nerve injuries was performed at Louisiana State University Health Science Center:[5]
  - They evaluated outcomes of 353 patients with buttock-level and thigh-level sciatic nerve injuries over a 24-year period.
  - Mechanisms of injury included injection injuries, hip surgeries, fracture dislocations, blunt ant penetration trauma, and compression.
  - Patients with partial nerve deficits without severe pain or with significant spontaneous recovery were treated with conservative management and achieved good recovery of motor and sensory function.
  - Patients with detectable nerve action potentials intraoperatively only underwent neurolysis.
  - Overall, they found thigh-level sciatic nerve injuries achieved better outcomes than buttock-level injuries (Table 1).
  - In addition, for peroneal nerve injuries, both primary repair and nerve grafting had worse outcomes in comparison to tibial nerve injuries.
  - It is postulated that worse outcomes for peroneal nerve injuries results from less robust blood supply and connective tissue padding between fascicles compared to the tibial nerve.[6,7]

COMPLICATIONS

- Neuropathic pain. There is a higher incidence of neuropathic pain with delayed repairs.[6]
- Development of complex regional pain syndrome (CRPS)
- Neuroma
- Rupture

Table 1 Percent of Patients Who Achieved At Least a Medical Research Council Strength of At Least 3

Level of Injury	All Patients	Suture Repair	Nerve Graft Repair
Buttock	87%	73	62
Thigh	96%	93	80
Tibial	71%	30	24
Peroneal	79%	69	45

Kim DH, et al. Management and outcomes in 353 surgically treated sciatic nerve lesions. *J Neurosurg*. 2004;101(1):8-17.

FEMORAL NERVE

DEFINITION

- Femoral nerve injuries are more common than sciatic nerve injuries.
- Most injuries are iatrogenic, resulting from abdominal and pelvic surgeries.
- In general, femoral nerve injuries have a better prognosis than other lower extremity nerve injuries.
- Most patients typically maintain the ability to ambulate with the use of orthotics.
- Early identification and treatment are critical for prevention of muscle atrophy and the need for long-term rehabilitation.

ANATOMY

- The femoral nerve forms in the pelvis from the ventral rami of L2, L3, and L4 spinal roots (see **TECH FIG 1B**).
- The nerve travels in the retroperitoneum, anterior to the psoas muscle and medial to the iliacus.
- It enters the thigh deep to the inguinal ligament and travels through the femoral triangle, which is bordered superiorly by the inguinal ligament, laterally by the sartorius, and medially by the adductor longus muscle.
- In the femoral triangle, it runs lateral to the femoral artery.
- Approximately 1 to 4 cm distal to the inguinal ligament, it divides into the anterior and posterior branches (**FIG 5**).
- The lateral circumflex femoral artery typical runs between the two divisions.[8]
- The anterior division provides motor innervation to the sartorius muscle and sensory innervation to the anterior and medial upper thigh.
- The posterior division provides motor innervation to the quadriceps muscles.

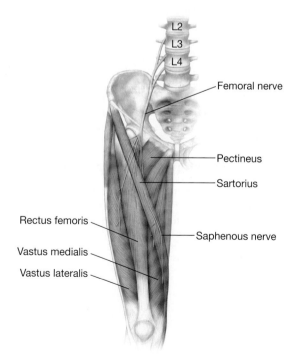

FIG 5 • Course of the femoral nerve in the anterior thigh.

- Its terminal division is the saphenous nerve, which runs with the greater saphenous vein and provides sensory innervation to the medial lower leg and foot.
- The blood supply to the femoral nerve is derived from the iliolumbar artery in the pelvis and the deep circumflex iliac artery and lateral circumflex femoral artery in the thigh.

Innervation/Function

- In the pelvis, it provides motor innervation of the psoas and the iliacus muscles, which contributes to flexion at the hip.
- It also gives off a branch in the pelvis or upper thigh to innervate the pectineus muscle that aids in adduction of the hip.[8]
- In the thigh, it provides motor function to musculature of the anterior compartment including the quadriceps (rectus femoris, vastus lateralis, vastus medialis, and vastus intermedius) and the sartorius muscle.
- The quadriceps functions to extend the knee, and the sartorius contributes in flexion, abduction and lateral rotation of the hip, as well as flexion of the knee.
- The femoral nerve does not provide any motor innervation below the knee.
- Sensory innervation of the femoral nerve includes the anterior thigh.
- Its terminal branch, the saphenous nerve, provides sensory innervation to the medial knee and medial lower leg, as well as the medial aspect of the foot.

PATHOGENESIS

- Majority of the published femoral nerve injuries are the result of iatrogenic injury from abdominal and pelvic procedures, primarily from compression by self-retaining retractors.[8]
- The saphenous nerve especially the infrapatellar branch can be injured during knee surgery. This can result in chronic pain after total knee arthroplasty.[9]
- At the inguinal ligament, the femoral nerve can become compressed particularly with flexion, abduction, and external rotation of the legs, such as in lithotomy position.
- Inadvertent injury during arterial cannulation for cardiovascular procedures has also been described.
- Retroperitoneal hematomas, pelvic lymphadenopathy, and colon or rectal malignancies can lead to femoral nerve compression in the pelvis.
- Femoral nerve stretch injuries can also be caused by hip hyperextension in dancers or yoga instructors.
- Ischemic injuries can lead to nerve devascularization, such as in aortic or iliac surgeries.

PATIENT HISTORY AND PHYSICAL EXAM

- Motor and sensory exam techniques are same as sciatic nerve.
- Evaluation of a patient with femoral nerve injury employs the same principles as for sciatic nerve injury.

- Injury to the intrapelvic femoral nerve results in weakness with hip flexion, knee extension, and an absent or diminished patellar reflex.
- Sensory deficits can include numbness, paresthesias, or hyperesthesia along anteromedial thigh and medial lower leg.
- Hip flexion should be tested by supporting and flexing the knee while requesting the patient to flex hip against resistance.
- Loss of quadriceps function can result in knee hyperextension if there is a functional tensor fascia lata or gracilis muscle.
- On reflex examination, the patient will have loss of knee jerk.
- The saphenous nerve can be compressed at the adductor hiatus: tenderness, Tinel, and positive scratch collapse at the adductor hiatus can help identify this.

IMAGING

- Similar evaluation as for sciatic nerve injury

NONOPERATIVE MANAGEMENT

- Contusions, compression, traction, or partial injuries are initially managed with conservative strategies to determine the amount of spontaneous recovery.
- Early ambulation is encouraged with the use of knee or knee to ankle orthotics for weakness of quadriceps muscles.
- All patients should participate in aggressive physical therapy to prevent muscle atrophy and the development of deep venous thrombosis.
- Joints can also be maintained supple by dynamic and static splinting to prevent contractures, in the event early ambulation cannot be performed.
- If there is no recovery of motor or sensory function within 3 months, surgical intervention is warranted.

SURGICAL MANAGEMENT

- Complete lacerations require early surgical exploration and repair.
- If the patient's medical condition is stable, neurorrhaphy should be performed within the first 3 to 7 days of injury.
- Primary repair should be attempted when possible, and autologous nerve grafts from the sural nerves is an alternative.
- For high femoral nerve palsies, a transfer of the obturator nerve has been described. These transfers have demonstrated good functional outcomes; however, there are limited data.[10]

■ Retroperitoneal Femoral Nerve Exposure: Pelvic Pathology

- The patient should be placed in the supine position.
- Surgical bumps should be placed under the hip to elevate the affected side.
- Dissection is carried down to the level of the external and internal oblique muscles.
- The muscle-splitting technique is utilized to separate the muscles in the direction of their fibers.
- The transversalis fascia is opened and the peritoneum retracted superiorly away from the retroperitoneal fat.

- The retroperitoneal fat is carefully mobilized for exposure of the femoral nerve, just lateral to the femoral artery.
- The iliac vessels and ureter will be coursing medially to the nerve.
- Dissection can be carried superiorly to the iliopsoas muscle for high exposure of the nerve.
- Care should be taken not to injure the lateral femoral cutaneous nerve and ilioinguinal or genitofemoral nerves.
- The inguinal ligament can be divided if needed to facilitate exposure.

■ Lower Femoral Nerve Exposure: Thigh-Level Pathology

- The patient is positioned supine with the knee flexed 30 to 45 degrees.
- The femoral artery is palpated midway between the anterior superior iliac spine and the pubic symphysis.

- A longitudinal incision is made lateral to the femoral artery or the midaspect of the inguinal ligament.
- The incision is carried inferiorly to the midthigh, following the course of the femoral nerve.

■ Painful Saphenous Neuroma

- The patient has had nerve blocked preoperatively, has had at least a 70% pain reduction, and is comfortable with the trade of decreased sensation for decreased pain.
- Identify area of pain and look for nerve proximally (**TECH FIG 2A**).

- If discrete nerve injury is identified, resect neuroma and reconstruct defect with allograft (**TECH FIG 2B**).
- If there is any question as to the extent of the zone of injury, it is advised to resect nerve proximally so it does not cross a joint and bury the end of the nerve within the muscle under no tension.

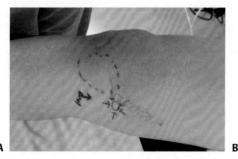 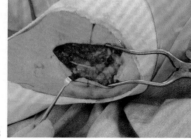

TECH FIG 2 • A. Patient with a painful neuroma in the saphenous nerve distribution after a laceration: *circle* denotes painful area and *dotted line* area of decreased sensation. **B.** Neuroma resected and defect reconstructed with nerve allograft. **A**   **B**

■ Nerve Repair

- The nerve is identified using the existing wounds or the approaches described above.
- The nerve can be directly coapted if a tension-free repair is possible.
- If there is tension on the repair, a bridging nerve graft is required.

- Nerve coaptation is done using microsurgical technique.
- Use 9-0 suture with minimal amount of sutures placed.
- Fibrin sealants can be used to seal the repair site and to hold cabled nerve grafts together.
- Repairs are protected for 3 weeks with splints/braces to limit mobility at adjacent joints.

PEARLS AND PITFALLS

Pathogenesis	■ Similar to sciatic nerve injury. ■ The femoral nerve travels with the femoral artery and femoral vein, and concomitant vascular injuries are common.
Surgical management	■ Vascular injury must be performed prior to nerve repair.

POSTOPERATIVE CARE

- Physical therapy should be initiated early focusing on ambulation with the use of braces and orthotics.
- Therapy should also focus on desensitization and scar management.

OUTCOMES

- There is a paucity of robust studies on outcomes of femoral nerve repairs.
- For the majority of compression, stretch, or partial lacerations, good outcomes in motor function have been reported; however, most patients have residual sensory deficits.[8,11]
- The Louisiana State University Health Science Center series published outcomes of 119 operative repairs of femoral nerve injuries over a 32-year period.[11]
- Mechanisms of injuries included iatrogenic, hip or pelvic fractures, gunshot wounds, and lacerations.
- They demonstrated good functional recovery regardless of mechanism of injury, level of the lesion, or primary vs nerve grafting.
- In addition, they reported that the majority of patients who had neurolysis regained almost complete function, for both thigh- and pelvic-level lesions.
- They concluded that femoral nerve injuries overall have a good prognosis, consistent in other smaller series.[6]

COMPLICATIONS

- Chronic pain
- Development of complex regional pain syndrome
- Neuroma
- Rupture

REFERENCES

1. Liu R, et al. Sciatic nerve course in adult patients with unilateral developmental dysplasia of the hip: implications for hip surgery. *BMC Surg.* 2015;15:14.
2. Wang JC, et al. Bilateral sciatic neuropathy as a complication of craniotomy performed in the sitting position: localization of nerve injury by using magnetic resonance imaging. *Childs Nerv Syst.* 2012; 28(1):159-163.
3. Topuz K, et al. Early surgical treatment protocol for sciatic nerve injury due to injection—a retrospective study. *Br J Neurosurg.* 2011; 25(4):509-515.
4. Burks SS, et al. Challenges in sciatic nerve repair: anatomical considerations. *J Neurosurg.* 2014;121(1):210-218.
5. Kim DH, et al. Management and outcomes in 353 surgically treated sciatic nerve lesions. *J Neurosurg.* 2004;101(1):8-17.
6. Secer HI, et al. The clinical, electrophysiologic, and surgical characteristics of peripheral nerve injuries caused by gunshot wounds in adults: a 40-year experience. *Surg Neurol.* 2008;69(2):143-152.
7. Aydin A, et al. The results of surgical repair of sciatic nerve injuries. *Acta Orthop Traumatol Turc.* 2010;44(1):48-53.
8. Moore AE, Stringer MD. Iatrogenic femoral nerve injury: a systematic review. *Surg Radiol Anat.* 2011;33(8):649-658.
9. Kinghorn K, et al. Case scenario: nerve injury after knee arthroplasty and sciatic nerve block. *Anesthesiology.* 2012;116(4):918-923.
10. Tung TH, Chao A, Moore AM. Obturator nerve transfer for femoral nerve reconstruction: anatomic study and clinical application. *Plast Reconstr Surg.* 2012;130(5):1066-1074.
11. Kim DH, et al. Intrapelvic and thigh-level femoral nerve lesions: management and outcomes in 119 surgically treated cases. *J Neurosurg.* 2004;100(6):989-996.

CHAPTER 42

Keystone and Related Perforator Flaps

Michael W. Findlay

DEFINITION

- Keystone flaps encompass a group of related fasciocutaneous flaps first devised by Behan that share a common geometric design (a keystone shape similar to the keystone of stone arches) but can vary in the following ways:[1]
  - Blood supply (perforator vs direct vs neurovascular vs composite)
  - Degree of islandization (complete vs incomplete, cutaneous or fasciocutaneous)
  - Method of transfer into the defect (advancement, transposition, combination)
  - Whether used alone or along with another keystone flap on the opposite side of the defect (double opposing keystone flaps).
- The classification of keystone flaps is based on the method of transfer and the number of keystone flaps involved (**FIG 1**).

ANATOMY

- Keystone flaps close defects by transferring fasciocutaneous tissue from an adjacent donor site to the defect while maximizing use of cutaneous arteries, superficial and deep venous drainage, and lymphatics without being defined by a specific form of the transfer (eg, transposition vs rotation).
- Human skin is well supplied with perforators and direct vessels for supply of keystone flaps with established patterns of cutaneous supply in the limbs (longitudinally oriented septocutaneous and musculocutaneous perforators), the trunk (segmental perforators with intercommunications in well-defined intermuscular planes), and the head and neck (profuse cutaneous supply dominated by direct cutaneous vessels in the head and perforators and direct vessels in the neck).[2]

- Conjoint supply to flaps refers to the incorporation of both cutaneous vessels and neurovascular supply within the flap (eg, incorporation of saphenous or sural nerves and their vasa nervorum) so as to augment blood supply. Codevelopment of arteries and nerves during development result in conjoint flaps that have a very strong axial blood supply that improves their robustness. An additional benefit is that blood supply from the vasa nervorum can be significant in some areas (eg, posterior thigh), further contributing to flap vascularity.
- Certain sites do not contain cutaneous perforators (eg, pretibial border, scalp) and hence represent problem areas for keystone flap elevation. Keystone flaps can be raised either side of the pretibial border for mobilization of tissue over a pretibial defect, but cannot reliably be designed directly over the pretibial skin as the basis for its blood supply due to the lack of direct cutaneous perforators.
- Superficial and deep venous drainage can be incorporated in most keystone perforator flaps through preservation of deep venous system along with arterial perforators and the subcutaneous veins by blunt dissection of subcutaneous tissues and islandization of the underlying fascia (if necessary) via the use of scissors through small windows in the subcutaneous tissue. Superficial veins are often numerous, and some may need to be divided to permit sufficient mobilization, but their division is performed sequentially, stopping once sufficient mobilization is achieved.
- The longitudinal orientation of fascial planes in many areas of the body (eg, limbs, paraspinous region) predispose to a longitudinal orientation for keystone flaps (slightly oblique orientations may help in limbs; see below), with the most appropriate mobilization of longitudinal keystone flaps

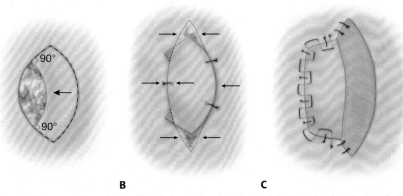

FIG 1 • Basic design and types of keystone flaps. **A.** An ellipse is formed as though the defect is to be closed primarily. Then, a keystone flap is designed beside it with sharp dissection undertaken through the skin and deep fascia. **B.** V-Y closure is performed at the flap margins during flap advancement. **C.** A skin graft may be used for closure of the secondary defect.

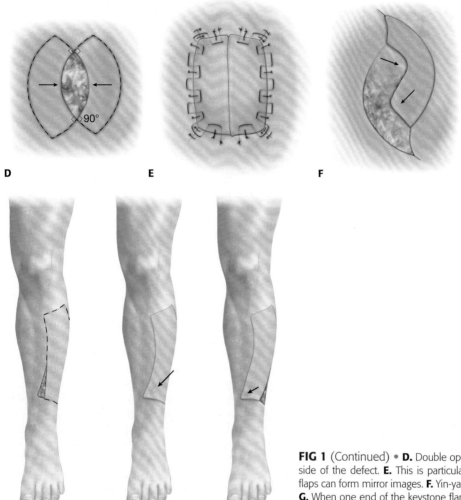

FIG 1 (Continued) • **D.** Double opposing keystone flaps may be used on either side of the defect. **E.** This is particularly useful for midline defects, for which the flaps can form mirror images. **F.** Yin-yang variant of double opposing keystone flaps. **G.** When one end of the keystone flap is transposed to fill a defect, skin grafting of the secondary defect may be necessary.

being in a transverse direction. That is, the longitudinal orientation of the paraspinous musculature makes medial and lateral movement of keystone flaps relatively easy to cover central back defects, whereas the fibrous attachments between the skin and underlying spinous processes make superior or inferior movement problematic.

- Where there is circumferential limitation for flap mobilization and direct closure of the secondary defect (eg, distal limbs), orienting keystone flaps oblique to the long-axis provides an oblique (longer) circumference, thereby maximizing available donor tissue for closure.
- Placement of incisions in relaxed skin tension lines where possible is very helpful. The keystone shape is one that naturally hides well. Caution should be exercised in selection of any island flap in patients prone to abnormal scarring (eg, hypertrophic/keloid scarring). Partial flap islandization is a good option where feasible in such individuals or in patients very sensitive about the scar burden.
- Undermining and skeletonization of the perforator/direct vessel pedicle to the flap can be undertaken but is unnecessary in the vast majority of cases, and therefore, only the division of structures felt absolutely necessary for elevation,

mobilization, and inset of the specific keystone flap are undertaken, thereby ensuring both surgical efficiency and safety.
- The design and flexibility in the blood supply, venous drainage, and mobilization of the keystone flap make it readily suitable for application in most areas of the body with local variation to optimize the outcome in specific areas.

PATIENT HISTORY AND PHYSICAL FINDINGS

- An understanding of the etiology of the defect to be reconstructed and relevant patient factors (health, comorbidities, activity levels, mobility, nutrition) help direct the most appropriate form of reconstruction in any potential flap case.
- As with all forms of flap reconstruction, particular interest should be focused on removal of the causative factor (eg, cancer, infection), identification and optimization of locoregional blood flow, selection of the best possible flap based on the needs of the defect and locoregionally available tissue, and optimization of the patient in the perioperative period.
- Any past history of conditions that affect local blood flow and wound healing should be elicited and mitigated where possible (eg, irradiation, peripheral vascular disease (micro

and/or macroangiopathy), diabetes mellitus, smoking, and previous surgery/trauma.

- Examination findings of note include quality of surrounding donor sites for skin and tissue quality (including presence of radiotherapy tattoos, scars, fibrosis).

IMAGING

- The vast majority of patients do not require preoperative imaging or the use of intraoperative Doppler ultrasound to achieve reliable and timely reconstruction using the keystone flap or its variants as long as normal design principles are followed (see **FIG 1**).
- Computed tomography, angiography, and similar imaging modalities are the most useful to answer what direct or perforating vessels are available to the locoregional tissues, and delayed views can show the venous drainage to the area of interest.
- Fluorescence microscopy is invaluable for pre- and intraoperative imaging of the perforators and direct vessels to the skin but is rarely indicated for keystone flap elevation and has anaphylaxis as a risk factor.
- Imaging can be of use where previous surgery or trauma may have damaged the normal blood supply of the donor skin, or if there is significant arterial disease, and therefore, the selection of the most appropriate local vessels is necessary to ensure success.

NONOPERATIVE MANAGEMENT

- As with any fasciocutaneous defect, careful consideration should be given to the potential of the defect to be closed directly (under physiologic tension and utilizing biological and mechanical creep as tolerated) or healed by secondary intention.
- The progression to flap reconstruction is considered where these options are either not possible or lead to unacceptable risks/complications.

SURGICAL MANAGEMENT

- Keystone flap reconstruction is reliable as long as a sequence of steps is undertaken in which the primary goal is sufficient mobilization of the flap to close the recipient and donor sites, while preserving as much arterial input, venous output, and lymphatic drainage as possible.
- No additional maneuvers are undertaken once recipient and donor-site closure can be achieved.
- If further mobilization of tissues is needed, then the flap can be fully islandized where the cutaneous vessels have been followed back through deep fascia and or freed where they exit muscles to facilitate mobilization; however, one must be cautious not to damaging perforating vessels as this can lead to tissue ischemia and necrosis.

Preoperative Planning

- The defect is assessed for its suitability for fasciocutaneous reconstruction, with a consideration of locally available tissue, including potential vascular pedicles, as the basis for the flap.

- Keystone flaps can be performed in irradiated tissue[1] or even in the setting of lymphedema,[2] but caution should be exercised with flap planning in these settings so as to ensure adequate perforators/direct vessels and avoid unnecessary tension across suture lines.
- Where primary closure is unachievable, consider a keystone design and determine the form of mobilization that will work best to close the defect and match the local tissue shape (eg, transposition flaps are best for convex surfaces and advancements are best for flat surfaces).
  - There are circumferential limitations in the limbs (where the defect size represents over 30% to 40% of the circumference of the limb), as these defects may require grafting of the secondary defect or an alternate form of reconstruction.
- Defects are marked out as though they are to be closed directly as part of an elliptical excision/closure, and keystone flaps can be designed on one or both sides of the ellipse with the best side (or sides) chosen based upon local tissue availability, suitability of local vessels, and the needs of the defect.
  - The ellipse does not need to be excised. It simply gives a guide to the best orientation for the flaps.
  - It is good practice to mark every excision or defect as though it will be closed by a keystone flap and then perform one if the defect cannot be closed primarily (if indicated). This maximizes experience with keystone planning.

Positioning

- Patient positioning is entirely dependent upon the ensuring easy access to the operative site. This is usually supine or lateral with circumferential draping in the limbs.
- Prone positioning is most useful for midline defects of the back that require bilateral keystone flaps.

Approach

- The design and mobilization of keystone flaps can be tailored to suit the needs of the defect and the area to be reconstructed, including variations in the following:
  - Design—eg, asymmetrical keystone in the calf
  - Mobilization—advancement, rotation, transposition, sliding
  - Grafting of the secondary defect
  - Single or double flaps—eg, yin-yang flap variant
  - Placement of V-Y points (best over convexities)
- Keystone flaps provide fasciocutaneous coverage of defects.
  - As a group, fasciocutaneous flaps are poorly suited to the reconstruction of complex three-dimensional defects where it is essential to obliterate dead space with filling with well-vascularized tissue.
- Keystone flaps are excellent at providing a simple and reliable approach to locoregional coverage and are sufficiently robust that they can be performed in conjunction with other flaps that will sit under the keystone flap (and can be tunneled under if necessary); thereby, providing vascularized soft tissue to fill a three-dimensional defect along with locally matching skin coverage.

■ Keystone Flap Reconstruction of the Lower Leg

Markings

- Mark out the planned design that incorporates local pedicles and consider how the design will capture suitable venous drainage for the flap (**TECH FIG 1**).
- Modify the design as required to maximize the potential for closure of both the defect and donor site (eg, the cone shape of the leg responds well to asymmetrical Keystone flaps (that are wider superiorly than inferiorly).
- Determine the nature of flap mobilization into the defect and plan in reverse around any pivot points.

Islandization of the Flap

- Apply a tourniquet to facilitate flap elevation where appropriate.
- Full islandization of the keystone flap promotes even tension across the flap (avoiding linear or point tension) and may augment cutaneous perfusion within the flap[3] but must be weighed against the added scar burden.
- Where significant skin elasticity is present, it may be possible to minimize incisions on the donor defect side of the flap while still performing V-Y advancement of the rest of the keystone flap.
- The skin is sharply incised while preserving underlying neurovascular structures (particularly venous drainage) (**TECH FIG 2A**).
- Blunt dissection and targeted release of fascial or skin retaining ligaments and similar fibrous structures are undertaken as necessary while maintaining the integrity of the vasculature and lymphatics (**TECH FIG 2B**).
- Islandization of the fascia is undertaken if necessary, by sharp incision with scissors through small windows in the subcutaneous tissue (**TECH FIG 2C**).
  - Islandization is undertaken only to the degree to which is it required to achieve flap mobilization and closure.
- Dissection of perforators is rarely necessary but, when performed, care to should be taken to divide supporting connective tissue structures that might otherwise impede blood flow following mobilization of the flap.

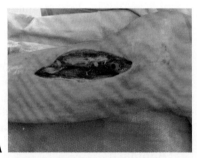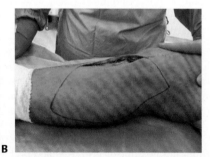

TECH FIG 1 • A. A complex defect of the left leg involving an exposed plate for fixation of a compound tibial plateau fracture. Flap reconstruction is planned following debridement, washout, and confirmation of minimal bacterial contamination through wound swabs for microscopy, culture, and sensitivity. The anterior tibial artery was injured in the fracture, but the peroneal and posterior tibial vessels were intact. There was obvious undermining superiorly and inferiorly to the defect. Lateral tissues would be most appropriate as the basis for a keystone flap in this setting. **B.** An asymmetrical keystone perforator flap is designed to take advantage of cutaneous perforators from the peroneal and posterior tibial vessels. The flap makes good use of the lateral calf tissue but does not cross the axis of knee movement superiorly (on the right) and the diameter of the flap is larger than the defect width to ensure capture of perforators and ready availability of soft tissue to close the wound.

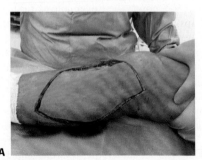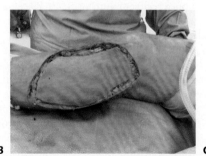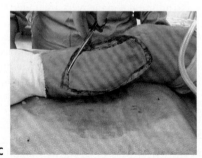

TECH FIG 2 • A. Islandization of the skin is performed by sharp incision while preserving the underlying soft tissues that contain important superficial venous drainage, lymphatics, and nerves. **B.** Blunt dissection is performed to retain important subcutaneous neurovascular structures (particularly superficial venous drainage seen on the right of the flap). The deep fascia is intact here with the exception of the existing defect. Flap closure of the defect was still not possible at this point; therefore, fascial islandization was performed. **C.** Fascial islandization is performed using partially open scissors and a pushing technique so as to minimize the risk of injuring nearby structures. This can be performed through small windows in the subcutaneous tissue so that neurovascular structures can be maintained. The leading edge of the flap is also mobilized (at the edge of the defect).

Assess Flap Viability and Achieve Definitive Hemostasis

- Following mobilization of the flap, the tourniquet is released so the viability of the keystone flap can be assessed.
  - The site and contribution of individual perforators can be assessed at tourniquet release as blood flows back into the flap.
- It is typical for keystone flaps to demonstrate hypervascularity initially and they may display a 3% to 5% increase in cutaneous perfusion secondary to changes in blood flow from the process of flap islandization.
- Initially, the flap may resemble venous congestion, but venous changes should not be present beyond 10 to 15 minutes following release of the tourniquet (as assessed by the presence of rapid capillary return).
- It is ideal to achieve hemostasis at this time and consider whether a drain should be placed.

Strategic Suturing

- Even physiological wound tension is one of the key elements to the success and good long-term aesthetic results seen with well-performed keystone flaps.

- Skin is normally under tension, and keystone flaps are typically under some tension upon closure.
  - Single lines of tension or point tension should be avoided as these are not tolerated well by the skin, including keystone flaps.
- Islandization can be helpful to ensure even tension across the flap.
- Excess flap tissue (common at the obtuse angles of the flap beside the defect) can be trimmed safely to facilitate wound closure.
- The generation of even tension begins with the placement of strategic sutures across both the defect and the donor site to induce creep across both wounds and the flap (**TECH FIG 3A,B**).
  - Creep results in some relaxation of the tissues and promotes a more even tension at final closure.
  - Mattress sutures are ideal as these provide for the induction of creep alongside wound eversion to improve the resulting scar.
- A fine continuous suture helps ensure eversion and even tension.
- The "hemming suture" (two horizontal mattress sutures followed by a simple suture) may be used as a means of closure (**TECH FIG 3C,D**).

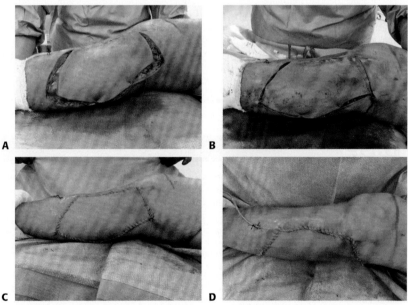

TECH FIG 3 • A. Following release of the tourniquet and hemostasis, strategic mattress sutures are placed, including tacking closure of the defect and the opposite side of the flap to induce creep and maximize even tension. The residual flap tissue at the leading edge of the flap has been trimmed. **B.** V-Y closure has been performed and further strategic mattress sutures have been placed to produce even physiological tension on the wound. **C.** A continuous skin suture (eg, Hemming mattress) is placed to ensure even tension and a nicely everted suture line for optimal aesthetic results. A suction drain is noted in the left of field, and this helped to minimize dead space in the otherwise planar defect. **D.** Anterior view of the flap at the point of V-Y closure to demonstrate even physiological tension and good contour following wound closure. Minor wound edge cones will resolve on the convex surface of the leg in the following weeks to months without the need for revision.

■ Keystone Flap Reconstruction of the Axilla

- **TECH FIG 4** is the case of a patient with medically refractory hidradenitis suppurative of the left axilla who

underwent excision of the involved axillary tissue and reconstruction with a lateral intercostal perforator-based keystone island flap (see **TECH FIG 4**).

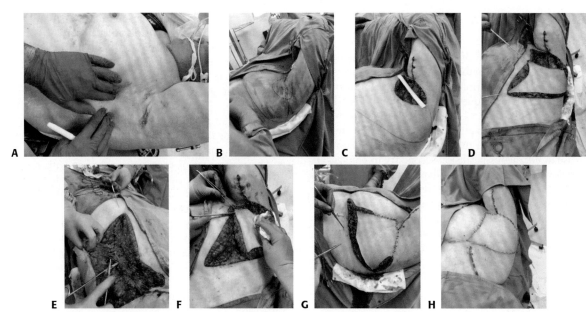

TECH FIG 4 • A. Medically refractory hidradenitis suppurative in the left axilla prior to excision. **B.** The area to be excised is marked along with a lateral intercostal perforator-based keystone perforator island flap. The breast base is marked anteriorly with a dotted line to ensure that the reconstruction does not involve the breast directly. **C.** Following excision, partial closure is performed in the arm, analogous to a brachioplasty, leaving a defect that is 15 cm by 10 cm and not able to be closed directly while still maintaining should movement. **D.** The skin of the flap is incised to form an island with elevation of the tissues as necessary to facilitate transposition into the defect. **E.** Blunt dissection is performed to the undersurface of the flap to divide fascial attachments to the lateral chest wall, yet preserving all neurovascular structures where possible. **F.** Placement of strategic deep sutures begins with those for closure of the primary defect. **G.** Strategic suturing around the periphery ensures even tension before skin sutures are placed. Potential delays in wound healing are anticipated in the axilla, so interrupted sutures are used in this area. **H.** Full closure is completed with deep dermal and subcuticular sutures for the rest of the wound. Note that all of suture lines run around the perimeter of the breast, including into the lateral aspect of the inframammary fold and V-Y closures in the periphery, have maintained good contour and shoulder movement despite the size of the primary defect.

PEARLS AND PITFALLS

Poor donor sites	▪ The subcutaneous border of the tibia has no perforators and few direct vessels. Keystone flaps may be designed on either side of pretibial defects, but should not be designed directly over the tibia if possible. The scalp has direct vessels, but no perforators, and therefore, is not generally suitable for keystone flaps.
Flap mobilization	▪ Understanding the underlying muscle and fascial arrangements will facilitate ease of flap movement into the defect (eg, coverage of spinal defects using flaps on either side of the spine, but not above or below).
Aesthetics	▪ Consider modification of keystone flap margins to lie in natural skin creases or within aesthetic units as this improves their appearance and minimizes scar burden.
Dissection	▪ Avoid overdissection of vascular structures. Only mobilize sufficiently to achieve wound and donor defect closure. Further dissection wastes time and puts important neurovascular structures at risk.
Skin grafting	▪ Retain all skin trimmed from the keystone flap until the end of the case as this can be useful as donor skin for any skin grafting that might be necessary toward the end of the case.
Design experience	▪ Plan a keystone flap for every defect but only use it if necessary and/or appropriate. This will rapidly increase experience with keystone flap planning.
Distal extremities	▪ Use an oblique flap orientation to increase the available circumference for closure and have a low threshold for skin grafting of secondary defects.
Contour	▪ Mobilization by transposition or elements of rotation produce a convexity, whereas advancement produces a more planar reconstruction. Consider matching the type of mobilization to suit the needs of the defect to enhance esthetics.
Documentation	▪ An operative note that includes a diagram or photo of the flap planning and eventual closure is very useful. ▪ In some circumstances, it may be difficult to identify the scars of keystone flaps, since scar generation is minimal in older individuals and the keystone design is not an obvious geometric pattern recognized by the human eye. ▪ Where the defect was from oncologic surgery, positive margins may require a thorough understanding of the nature of flap mobilization so that further resection can be performed effectively if necessary.

POSTOPERATIVE CARE

- Following closure, if movements across joints adversely impact the integrity of the flap closure, then splinting is recommended.
- Splinting is rarely needed for more than 3 to 5 days.
- If the reconstruction is associated with an underlying musculoskeletal injury that requires immobilization, this takes precedence.
- Keystone flaps are very robust and are tolerant of being dependent for short periods in the immediate postoperative setting.
- Keystone flaps are suitable to ambulatory surgery.
- Encourage elevation of the limb to limit postoperative swelling, but it is rare to need to immobilize patients.
- If closure is tight, then splinting will limit the risk of wound dehiscence during the period of postoperative edema (3 to 5 days).
- Keystone flaps do not require specific monitoring in general.

OUTCOMES

- Keystone flap reconstruction is a straightforward approach to fasciocutaneous reconstruction that is well tolerated by patients and has a low complication profile relative to other forms of flap reconstruction.
- A retrospective analysis of 200 consecutive keystone flaps for head and neck reconstruction demonstrated a 2% flap revision rate for partial flap necrosis and a single complete flap loss.[4] This compares very favorably to other forms of fasciocutaneous flap reconstruction in the head and neck.

COMPLICATIONS

- Keystone flaps are robust as evidenced by their relatively low partial and total flap loss rates.
- Minor complications can occur in up to 15% of cases in the head and neck with local wound issues including suture abscess, cellulitis, and wound dehiscence being the most common forms.[4]
- Donor site morbidity is very low, secondary to the conservative nature of flap dissection, including minimal dissection of muscle.

REFERENCES

1. Behan F, Sizeland A, Porcedu S, et al. Keystone island flap: an alternative reconstructive option to free flaps in irradiated tissue. *ANZ J Surg.* 2006;76(5):407-413.
2. Behan FC, Lo CH, Shayan R, Findlay M. The keystone technique for resolution of chronic lower limb wound with lymphoedema. *J Plast Reconstr Aesthet Surg.* 2009;62(5):701-702.
3. Rubino C, Coscia V, Cavazzuti AM, Canu V. Haemodynamic enhancement in perforator flaps: the inversion phenomenon and its clinical significance. A study of the relation of blood velocity and flow between pedicle and perforator vessels in perforator flaps. *J Plast Reconstr Aesthet Surg.* 2006;59(6):636-643.
4. Findlay MW, Sinha S, Rotman A, et al. The Keystone perforator island flap in head and neck reconstruction: indications and outcomes from 200 flaps. *Plast Reconstr Surg.* 2013;132(4S):8-9.

43

CHAPTER

Section V: Amputation and Replantation

Amputation of the Lower Extremity: Toes, Foot, Ankle

Kedar S. Lavingia and Jason T. Lee

INTRODUCTION

- Partial foot amputation (PFA) is a common sequel to advanced vascular disease secondary to diabetes and its complications.[1]
- PFA may also occur due to injury, infection, cancer, or birth defect.
- PFA affects approximately 2 per 1000 patients in western countries, making it the most common type of amputation surgery.[2]
- PFA is associated with a significant failure rate and numerous complications including skin breakdown, ulceration, and equinus contracture, which can lead to subsequent and more proximal amputation.
- Thoughtful patient selection, early involvement of neuropsychiatry and physical medicine and rehabilitation (PM&R) are fundamental to a successful outcome.

BACKGROUND/CONSIDERATIONS

Forefoot Amputation

- Toe disarticulations are quite challenging when dealing with the remaining cartilage of the involved metatarsal head and possible complications of residual osteomyelitis.
- Ray amputation, which involves the excision of the toe and part of the metatarsal, provides a more viable option of ensuring an adequate surgical debridement of the septic margins if that is the indication.
- Indications may include a wet or dry gangrene of a toe, osteomyelitis of the metatarsal head and/or proximal phalanx, septic arthritis of the metatarsophalangeal joint, and gross infection of the toe.
- Suggested inclusion criteria by a variety of authors for this type of amputation may include one or two palpable pedal pulses, ankle brachial index (ABI) $\geq$ 0.8, and toe brachial index $\geq$ 0.7.[3]
- In recent studies, absence of pulses, delayed capillary filling, high erythrocyte sedimentation rate, high creatinine, and high neutrophil counts were found to be predictive factors for a poor clinical outcome.[4]
- Indications for transmetatarsal amputation may include wet or dry gangrene involving only the forefoot and/or infection involving the forefoot, whereas the inclusion criteria are the same as those mentioned above required for a ray amputation.
- Amputation at the metatarsal level causes a muscular imbalance due to resultant equinovarus deformity from unopposed action of gastrocnemius, tibialis anterior, and tibialis posterior tendons, which is coupled with the deficiency of the muscular tension of the extensor tendons.[5,6]

Midfoot Amputation

- Lisfranc disarticulation is a disarticulation through the tarsometatarsal joint, whereas Chopart disarticulation is a disarticulation through the talonavicular and calcaneocuboid joints leaving only the hindfoot (talus and calcaneum) behind (**FIG 1**).
- These amputations are rarely performed in diabetic foot infections due to high failure rate and the proximity of infected tissue to the heel pad.[7]

Hindfoot/Ankle Amputation

- This category included the amputations such as Syme amputation and has the indications and inclusion criteria as mentioned in the forefoot amputation category (**FIG 2**).
- Syme amputation has been advocated for trauma cases; however, Syme amputation can give good results in patients with diabetic foot infections.[8]
- Syme amputation should be reserved for patients with at least a palpable posterior tibial pulse and an ankle-brachial index of more than 0.5.

SURGICAL MANAGEMENT

Preoperative Planning

- All patients undergoing an amputation should be evaluated by both neuropsychiatry and PM&R early.
- Prevention and early detection of future disease should be discussed with the patient.
- Education on pressure-area pathogenesis is important as part of a strategy to encourage the patient to prevent further problems.
- Cardiac optimization is important given the high incidence of cardiac disease among this patient population.
- If discussing limb viability from trauma, a multidisciplinary approach involving vascular, orthopedics, and plastics should take place prior to proceeding with amputation.

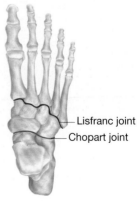

FIG 1 • Midfoot amputation.

— Lisfranc joint
— Chopart joint

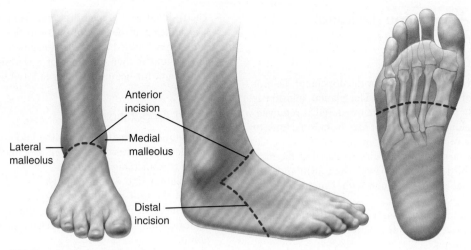

FIG 2 • Hindfoot/ankle amputation.

TECHNIQUES

Toe Amputation

- Place the patient supine with a small bump under the ipsilateral foot if desired.
- Incision lines are marked on the skin as appropriate for the planned amputation.
- For a partial toe amputation, a plantar-based flap is commonly used. However, several other possibilities exist (eg, dorsal flap, side-to-side flap, and fish-mouth flap).[9]
- The most important principles are to ensure that the flap is viable before closure and to perform a tension-free repair.
- All necrotic tissue is debrided. If infection is present, the tendon sheaths must be drained of any purulent material, which often tracks along them.
- Microbiology samples may be sent for culture and sensitivity testing.
- Neurovascular bundles are ligated or cauterized as they are dissected.
- If the wound is left open, many dressing options are available. Commonly, the wound is loosely packed with gauze soaked in saline or povidone-iodine. Generous amounts of cotton dressing and ACE bandages are then applied.
- If conducting an osteotomy, dissection is carried down to the periosteum, and a bone cutter or pneumatic saw is used to perform the osteotomy at the appropriate level.
- It is important to be mindful of tendon insertions and to consider the biomechanical effects that sacrificing these

will have; disruption may predispose to further surgical intervention in the future.

Transmetatarsal Amputation

- A curved fish-mouth incision is made just proximal to the infected tissue of the foot (**TECH FIG 1**).
- The incision runs from the midshaft of the fifth metatarsal laterally to the midshaft of the first metatarsal medially through a midplane axis and carried circumferentially. The plantar flap is left longer to allow for closure. Also, the residual flap should be little longer on the medial side than on the lateral side again to aid with closure.[9]
- The incision is again circumferential and extended downward to bone. As the incision is deepened, hemostasis is achieved by means of cautery and/or vessel ligation with ties. The bony landmarks of the metatarsals are identified and presented by means of a periosteal elevator. The metatarsals are cut with a saw, and the bony ends are rounded with a bone file.[10]
- The wound is copiously irrigated and adequate hemostasis is achieved.
- Standard synthetic braided suture is used for closure of muscular and subcutaneous layers. Skin closure with synthetic nonbraided suture results in low skin tension and good approximation. Staples may also be added and dressing applied.

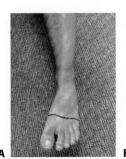
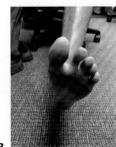
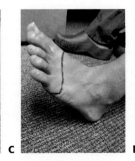
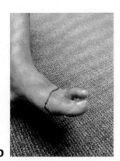

TECH FIG 1 • **A–D.** Transmetatarsal amputation.

TECHNIQUES

■ Midfoot Amputation (Lisfranc/Chopart)

Lisfranc Amputation

- The proximal incision passes over the dorsum of the foot at the base of the metatarsals. The plantar incision is placed distally so that the infected material is removed, but the flap is long enough that it may be tailored later to cover the ends of the resected bones.
- The tarsometatarsal joints are disarticulated at the first, second, and third metatarsal bases. The fourth and fifth metatarsal bases are cut through with a motorized saw and left in the residual foot.
- On occasion, it may be necessary to leave the third metatarsal base in place to provide a better surface to support the local soft tissues.

- The residual foot is then dissected from the plantar surface, starting at the level of the short flexor muscles. The flap is then beveled to the distal edge.
- The wound is then checked for any residual infectious tissues and for hemostasis. It is tailored to close without tension.

Chopart Amputation

- Amputation of the forefoot at the talonavicular and calcaneocuboid joints closely resembles that of amputation at the tarsometatarsal joints.
- The plantar flap is long enough to fold up to the dorsum of the foot. In infected cases, no bone trimming is performed. In noninfected cases, the distal surfaces of the calcaneus are rounded to relieve potential pressure points.

■ Ankle Amputation (Syme Amputation)

- The anterior incision of the Syme amputation extends across the ankle just distal to the tip of each malleolus.
- The posterior incision extends from the malleoli vertically and also transversely across the heel.
- The extensor tendons are all divided at the level of the skin incision.
- The dorsalis pedis artery and vein are then identified, ligated, and divided.
- The ankle joint capsule is incised while plantar-flexing the foot. The medial and lateral ankle ligaments are divided.
- The tendons of the posterior tibialis and flexor hallucis longus are transected, taking care to avoid injury to the posterior tibial artery. This will be the sole blood supply to the flap.[11]

- The heel fat pad is carefully dissected by staying close to the calcaneus to avoid creating a buttonhole, which can doom the operation. The ankle joint is disarticulated and the foot is passed from the table.
- In a single-stage amputation, the malleoli are divided with a saw at the level of the articular surface of the tibia and the width is reduced by vertical bone excision. Holes are drilled in the medial, anterior, and lateral parts of the distal tibia and fibula to secure the heel pad directly under the tibia.[12]
- In a two-stage Syme amputation, the wound is closed by suturing the heel flap to the dorsal fascia. Six weeks later, the malleoli are removed through separate vertical incision.[13]

PEARLS AND PITFALLS

Indications	A careful and complete history and physical examination are essential. Preoperative studies are necessary to plan the resection and reconstruction. Vascular supply to planned reconstruction and amputation must be assessed prior to procedure.
Surgical incision	A long plantar flap leads to a better end-bearing stump. Leaving a flap to short will lead to complications and wound break down.
Infections/flap necrosis	Intravenous antibiotics and surgical debridement may be necessary to treat deep infections. Early diagnosis and treatment can affect outcome. Do not delay treatment if suspected infection after amputation.
Postoperative management	Keep the wound wrapped in sterile soft dressings and a pressure wrap for 3–5 days and physical therapy and rehab should be consulted early in the course.

POSTOPERATIVE CARE

- Keep the wound wrapped in sterile soft dressings and a pressure wrap for 3 to 5 days.
- Staples/sutures will remain in place for approximately 2 weeks.
- Physical therapy and PM&R should be consulted early.

REFERENCES

1. Dillingham TR, Pezzin LE, MacKenzie EJ. Limb amputation and limb deficiency: epidemiology and recent trends in the United States. *South Med J.* 2002;95:875-883.
2. Heikkinen M, Saarinen J, Suominen VP, et al. Lower limb amputations: differences between the genders and long-term survival. *Prosthet Orthot Int.* 2007;31:277-286.
3. Humzah MD, Gilbert PM. Fasciocutaneous blood supply in below-knee amputation. *J Bone Joint Surg (Br).* 1997;79:441-443.
4. Fisher DF Jr, Clagett GP, Fry RE, et al. One-stage versus two-stage amputation for wet gangrene of the lower extremity: a randomized study. *J Vasc Surg.* 1988;8:428-433.
5. Desai Y, Robbs JV, Keenan JP. Staged below-knee amputations for septic peripheral lesions due to ischaemia. *Br J Surg.* 1986;73:392-394.
6. Scher KS, Steele FJ. The septic foot in patients with diabetes. *Surgery.* 1988;104:661-666.
7. Bunt TJ. Physiologic amputation. Preliminary cryoamputation of the gangrenous extremity. *AORN J.* 1991;54:1220-1224.
8. Choksy SA, Lee Chong P, Smith C, et al. A randomised controlled trial of the use of a tourniquet to reduce blood loss during transtibial amputation for peripheral arterial disease. *Eur J Vasc Endovasc Surg.* 2006;31:646-650.
9. Blanc CH, Borens O. Amputations of the lower limb—an overview on technical aspects. *Acta Chir Belg.* 2004;104:388-392.
10. Burgess EM, Romano RL, Zettl JH, Schrock RD Jr. Amputations of the leg for peripheral vascular insufficiency. *J Bone Joint Surg Am.* 1971;53:874-890.
11. Allcock PA, Jain AS. Revisiting transtibial amputation with the long posterior flap. *Br J Surg.* 2001;88:683-686.
12. Smith DG, Fergason JR. Transtibial amputations. *Clin Orthop Relat Res.* 1999;(361):108-115.
13. Tisi PV, Than MM. Type of incision for below knee amputation. *Cochrane Database Syst Rev.* 2014;(1):CD003749.

44 CHAPTER

Amputation of the Lower Extremity: Above-Knee Amputation, Below-Knee Amputation, Through-Knee Amputation

Anahita Dua and Jason T. Lee

INTRODUCTION

- Approximately 1.7 million Americans are living with the loss of a limb, and this number is expected to nearly double by 2050.[1]
- Amputations of the lower extremity may be performed for a myriad of reasons including infection, trauma, cancer, and pain.
- Thoughtful patient selection, early involvement of neuropsychiatry, and physical medicine and rehabilitation (PM&R) are fundamental to a successful outcome.

APPROACH CONSIDERATIONS

- Before considering an amputation, the patient should be evaluated by vascular surgery to ensure no other options (endovascular or open) exist.
- Patients who are suited for an above-knee amputation (AKA) include those who have limited or no mobility, a nonfunctional limb, infection that has progressed above the knee, inadequate overlying skin/muscle to provide stump coverage, and those patients who do not have adequate blood flow to heal a below-knee amputation (BKA) incision (popliteal pressures less than 50 mm Hg).
- BKA is suited in patients who wish to ambulate with a prosthesis, do not have extensive infection above the knee joint, and have popliteal pressures greater than 50 mm Hg to heal the stump.
- Knee disarticulations (through-knee amputations) represent less than 2% of all amputations and are typically performed for trauma; they are best suited for patients who are unlikely to ambulate.
- AKA is also suitable for patients unlikely to ambulate, but cannot be performed in patients with inadequate femoral artery blood flow as the AKA stump will not heal.
- Severe infection that involves the femoral head or proximal femur also preclude AKA.[2]

PREOPERATIVE PLANNING

- All patients undergoing an amputation should be evaluated early by both neuropsychiatry and PM&R.

- Thorough physical exam and arterial pressures should be used to determine which level (AKA or BKA) is best for the patient (**FIG 1**).
- Cardiac optimization is important given the high incidence of cardiac disease among this patient population.
- If discussing limb viability status post trauma, a multidisciplinary approach involving vascular, orthopedic, and plastic surgery services should take place prior to proceeding with amputation.

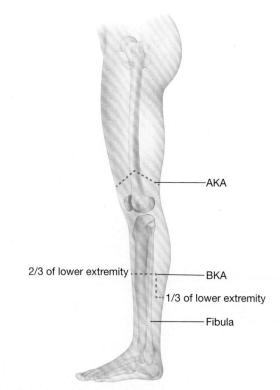

FIG 1 • Incisions for above-knee (AKA), below-knee (BKA), and through-knee amputation.

■ Above-Knee Amputation

- Place the patient supine with a small bump under the ipsilateral hip to internally rotate the leg.
- Outline the circumferential incision (fish mouth configuration)—amputation level should be at the proximal femur, midfemur, or supracondylar.
- Sharply dissect the skin, soft tissue, and muscle down to the femur.
- Identify the vascular bundle and individually suture ligate the artery, vein, and nerve—nerve should be transected as proximally as possible.
- Using a periosteal elevator, elevate the femoral periosteum.

- Transect the bone using a Gigli saw or battery-operated oscillating saw.
- Bevel the femoral edge using the saw.
- Utilize a rasp to smooth the bone edge.
- Irrigate the wound thoroughly.
- Complete the amputation with the amputation knife.
- Approximate the anterior and posterior flaps with 0-Vicryl for deep fascia and 2-0 Vicryl for superficial tissue using interrupted figure of eights.
- Staple or suture the skin with 2-0 nylon.
- Cover skin wound with antibiotic ointment, petroleum jelly dressing, and cotton dressings for padding. Wrap a circumferential compressive elastic dressing for the stump.

■ Below-Knee Amputation

- Place the patient supine with a bump under the ipsilateral thigh and place a thigh tourniquet.
- Prep the lower extremity circumferentially up to the midthigh.
- The anterior incision is placed 10 cm distal to the tibial tubercle (anterior incision 2/3 total circumference), and the posterior incision (1/3 total circumference) should be long enough to ensure flap coverage (typically 1.5 times the length of the anterior flap).
- Carry down the anterior incision sharply to the tibia.
- Carefully tie off the anterior tibial vessels with 2-0 silk suture.
- Dissect through the lateral and superficial posterior compartments of the leg.
- Using a periosteal elevator, remove the periosteum and soft tissue to expose a clean segment of bone to be transected.

- Using a Gigli saw or battery-operated saw, transect the tibia—bevel distal tibia cut at 45 degrees.
- Transect the fibula 2 cm proximal to the tibia.
- Remove the muscle and soft tissue with an amputation knife.
- In the posterior compartment, identify and ligate the peroneal and posterior tibial vessels with 2-0 silk.
- Tie all nerves with 2-0 silk and transect sharply as proximally as possible.
- Utilize a rasp to smooth the edges of the tibia.
- Deflate the tourniquet and coagulate or tie off any bleeding vessels.
- Close pretibial fascia with 2-0 Vicryl figure of eights in an interrupted fashion.
- Staple or suture the skin.
- Cover skin wound with antibiotic ointment, petroleum jelly dressing, and cotton dressings for padding. Wrap a circumferential compressive elastic dressing for the stump.

■ Through-Knee Amputation

- Mark the leg at knee level with a posterior soft tissue flap of sufficient length to close the incision without tension.
- Proximal thigh tourniquet is placed, the patient is prepped and draped, planned incisions are remarked, and the tourniquet is inflated without exsanguination.
- Incisions are created with sharp dissection and carried down circumferentially to the level of the knee, through the joint, and along the drawn posterior flap.
- Distal leg is removed from the operative field.
- Distal end of femur is shaved down from distal to proximal using a sagittal saw anteriorly, posteriorly, medially, and laterally.
- Do not manipulate the insertion of the adductor magnus muscle.

- Preserve cruciate ligaments and posterior capsule.
- Posterior articulating surface is shaved to cancellous bone.
- Identify the patella and advance it to cover the distal surface of the femur.
- Sew the quadriceps tendon to the cruciate ligament and posterior joint capsule so that the posterior surface of the patella is in direct contact with the distal end of the femur.
- Sew the hamstring muscles to the quadriceps tendon and posterior capsule using 2.0-polydioxanone (PDS) so the distal femur is covered.
- Place a closed-suction drain, such as a Jackson Pratt (JP) drain over the myodesis, and trim the posterior flap so it can be sewn to the anterior flap using 2.0-Prolene vertical mattress suture.[3]

PEARLS AND PITFALLS

Posterior flap creation	▪ Ensure that the flap length is adequate for coverage without being too tight as a tight flap can result in necrosis of the closure.
Stump edema	▪ Swelling of the stump post operatively can result in wound healing complications as it places tension on the suture line. Wrapping the stump in a sterile ACE bandage for at least the first three days post operatively will assist with keeping the edema to a minimum.
Knee immobilizer	▪ A knee immobilizer is a good adjunct to help keep the knee joint straight during recovery. A straight and flexible knee joint is imperative to being able to use a prosthesis for ambulation. A knee immobilizer has to be used with caution as it can cause pressure wounds to the knee area of the stump. It should be removed under supervision daily during physical therapy to prevent pressure wounds.

POSTOPERATIVE CARE

- Keep the wound wrapped in sterile soft dressings and a pressure wrap for 3 to 5 days.
- Staples/sutures will remain in place for a minimum of 4 weeks.
- Drains may be removed when 24-hour output is less than 30 mL.
- Ensure no contractures by placing a knee immobilizer in patients with a BKA.
- Physical therapy and PM&R should be consulted early.
- Nonweight bearing for 2 weeks.
- Fit for prosthesis and advance rehabilitation in 3 to 6 months.[4]

REFERENCES

1. Ziegler-Graham K, MacKenzie EJ, Ephraim PL, et al. Estimating the prevalence of limb loss in the United States: 2005 to 2050. *Arch Phys Med Rehabil.* 2008;89(3):422-429.
2. Morris CD, Potter BK, Athanasian EA, Lewis VO. Extremity amputations: principles, techniques, and recent advances. *Instr Course Lect.* 2015;64:105-117.
3. Albino FP, Seidel R, Brown BJ, et al. Through knee amputation: technique modifications and surgical outcomes. *Arch Plast Surg.* 2014;41(5):562-570.
4. Perkins ZB, De'Ath HD, Sharp G, Tai NR. Factors affecting outcome after traumatic limb amputation. *Br J Surg.* 2012;99(suppl 1):75-86.

Lymphaticovenous Anastomosis

Ann-Charlott Docherty Skogh and Martin Halle

DEFINITION

- Lower extremity lymphedema can either be primary, occurring as a structural or anatomical birth defect, or secondary following surgery and/or radiotherapy, trauma, infection, and other causes.
- Chronic lymphedema is a progressive condition where tissue remodeling lead to fibrosis and fat deposition if not treated adequately.
- Lymphedema can be severely disabling and affect the patient's daily life with difficulties in range of motion, fitting into normal clothing, and can also cause psychological distress.

ANATOMY

- The lymphatic system is composed of collecting vessels and lymph nodes.
- The lymphatic system of the lower extremities includes a superficial and a deep system divided by the muscle fascia-aponeurosis. Perforating lymphatic vessels interconnect both systems.
- The superficial system includes the interfascial and epifascial subsystems, where the latter is the most superficial one, located between the skin and the saphenous fascia (**FIG 1**).

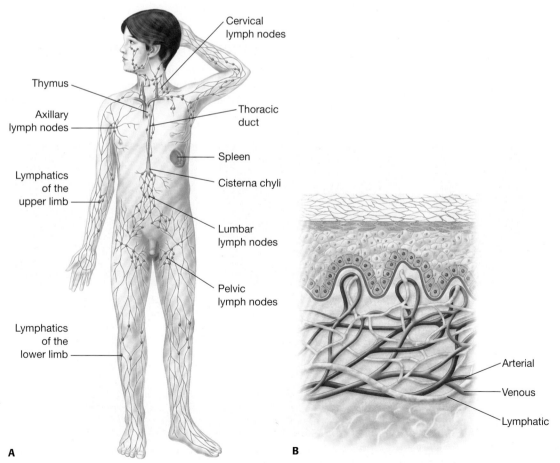

Cervical lymph nodes

Thymus

Axillary lymph nodes

Lymphatics of the upper limb

Lymphatics of the lower limb

Thoracic duct

Spleen

Cisterna chyli

Lumbar lymph nodes

Pelvic lymph nodes

Arterial

Venous

Lymphatic

A

B

FIG 1 • **A.** The lymphatic vessels of the lower limb drain into the inguinal and pelvic system and proximally to cisterna chyli. **B.** The sub- and intradermal lymph capillaries drain into deeper lymphatic collectors located below the dermis.

PATHOGENESIS

- Lymphedema can be primary, occurring as a structural or anatomical birth defect in which genetics seem to play a major role. Secondary lymphedema may occur after surgery and/or radiotherapy, trauma, infection, and other causes. Lymphatic filariasis following infection of invading pathogens is globally the most common cause of secondary lymphedema.[1]
- The transport capacity of lymphatic drainage may be reduced by damage that further affects the homeostasis of the interstitium, including both the cellular and extracellular compartments.
- Lymphostasis with fluid accumulation in the tissues leads to inflammation and subsequent tissue remodeling of skin and subcutaneous tissues with fibrosis and fat deposition.

NATURAL HISTORY

- Untreated lymphedema tends to deteriorate with time, leading to fibrosis and fat deposition that occur at later stages. Inflammatory changes make the patient susceptible to recurrent episodes of erysipelas and cellulitis.

PATIENT HISTORY AND PHYSICAL FINDINGS

- Initially, there is a phase with reduced transport capacity without clinical swelling.
- Stage 1 lymphedema includes pitting edema that subsides with limb elevation, whereas elevation is not effective in stage 2, when fibrosis of the tissues may already be seen.
- Stage 3 includes increasing volume of the extremity with congestive dermatitis, trophic skin, and fat deposition.[2]
- A pitting test shall be performed with pressure applied to the affected area (ideally over the tibial bone) for at least 60 seconds with the examiners fingers. The absence of pitting

confirms tissue remodeling and fat deposition, where lymphaticovenular anastomoses may be less successful and suction-assisted lipectomy shall be considered.[3]

IMAGING

- Imaging methods for lymphedema include radionuclide lymphoscintigraphy, indocyanine green (ICG) lymphography, and magnetic resonance lymphangiography.
- Lymphoscintigraphy can indicate the location of lymph collectors, but does not provide information about specific areas of occlusion.[2]
- ICG lymphography, on the other hand, visualizes real-time superficial lymph flow without radiation exposure.[4]
- ICG lymphographic patterns are categorized from normal linear pattern (stage 0) to abnormal dermal backflow patterns; splash (stage I), stardust (stages II–IV), and diffuse stardust (stage V) patterns with lymphedema progression of the lower extremity[5] (**FIG 2**).

DIFFERENTIAL DIAGNOSIS

- Venous insufficiency
- Deep vein thrombosis
- Thrombophlebitis
- Erysipelas
- Renal failure
- Cardiac failure
- Neurofibromatosis
- Lymphangioma
- Others

NONOPERATIVE MANAGEMENT

- Decongestive physiotherapy and compression garments have been the most common nonsurgical treatment methods in reducing edema volumes, although they are not curative.

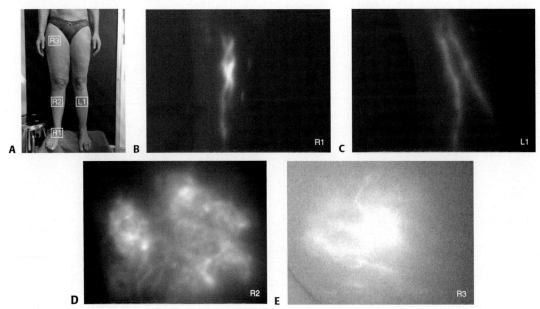

FIG 2 • **A.** Right leg lymphedema. **B,C.** ICG images illustrating different flow patterns. Linear pattern **(D)**, stardust pattern **(E)**, and diffuse pattern as described by Narushima M, Yamamoto T, Ogata F, et al.

SURGICAL MANAGEMENT

- Surgical treatment of lymphedema includes debulking surgery, suction-assisted lipectomy, vascularized lymph node transfer, and lymphaticovenular, lymphaticovenous, and lymphatico-lymphatic anastomosis.[6]
- Suction-assisted lipectomy is usually performed for late lymphedema, when edematous tissues has remodeled to adipose tissue, without remaining signs of pitting edema. However, there is still a lack of consensus whether vascularized lymph node transfer or lymphaticovenous anastomosis is the primary choice in pitting lymphedema.
- Surgical treatment of lymphedema with lymphaticovenular anastomosis has recently gained popularity due to better imaging systems together with recent technical advances in supramicrosurgery, including high magnification operative microscopes and supramicrosurgical instruments.[7,8]

Preoperative Planning

- Positive pitting test is of paramount importance for the prognosis, because the absence of pitting may reveal a certain degree of irreversibility of the lymphedema.

- Lymphoscintigraphy facilitates confirmation of the diagnosis.
- ICG lymphography is commonly performed using a photodynamic eye (PDE) camera (Hamamatsu Photonics, K.K, Hamamatsu, Japan), ideally in an outpatient setting for patient selection and subsequently repeated perioperatively.
- Preoperative markings of linear flow as well as dermal backflow areas, based on ICG imaging, facilitate selection of anatomical sites for multiple LVAs.

Positioning

- The patient is usually positioned supine or in a unilateral "frog-leg" position for better access to medial structures, depending on results from preoperative ICG imaging.

Approach

- The procedure may be performed under local anesthesia, whereas general anesthesia is recommended if any movement during surgery is to be avoided.
- The use of two or three microscopes can facilitate the performance of multiple anastomoses.

■ Lymphaticovenous Anastomosis

- A volume of 0.3 to 1.0 mL ICG (Pulsion Medical Systems SE, Feldkirchen, Germany, 5 mg/mL) is injected intradermally into the first web space of the affected leg to locate lymphatic vessels suitable for anastomosis (**TECH FIG 1A,B**). Similarly, the technique can be used for upper extremity lymphedema, performed with intradermal injection into the first and fourth web space.
- A linear flow pattern segment confirmed by ICG lymphangiography is chosen (**TECH FIG 1C,D**).
- A 15- to 30-mm incision transverse to the selected lymph vessel is performed into the deep layer of dermis. The remaining thickness of the dermis is gently dissected under meticulous hemostasis, avoiding injury to the subdermal lymphatic vessels and venules (**TECH FIG 1E**).
- If lymphatic vessels are difficult to locate, a complementary injection of 0.3- to 1.0-mL patent blue (Patentblau,

Guerbet, Germany V, 25 mg/mL) can be administered intradermally, a few centimeters distal to the skin incision.
- Suitable subdermal venules (around 0.5 mm in diameter) are explored adjacent to the chosen lymphatic vessel (**TECH FIG 1F**).
- Preparation and alignment of vessels (**TECH FIG 1G,H**).
- A stent using 6-0 nylon suture that is placed into the lumen of the vessels may be used to facilitate anastomosis of the vessels, which range from 0.3 to 0.8 mm (**TECH FIG 1I,J**).
- Patent blue or ICG lymphography can be used to confirm patency of LVA (**TECH FIG 1K**).
- The venules of choice may differ in diameter compared to the lymphatic vessels, where different types of anastomoses may be applied. The first choice is an end-to-end anastomosis. If a Y-shaped venule is available, both afferent and efferent lymphatic flow can be diverted into the same venule[9] (**TECH FIG 1L–P**).

TECHNIQUES

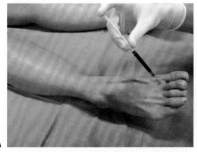 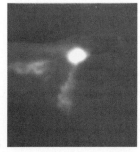 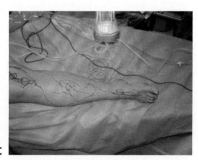

TECH FIG 1 • **A.** Injection of indocyanine green into the first web space of the foot. **B.** ICG staining of lymphatic vessels in the foot as seen with PDE camera. **C.** Markings on the skin of the leg after injection of ICG.

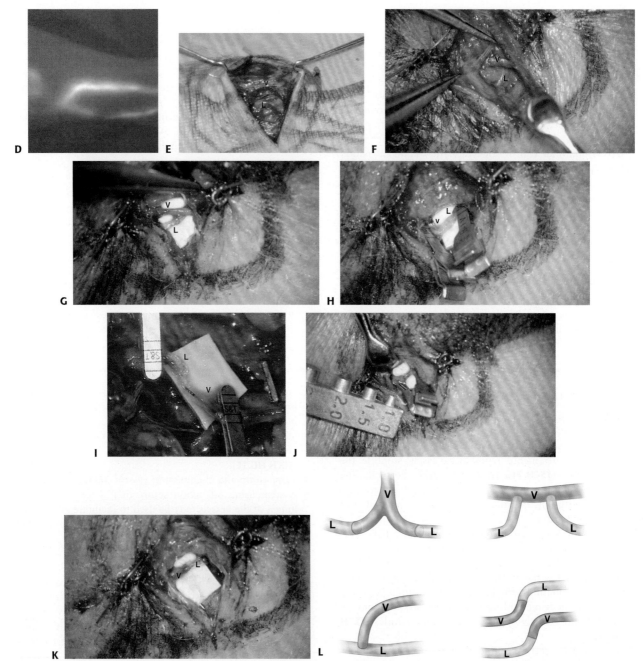

TECH FIG 1 (Continued) • **D.** ICG staining of linear lymphatic vessels in the leg as seen with PDE camera. **E.** Incision of the skin showing subdermal venule (*V*) and lymphatic vessel (*L*). **F.** Preparation of venule (*V*) and lymphatic vessel (*L*) stained with patent blue. **G.** Preparation of venule (*V*) and lymphatic vessel (*L*) stained with patent blue with background to facilitate anastomosis. **H.** Aligning of vessels before suturing. **I.** Stent using 6-0 nylon suture to prevent back wall stitches. **J.** End-to-end lymphaticovenular anastomosis with 12-0 nylon sutures. Vessels with luminal diameter of approximately 0.5 mm. **K.** Lymphatic flow over anastomosis as shown by patent blue staining in lymphatic vessel and venule. **L.** Different types of lymphaticovenous anastomoses according to Narushima et al.[9] (*V*) Venule or vein, (*L*) lymphatic vessel.

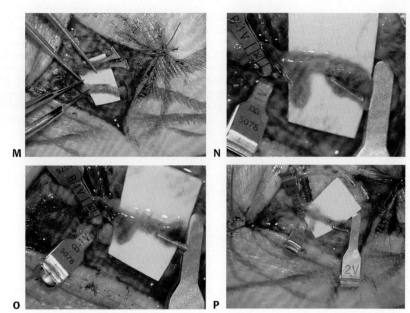

TECH FIG 1 (Continued) • **M.** Preparation of Y-shaped vein and lymphatic vessel. **N,O.** Coaptation of vein and lymphatic vessel with antegrade and **(P)** retrograde flow.

PEARLS AND PITFALLS

- Choose small venules to avoid venous backflow.
- Tension-free anastomosis is of great importance due to the low-flow nature of lymphatic vessels and venules.
- Perioperative antibiotics are indicated due to long surgery time and an increased risk for erysipelas in lymphedema patients.
- The dorsum of the foot and lower leg are usually good locations to perform LVAs in the lower extremity. The lymphatic vessels are usually easy to find after examination with ICG, complemented with patent blue if necessary. The upper extremity presents a similar pattern, where it is easier to find suitable vessels on the dorsum of the hand and in the forearm compared to the upper arm.
- LVAs may be more difficult to perform in the thigh area due to the greater width of the epifascial compartment.

POSTOPERATIVE CARE

- Low molecular weight heparin is indicated the first postoperative week due to immobilization during surgery.
- Postoperatively, the leg is kept slightly elevated at night and a low-pressure bandage is applied the day after surgery to avoid interstitial swelling.
- Postop day 1, the patient is allowed to ambulate with full weight bearing with a low-pressure bandage applied (about 30 mm Hg), but with reduced physical activity.
- Normal physical activity can be resumed after 3 weeks.

OUTCOMES

- Several case reports of successful treatment of lower extremity lymphedema with LVAs are available, and multiple LVAs seem to be favorable.[10]
- Reduced number of episodes of erysipelas after LVAs has been reported.[11]
- The outcome of lower extremity LVAs has been less investigated as compared to upper extremity LVAs, and data from prospective, controlled studies are scarce.

COMPLICATIONS

- Infections may occur in the postoperative period and shall be treated with antibiotics.
- Temporary local redness can occur due to venous backflow into the anastomosis.
- Deterioration of the lymphedema is a very rare complication, but can occur, after LVA surgery.

REFERENCES

1. Olszewski WL. The pathophysiology of lymphedema—2012. *Handchir Mikrochir Plast Chir.* 2012;44:322-328.
2. Murdaca G, Cagnati P, Gulli R, et al. Current views on diagnostic approach and treatment of lymphedema. *Am J Med.* 2012;125:134-140.
3. Brorson H, Ohlin K, Olsson G, et al. Controlled compression and liposuction treatment for lower extremity lymphedema. *Lymphology.* 2008;41(2):52-63.
4. Ogata F, Narushima M, Mihara M, et al. Intraoperative lymphography using indocyanine green dye for near-infrared fluorescence labeling in lymphedema. *Ann Plast Surg.* 2007;59(2):180-184.
5. Narushima M, Yamamoto T, Ogata F, et al. Indocyanine green lymphography findings in limb lymphedema. *J Reconstr Microsurg.* 2016;32(1):72-79.

6. Granzow JW, Soderberg JM, Kaji AH, Dauphine C. Review of current surgical treatments for lymphedema. *Ann Surg Oncol.* 2014;21(4):1195-1201.

7. Koshima I, Inagawa K, Urushibara K, Moriguchi T. Supermicrosurgical lymphaticovenular anastomosis for the treatment of lymphedema in the upper extremities. *J Reconstr Microsurg.* 2000;16(6):437-442.

8. Koshima I, Nanba Y, Tsutsui T, et al. Long-term follow-up after lymphaticovenular anastomosis for lymphedema in the leg. *J Reconstr Microsurg.* 2003;19(4):209-215.

9. Narushima M, Mihara M, Yamamoto Y, et al. The intravascular stenting method for treatment of extremity lymphedema with multiconfiguration lymphaticovenous anastomoses. *Plast Reconstr Surg.* 2010;125(3):935-943.

10. Maegawa J, Hosono M, Tomoeda H, et al. Net effect of lymphaticovenous anastomosis on volume reduction of peripheral lymphoedema after complex decongestive physiotherapy. *Eur J Vasc Endovasc Surg.* 2012;43(5):602-608.

11. Mihara M, Hara H, Furniss D, et al. Lymphaticovenular anastomosis to prevent cellulitis associated with lymphoedema. *Br J Surg.* 2014;101(11):1391-1396.

Lymphedema: Lymph Node Transfer

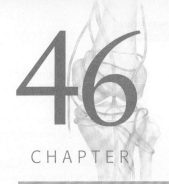

46

CHAPTER

Adrian S. H. Ooi and David W. Chang

DEFINITION

- The lymphatic system is responsible for reabsorption of excess interstitial fluid, protein, and waste products, as well as filtration and removal of foreign material from interstitial fluid and absorption of lipids from intestines. Up to 50% of the body's circulating albumin is processed through the lymphatic system every day.
- Lymphedema is an abnormal accumulation of protein-rich fluid in the interstitial compartment resulting in edema formation.
- It occurs when the generalized or regional lymphatic load exceeds its transport capacity.
- Long-standing lymphedema leads to chronic inflammation, adipose tissue hypertrophy and fibrosis, and eventually lymphatic channel fibrosis.
- Lymphedema is a problem that affects about 200 million people worldwide.
- Distribution: Lower limb 90% greater than upper limb 10% greater than genitalia 1%.

ANATOMY

- Endothelial cells bud off from veins during early embryonic development and transdifferentiate to form the lymphatic vasculature.
- The lymphatic primary plexus is composed of capillary-like vessels and is further remodeled to form pre-collecting, collecting, and ductal components. The major lymphatic ducts are formed by two paired lymph sacs (jugular and iliac) and two unpaired sacs (retroperitoneal and cisterna chyli).
- Lymphatic channels are thin-walled vessels composed of endothelial cells connected by discontinuous junctions and surrounded by smooth muscle. The basement membranes of the larger, deeper lymphatic vessels have multiple intercellular gaps, which form valves through which fluid flows unidirectionally.
- The superficial dermal lymphatics are unvalved and drain into the valved subfascial deep dermal system, which run with the superficial veins.
- Lymphatic fluid is then transported through afferent lymphatic channels to lymph nodes, which are gathered in basins throughout the body. After undergoing immunological processes within the lymph nodes, the fluid flows out through efferent lymphatic channels and ultimately into the thoracic ducts and subclavian veins where they rejoin the venous circulation.
- Lymph nodes are bean-shaped structures distributed along the lymphatic channels. They consist of a capsule, an outer cortex and an inner medulla. Multiple afferent lymphatics can enter via the outer cortex, and a lymph node is supplied by an artery and a vein at the hilar region, which accompany a single efferent lymphatic vessel. The lymph nodes contain lymphocytes and macrophages, which are responsible for removal of organisms, foreign substances, and tumor cells.
- Lymph nodes are distributed deep in the body along the respiratory and gastrointestinal tract and superficial in the cervical, thoracic, and inguinal regions.
- Lymphatic fluid transportation is under humoral influences and is propelled by a combination of:
  - Smooth muscle surrounding the collecting vessels that have an intrinsic autocontractile mechanism
  - Extrinsic compression by neighboring skeletal muscles
  - Negative intrathoracic pressure

PATHOGENESIS

- Lymphatic homeostasis is a function of filtration of plasma across the capillary walls into the interstitial compartment and absorption by the lymphatic system. This rate of filtration is governed by the Starling equation whereby net filtration is determined by intra- and extracapillary hydrostatic and oncotic forces.
- Lymphedema arises when the rate of filtration exceeds absorption by 2 to 4 L/d.
- This disruption can occur at the level of the lymphatic vasculature or the lymph nodes and can arise due to a primary or secondary disease process.
- True primary lymphedema can be classified as congenital (Milroy disease), pubertal/praecox (Meige disease), and tarda, which occurs in the adult age group. Lymphedema praecox is the most common form of primary lymphedema.
- Lymphedema can also arise secondary to acquired damage to the lymphatic system. These include infection, trauma, malignancy, surgery, and radiation.
- The most common cause worldwide is filariasis, caused by the parasite *Wuchereria bancrofti*. In the developed world, it is most commonly due to treatment for cancer.
  - For breast cancer treatment, it occurs in up to 40% of cases with lymph node dissection and radiation and 5% of cases with sentinel lymph node biopsy.
  - 41% after gynecological cancer treatment.
  - 12% to 55% after groin lymph node dissection.

NATURAL HISTORY

- When there is disruption in the lymphatic system and as lymphatic pressure builds, flow within the lymph vessels stagnates, leading to valvular incompetence and dermal backflow.

- Lymphedema is confined to the subcutaneous compartment as the deeper lymphatics are driven by the skeletal muscle pump.
- Over time, macromolecular protein and hyaluronan are deposited in the interstitium leading to increased tissue colloid osmotic pressure.
  - Fibroblast, monocytes, adipocytes, and keratinocytes also increase within the tissue, leading to increased collagen deposition, degeneration of elastic fibers, and fibrovascular proliferation.
  - The basement membranes of lymphatic vessels are obliterated and the vessels become fibrotic.
  - This combination results in nonpitting edema, and eventually a chronic inflammatory state ensues.
- The cytokines arising from the inflammation and the disruption in lymphatic flow of lipids leads to adipose deposition and hypertrophy in the interstitium.
- The verrucous appearance of long-standing lymphatic extremities is caused by hyperplasia of skin at the dermal-epidermal junction.
- Lymphatic stasis and decreased immunological function predispose the patient to an increased risk of local skin infections, erysipelas, and later, lymphangitis. The excess tissue can lead to symptoms of pain, heaviness, and decreased mobility. Long-standing chronic lymphedema can lead to development of lymphangiosarcoma (Stewart-Treves syndrome). Lymphedema has significant adverse impact on patients' quality of life and psychosocial health.
- The International Society of Lymphangology (ISL) has classified lymphedema into three stages:
  - 0: Latent/subclinical period
  - I: Pitting edema which is reversible on elevation
  - II: Tissue fibrosis and edema, which is nonreversible on elevation
  - III: Elephantiasis and trophic skin changes

PATIENT HISTORY AND PHYSICAL FINDINGS

- The history is targeted at determining the diagnosis and etiology of lymphedema, duration, symptoms, and complications, and how the patient has been managing it.
  - Elucidating diagnosis and etiology include asking about risk factors for malignancy, travel history, prior surgical procedures, history of radiation therapy, trauma and infection, and family history. Obesity can contribute to lymphedema through the overload of lipids in the body. Other causes of extremity swelling such as congestive cardiac failure, venous insufficiency, and deep vein thrombosis have to be excluded (see differential diagnosis).
  - Important symptoms and complications to ask about include pain and infections in the affected extremity, a feeling of heaviness and difficulty in movement.
- The examination of the patient with lymphedema should include a general physical and a targeted examination of the affected part. The general examination is aimed at excluding any active infection or malignancy and general causes of extremity edema.
- Lymphedema is typically unilateral, with the swelling beginning distally and progressing over months to years.
  - The edema starts off soft and pitting and eventually becomes nonpitting as interstitial fibrosis sets in.

- There is minimal pigment change or ulceration and peau d'orange indicating dermal fibrosis can be present.
- Late changes in the extremity include hyperkeratosis, papillomatosis, and the development of a positive Stemmer sign in which the skin on the dorsum of the second web space of the foot cannot be pinched as a fold.
- Reproducible measurements of the limb should be taken to help with accurate follow-up. These can include circumference measurements and volumetric measurements such as water displacement tests, perometry, and bioimpedance testing. Digital photographs are also useful for comparative analysis.
  - Circumference measurements are typically taken at 4- to 10-cm intervals from consistent landmarks such as the patella in the lower extremity and the olecranon in the upper extremity. Figures that are used in the diagnosis of lymphedema include the following:
    - Greater than 2 cm difference from the nonaffected limb.
    - Severity can be graded as mild (greater than 10% difference), moderate (greater than 20%), and severe (greater than 30%).
  - Water displacement has been the standard for volume measurement and is highly accurate but cumbersome. Lymphedema is diagnosed if the volume differential of the affected limb is greater than 10% of the normal limb.
  - Perometry utilizes an infrared optical electronic scanner to calculate volume.
  - Bioimpedance testing calculates the fluid composition of an affected limb using resistance to an electrical current.

IMAGING

- Lymphangiography is the visualization of lymphatic vessels using contrast medium. Vessels can be classified as anaplastic, hypoplastic, or hyperplastic. There are the direct and indirect forms of lymphangiography.
  - Direct lymphangiography involves transecting distal lymphatic vessels and directly injecting water-soluble iodide contrast medium into them. This has largely been abandoned because of patient discomfort and damage to the lymphatic channels.
  - Indirect lymphangiography injects contrast medium distally into the subepidermis and uses radiographic imaging to delineate the lymphatic system.
- Isotopic lymphoscintigraphy is the current standard for lymphatic imaging. It injects Technetium-99–labeled albumin into the subepidermis of the distal affected extremity and timed post injection imaging to determine lymphatic anatomy and function. It has a sensitivity of 97% and specificity of 100%. However, when done awake, the injection can be painful, and the length of time required can be distressing to the patient.
- The injection of indocyanine green (ICG) and imaging using an infrared camera have become widely used in the imaging of lymphatic vessels and are particularly useful intra-op when needing to delineate the superficial lymphatic system. A classification based on the appearance of the ICG has been developed and correlated with the Campisi classification (Table 1).[1]
- Computed tomography (CT) and magnetic resonance imaging (MRI) scanning are useful in determining the architecture of the affected limb and elucidating any underlying

Table 1 Indocyanine Green Appearance to Classify Severity of Lymphedema

Stage	Description
0	No dermal backflow
I	Splash pattern around the axilla/groin region
II	Stardust pattern proximal to the patella/elbow
III	Stardust pattern distal to the patella/elbow
IV	Stardust pattern in the entire limb
V	Diffuse pattern

cause such as neoplasm. There is commonly a "honeycomb" appearance above the deep subcutaneous fascia. MRI with contrast has proven promising in outlining lymphatic vasculature.[2]

DIFFERENTIAL DIAGNOSIS

- Venous insufficiency
- Deep venous thrombosis
- Vascular malformations
- Lipedema
- Myxedema
- Fluid overload
  - Congestive cardiac failure
  - Renal failure
  - Liver failure
- Hypoalbuminemia
- Soft tissue tumors
- Morbid Obesity

NONOPERATIVE MANAGEMENT

- Nonoperative management is aimed at reducing the amount of swelling and treating any resulting complications. The former is accomplished by compression and massage therapy, whereas the latter involves adequate skin care and early detection of infection and treatment with the appropriate antibiotics. In a compliant patient, this helps to slow down the progress of lymphedema.
- Patients should be educated about lymphedema and its complications, and given responsibility for their own care.
- Conservative treatment of lymphedema has been well researched and the regimen described is complete decongestive therapy (CDT). This should be started early to have the most benefit and is useful in cases of lesser than stage III lymphedema. Analyses have shown up to 40% to 60% reduction in lymphedema volume. It consists of two phases:
  - Initial reductive phase (up to 8 weeks) consisting of:
    - Manual lymphatic drainage—Circular tissue stretching massage with varying degrees of pressure
    - Compression therapy during waking hours
    - Regular skin care
    - Targeted exercise
  - Maintenance phase consisting of
    - Self-conducted lymphatic drainage
    - Continuation of compression garments
- Weight loss may help with lymphedema by reducing the flow of fatty acids through lymphatic channels and decreasing fatty deposition in the subcutaneous tissue.

- Exercises such as swimming can be useful in reducing the severity of lymphedema.
- Unsubstantiated nonoperative measures include coumarin (5,6 benzo-a-pyrone), diuretic use, microwave heating, and intra-arterial injection of lymphocytes.

SURGICAL MANAGEMENT

- Although significant advances have been made in the surgical treatment of lymphedema, no surgical technique offers a cure, and an aggressive trial of nonsurgical therapy should first be done.
- Indications for surgical treatment include failed conservative therapy, grossly impaired limb function, debilitating extremity size and weight, recurrent lymphangitis (greater than 3 episodes of infection per year), and uncontrolled pain.
- Surgical techniques for the treatment of lymphedema are classified as excisional and physiological.
- Excisional techniques aim to reduce the amount of lymphatic tissue and tighten the skin envelope. They are described elsewhere in this book and include but are not limited to excision and skin grafting (eg, Charles procedure), staged excision, liposuction, and, more recently, radical resection with preservation of perforators (RRPP).[3] Unfortunately, as the primary disease process is not addressed, there is a high risk of recurrence with these techniques, and the appearance can be undesirable.
- Physiological techniques attempt to replicate the normal lymphatic flow in the affected extremity. Procedures that have been developed and described elsewhere include buried dermal flaps, lymphovenolymphatic bypass, lymphatic bypass, and lymphovenous anastomosis (LVA).[4]
- The vascularized lymph node transfer (VLNT) is a physiological technique that transfers intact autologous lymph nodes from a nonlymphedematous region of the body to the affected extremity. In a sense, this is the most physiological method of addressing the problem in a patient whose lymphedema is due to damage to or paucity of lymph nodes in a particular basin.
- The lymph nodes are microsurgically anastomosed to the chosen recipient site vessels and allowed to develop collateral blood supply. Over time, reported mechanisms of lymphedema reduction include reduction of scarring at the recipient site, hydrostatic "pumping" of intraflap lymph via arterial inflow and venous outflow, and lymphangiogenesis aided by the production of VEGF-C by the transplanted lymph nodes.
- Though not curative, physiological techniques have proven to alleviate symptoms and reduce lymphedema volume.

Preoperative Planning

- Preoperative workup should include elucidating etiology of the lymphedema, comorbidities, the patient's treatment to date, limb measurements, weight fluctuations, and ability to comply with therapy.
- Severity of lymphedema should be clinically staged according to the ISL grading system, and treatment planned accordingly:
  - Patients with mild to moderate stage 1 or 2 lymphedema are best candidates for physiologic procedures such as VLNT and/or LVA.

- Patients with stage 3 fibrofatty lymphedema or elephantiasis may benefit from excisional procedures prior to physiologic procedures in order to offset the lymphatic load and optimize the result of physiologic procedures.
- Specific history to note with regard to vascularized lymph node (VLN) harvest includes previous surgery in the region of planned harvest or pre-existing lymphedema if harvest is planned from the groin. Scars and surface anatomical landmarks should be noted. Active infection in the affected extremity should be ruled out.
- Definitive diagnosis of lymphedema is made with lymphoscintigraphy, which evaluates lymphatic function.
- ICG imaging of the affected extremity prior to surgery aids in lymphatic mapping for the simultaneous performance of LVA.
- If groin VLNT is planned, reverse lymphatic mapping should be performed to determine the crucial deep groin lymph node basin of the lower extremity, which should be avoided in groin VLNT harvest.
    - This involves the preoperative injection of technitium-99–labeled albumin subcutaneously into the inner thigh and a gamma probe used intraoperatively to detect the sentinel lymph node of the deep groin lymph node basin.[5]
    - Harvest of this lymph node should be avoided at all costs to prevent postoperative lower extremity lymphedema.

Positioning

- For most VLN harvest, the patient is placed in a supine position.
- For TAP flap or split LD flap with LNT, the patient is placed in lateral decubitus position.
- If the lymph nodes are intended to be placed in the axilla, the arm is extended at right angles to the torso to access and prepare the recipient site.
- For specific points for each source of VLN, refer to the subheadings below.

Approach

- For harvest of VLN, the common sources are the submental, supraclavicular, thoracic, inguinal, and omental lymph nodes. The advantages, disadvantages, and potential complications of each are listed in Table 2.
- For recipient sites in the limbs, placement location and the need for a skin paddle for the VLNT are debated.
    - Some surgeons prefer proximal placement of the lymph nodes, whereas others prefer distal placement. This is dependent on which mechanism the lymph nodes are thought to work.
        - For the "pumping" mechanism, distal sites such as the ankle and wrist are chosen as gravitational forces aid in the flow of lymphatics.
        - For the argument that VLNT works by promoting lymphangiogenesis, more proximal sites near the vicinity of lymph node damage are chosen. It is thought that dual effect of scar release and placement of well-vascularized lymph nodes enhance the restoration of lymphatic flow.
    - It is likely that both mechanisms contribute simultaneously to the resolution of lymphedema. A conservative approach to recipient site selection is therefore the best approach.[6]
    - The proximal site is chosen when there is a definite area of scarring from previous surgery or radiation.
        - When it is difficult to access or remove scars, the VLNT can be done distal to the site of obstruction. An example is in patients whose pelvic lymph nodes were removed via intra-abdominal surgery.
        - In patients who have no definite site of injury, placement of the VLNs directly proximal to the area of the swelling is effective.
    - VLNT should be monitored if possible in most cases as in any other free tissue transfers. A skin paddle can be helpful when closure of native skin over the lymph nodes is tight, such as at the wrist, but is not cosmetically appealing. This can be resolved by excision of the skin paddle at a second stage.
- Our preference is to harvest supraclavicular lymph nodes without a skin paddle, and place them at the axilla for the upper extremity and the groin for the lower extremity.
    - We use an implantable Doppler probe postoperatively to monitor the microanastomotic patency.

Table 2 Comparison of Different Vascularized Lymph Node Transfer Donor Sites

Donor site	Average Number of Lymph Nodes	Advantages	Disadvantages
Supraclavicular	2–3	• Inconspicuous donor site • Low risk of causing donor site lymphedema	• Variable anatomy • Need for meticulous harvest technique
Submental	3–4	• Consistent anatomy • Low risk of causing donor site lymphedema	• Visible donor site scar • Risk of injury to the marginal mandibular nerve
Thoracic	Variable	• Ability to harvest with latissimus dorsi or thoracodorsal artery perforator flap • Inconspicuous donor site scar	• Risk of upper extremity lymphedema
Inguinal	5–8	• Ability to harvest with abdominally based flap • Inconspicuous donor site	• Risk of lower extremity lymphedema
Omentum	Unknown	• No risk of causing donor site lymphedema • If harvested laparoscopically, minimal donor site scar	• Need to enter abdominal cavity • No skin paddle possible

TECHNIQUES

■ Supraclavicular Vascularized Lymph Node Harvest

- Based on the transverse cervical (TC) artery.
  - The flap can be harvested with or without a skin paddle.
- Surface landmarks (**TECH FIG 1A**) are a triangle formed by the clavicle (inferior border), lateral edge of the sterno-cleidomastoid muscle (SCM; medial border), and external jugular vein (lateral border).
- Lymph node harvest from the right neck is preferable to avoid the risk of damaging the thoracic duct in the left side of the neck. Lymph nodes are harvested from the left neck if the lymphedema involves right arm.
- In the supine position, the patient's head is tilted 45 degrees away from the side of harvest.
- A longitudinal skin incision is made 1 to 2 cm above the superior border of the clavicle between the medial and lateral borders (**TECH FIG 1B**).
  - If harvesting a skin paddle, the perforator to the skin should be marked with a Doppler probe prior to harvest and an ellipse marked encompassing the perforator along the line of the recommended skin incision.
- The platysma is breached with sharp dissection, and the omohyoid muscle or tendon is identified and cut to reveal fat and lymphatic tissue posteriorly (**TECH FIG 1C**).

- Medial dissection proceeds along the lateral border of the SCM. The internal jugular vein (IJV) is next identified, and the tissue within the triangle gently dissected off. The anterior scalene muscles are identified at the base.
- Proceeding inferiorly from the medial border, the TC artery can usually be identified arising from the thyrocervical trunk (**TECH FIG 1D**).
  - Pedicle length should be maximized by dissecting down to the source vessel.
  - There is usually an accompanying vein supplying the flap arising from the IJV or subclavian vein.
- The distal ends of the TC vessels are identified and ligated.
- Using the EJV as the lateral landmark, lateral dissection then proceeds in a natural plane medial to the trapezius muscle and stops once the anterior scalene muscles are identified at the base.
- Once the borders have been dissected, the supraclavicular VLN flap can be lifted off the anterior scalene muscles and the flap isolated on its vascular pedicle (**TECH FIG 1E**).
  - The phrenic nerve should be identified and preserved.
- When the recipient site is ready, the pedicle can be ligated.
- Donor site closure is done over a suction drain placed away from the IJV. The platysma is approximated with interrupted absorbable polyfilament sutures, and the skin is closed with a running subcuticular suture.

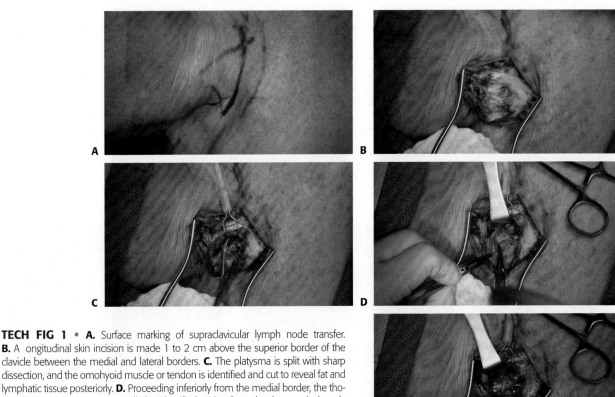

TECH FIG 1 • A. Surface marking of supraclavicular lymph node transfer. **B.** A ongitudinal skin incision is made 1 to 2 cm above the superior border of the clavicle between the medial and lateral borders. **C.** The platysma is split with sharp dissection, and the omohyoid muscle or tendon is identified and cut to reveal fat and lymphatic tissue posteriorly. **D.** Proceeding inferiorly from the medial border, the thoracodorsal (TD) artery can usually be identified arising from the thyrocervical trunk. **E.** Once the borders have been dissected the supraclavicular VLN flap can be lifted off the anterior scalene muscles and the flap isolated on its vascular pedicle. (From Ooi AS, Chang DW. 5-Step harvest of supraclavicular lymph nodes as vascularized free tissue transfer for treatment of lymphedema. *J Surg Oncol.* 2017;115:63-67.)

■ Submental Vascularized Lymph Node Harvest

- Based on the facial artery and its submental branch.
  - The flap can be harvested with or without a skin paddle.
- Surface landmarks are the symphysis, body and angle of the mandible, and facial artery.
- The facial artery is palpated and marked as it crosses the inferior border of the mandible. The skin incision is made 1 cm posterior to the lower border of the mandible.
  - If a skin paddle is desired, a handheld Doppler probe is used to detect the perforators from the submental artery (SMA). An ellipse encompassing the perforators is designed extending from the symphysis medially to the angle of the mandible laterally, with the upper margin along the lower border of the mandible from the mandible angle to the symphysis. The initial skin incision is then initiated at the upper margin of the ellipse.[7]

- The incision is deepened through the platysma, and the SMA is identified at its junction with the FA. The marginal mandibular branch of the facial nerve is identified as it crosses the FA and must be preserved. The SMA is dissected proximal to distal end along its axis.
- The submental lymph nodes are found at the junction of the SMA and FA, and the soft tissue at this region is included to preserve the maximal amount of lymphatic tissue.
- If a skin paddle is included, the septocutaneous perforator from the SMA to the skin paddle must be preserved. To aid with this, the anterior belly of the digastric muscle can be included with the perforator.
- The distal ends of the facial vessels are ligated, and the submental lymph nodes are harvested with the submental vessels and the proximal facial vessels to maximize pedicle length.
- The donor site is closed primarily over a suction drain. The platysma is approximated with interrupted absorbable polyfilament sutures, and the skin is closed with a running subcuticular suture.

■ Thoracic Vascularized Lymph Node Harvest

- Based on the thoracodorsal (TD) vessels or the lateral thoracic (LT) vessels:
  - The thoracic lymph nodes can be harvested as part of a muscle-sparing latissimus dorsi (LD) or thoracodorsal artery perforator (TAP) flap, which can be used for simultaneous pedicled breast reconstruction.
- A longitudinal line just anterior to the LD muscle and lateral to the breast is marked and incised (**TECH FIG 2A**).
- The TD pedicle is located as it enters the LD muscle, and the LT vessels can be identified just anterior to this as it hugs the serratus anterior muscle fascia.
- The lymph nodes to be harvested are located inferior to the lateral border of the pectoralis minor muscle

(**TECH FIG 2B**). These are the level 1 lymph nodes of the axillary region, and harvest of these will avoid damage to the draining lymphatics of the arm.
  - If the lymph nodes alone are harvested, the LT pedicle is preferred as they are the preferential supply.[8]
  - If a pedicled LD or TAP flap is desired for breast reconstruction, the lymph nodes are captured as an anterior extension of the flap skin paddle. As the flap is transposed into the breast anteriorly the lymph nodes are swung upward and placed in the axilla (**TECH FIG 2C**).
- The donor site is closed primarily over a suction drain. The superficial fascia is approximated with strong absorbable polyfilament sutures, and the skin is closed with a running subcuticular suture.

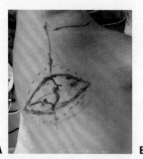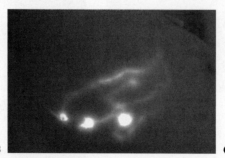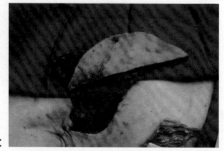

TECH FIG 2 • A. A longitudinal line just anterior to the LD muscle and lateral to the breast is marked and incised. **B.** The lymph nodes to be harvested are located inferior to the lateral border of the pectoralis minor muscle. **C.** As the flap is transposed into the breast anteriorly the lymph nodes are swung upward and placed in the axilla. (From Ooi AS, Chang DW. 5-Step harvest of supraclavicular lymph nodes as vascularized free tissue transfer for treatment of lymphedema. *J Surg Oncol.* 2017;115:63-67.)

▪ Inguinal Vascularized Lymph Node Harvest

- Based on the superficial circumflex iliac artery (SCIA) or occasionally on the superficial inferior epigastric artery (SIEA).
  - The lymph nodes can be harvested alone or as part of an abdominal flap for simultaneous breast reconstruction and VLNT.
  - For lymph nodes alone, the flap can be harvested with or without a skin paddle.
- Surface landmarks (**TECH FIG 3A**) are the anterior superior iliac spine (ASIS), pubic symphysis, inguinal ligament, and the femoral canal.
- Reverse lymphatic mapping is done for the side that lymph nodes are to be harvested from. This first involves the preoperative injection of technitium-99–labeled albumin into the medial thigh.
- The skin incision is made 2 cm superior to the inguinal ligament and deepened to the level of the cribriform fascia.
  - If a skin paddle is desired, a handheld Doppler probe can be used to detect the perforators from the SCIA, along a line 1 to 2 cm inferior to the inguinal ligament.

- The SCIA and SIEA are identified. The lymph nodes are located in the fat lateral to the SIE vessels and around the SCI vessels, superior to the inguinal ligament (**TECH FIG 3B**). Their superficial border is the Scarpa fascia and the deep boundary is the muscular aponeurosis.
- A gamma probe is used to locate the sentinel lymph node in the leg via reverse lymphatic mapping.
  - It is imperative that the sentinel lymph nodes along with the deeper lymph nodes that drain the leg are not included in the flap.
- Once the deep lymph nodes have been identified and kept away from the dissection, lymph node harvest can be completed.
- If an abdominal flap for breast reconstruction is planned together with the VLNT, the lymph nodes should be harvested in continuity with the abdominal tissue along the SIE and/or SCI vessels. The pedicle of the abdominal flap (be it a perforator or muscle-sparing flap) is then anastomosed to the internal mammary vessels, with supercharging of the lymph node vein to an axillary recipient vein (**TECH FIG 3C**).[9]
- The donor site is closed over a suction drain, ensuring that Scarpa fascia is approximated before a running subcuticular suture for the skin. If an abdominal flap is taken, this is closed in the usual fashion.

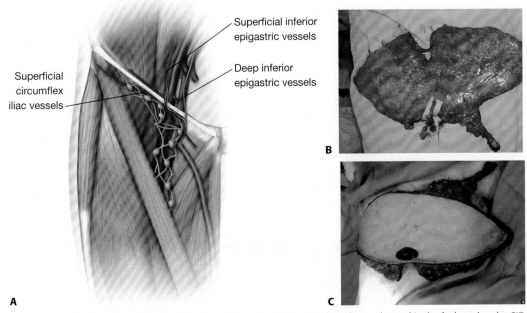

TECH FIG 3 ▪ **A.** Surface landmarking of inguinal lymph node transfer. **B.** The lymph nodes are located in the fat lateral to the SIE vessels and around the SCI vessels, superior to the inguinal ligament. **C.** The pedicle of the abdominal flap is then anastomosed to the internal mammary vessels, with supercharging of the lymph node vein to an axillary recipient vein. (**B,C:** From Ooi AS, Chang DW. 5-Step harvest of supraclavicular lymph nodes as vascularized free tissue transfer for treatment of lymphedema. *J Surg Oncol.* 2017;115:63-67.)

■ Omental Vascularized Lymph Node Harvest

- The omentum has been called the guardian of the abdomen due to its lymphatic and immunological capability.
- The omental flap is based on the right gastroepiploic artery and can be harvested via an open or laparoscopic approach. A skin paddle is not possible.
  - For the open approach, an upper minilaparotomy incision is used.
  - For the laparoscopic approach, the abdomen is accessed with four ports.
- The lymphatic territory of the omentum can be identified with methylene blue dye injection preoperatively. This can be done using upper gastrointestinal endoscopy or via direct injection using the open or laparoscopic approach.
- The free border of the omentum is first identified. This is then dissected along its natural anatomical plane toward the greater curve of the stomach. Gentle manipulation of the omentum is required throughout the harvest.
- The lesser sac is entered and the short gastric and left gastroepiploic vessels are identified and ligated, and the flap is dissected off the greater curve of the stomach with meticulous cautery.
- The flap is harvested in its entirety based on the right gastroepiploic artery, which is dissected to its origin. It can be debulked by up to 40% to aid in inset.
  - Preoperative dye mapping aids in preserving the critical lymphatic tissue.[10]
- Once the flap is rendered ischemic, delivery of the flap extra-abdominally can be done via the minilaparotomy incision or, in the case of the laparoscopic approach, a 3-cm infraumbilical extension of the umbilical port.
- The laparotomy or laparoscopic wounds are closed in the usual fashion.

■ Recipient Site Preparation and Microanastomosis

- As mentioned previously, recipient site is dependent on clinical indication and surgeon preference. The advantages and disadvantages of each are summarized in Table 3.
- In the upper extremity, the lymph nodes are commonly placed in the axilla or at the dorsal wrist.
- In the lower extremity, the lymph nodes are commonly placed in the groin, anterior ankle and less commonly, the popliteal region.

Axilla

- A skin paddle is usually not required for VLNT to this region.
- If available, a previous axillary scar is used for the skin incision.
- The incision is deepened toward the axillary fat, releasing and removing any scar tissue. Care must be taken to avoid injury to vital structures within the axilla.

- The TD or LT vessels are identified and preserved. Arterial and venous anastomosis is done end to end (ETE) to these vessels. The flap is placed in the pocket created.
- The axillary wound is closed over a suction drain. An implantable Doppler probe can be used for monitoring of anastomotic patency.

Medial Elbow

- The VLN flap is usually harvested with a skin paddle for this recipient site.
- A curvilinear skin incision is made on the medial volar elbow area at the level of the epicondyle.
- A pocket is created for the flap placement.
- The anterior recurrent ulnar artery and the basilic vein are identified and used for ETE anastomosis.
- The flap is inset loosely over nonsuction drains.

Dorsal Wrist

- The VLN flap is usually harvested with a skin paddle for this recipient site.

Table 3 Advantages and Disadvantages of Different Vascularized Lymph Node Transfer Recipient Sites

		Advantages	Disadvantages
Upper extremity	Axilla	Hidden incision/scar Scar tissue release Multiple recipient vessels	Buried flap requiring implantable Doppler probe for monitoring of anastomotic patency
	Elbow	Hidden donor site scar medially	Difficult dissection of recipient vessels Interruption with elbow flexion
	Wrist	Tension-free closure with skin paddle Ease of monitoring	Aesthetically displeasing skin paddle May require skin graft
Lower extremity	Groin	Hidden incisional scar Scar tissue release	Potentially deep dissection Buried flap requiring implantable Doppler probe for monitoring of anastomotic patency
	Posterior knee	Hidden incisional scar	Difficulty with positioning and microanastomosis
	Ankle	Tension-free closure with skin paddle Ease of monitoring	Aesthetically displeasing skin paddle May require skin graft Difficulty with footwear

TECHNIQUES

- A transverse skin incision is used to create a pocket within which the flap can be partially inset.
- Arterial microanastomosis is done ETE to a superficial branch of the radial artery at the anatomical snuffbox.
- Venous microanastomosis is done ETE to a branch of the cephalic vein.
- The skin of the VLN flap is loosely approximated to the wrist skin over nonsuction drains to avoid compression.

Groin

- A skin paddle is usually not required for VLNT to this region.
- A vertically oriented linear skin incision is made at the medial groin beneath the inguinal ligament and just above the femoral pulse.
- Dissection proceeds toward the superficial femoral vessels, carefully preserving any skin perforators or branches of the greater saphenous vein.
- Any scar tissue is aggressively released and removed to create a pocket for the VLNT.
- Arterial microanastomosis can be done ETE to a branch of the superficial femoral artery or an adequate skin perforator or end to side (ETS) to the superficial femoral artery.
- Venous anastomosis can be done ETE to a branch of the accompanying femoral vein or a branch of the greater saphenous vein.
- The axillary wound is closed over a suction drain. An implantable Doppler probe can be used for monitoring of anastomotic patency.

Posterior Knee

- For the rare occasions where the flap is to be placed at the posterior knee, a skin paddle is usually not required.
- A vertical skin incision is made medially just below the popliteal region.
- A pocket is created for placement of the VLN.
- Microanastomosis can be done ETE to the medial genicular branches or ETS to the posterior tibial vessels.
- Closure of the wound is done over a suction drain.

Dorsal Ankle

- The VLN flap is usually harvested with a skin paddle for this recipient site.
- A curvilinear incision is made on the dorsal ankle and deepened to the deep fascia.
- The superior and inferior skin envelopes are undermined to allow for the inset of the VLN flap.
- The dorsalis pedis (DP) vessels are identified and preserved for microanastomosis. This can be done in an ETE or ETS fashion for both the flap artery and vein.
- The flap skin paddle is then loosely inset into the skin pocket over nonsuction drains.
- A split-thickness skin graft may be required in cases in which the sides of the flap are too large to fit into the created skin pocket.

PEARLS AND PITFALLS

Assessment	▪ Confirm the diagnosis of lymphedema and find out what therapy has been tried. ▪ Exclude smoking, hypercoagulable states, or bleeding tendencies.
Donor site selection and harvest	▪ The surgeon should be comfortable with harvesting from the chosen donor site. ▪ Avoid harvesting the deep lymphatic chain of the thoracic and groin lymph node basins to prevent donor limb lymphedema.
Recipient site selection	▪ Selection of proximal or distal recipient sites is dependent on surgeon preference, familiarity, and comfort; also, the area of the lymphedema, as well as discussion with the patient. ▪ Release of scar tissue and the introduction of well-vascularized lymph nodes can promote angiogenesis.
Postoperative care	▪ The vascularized lymph node transfer is a free flap, and monitoring should proceed accordingly. ▪ Compression therapy should be continued postoperatively.

POSTOPERATIVE CARE

- Immediate postoperative care would include monitoring of the free VLNT recipient site for anastomotic patency and local wound complications, as well as monitoring of the donor site. Postoperative free flap care is unit dependent, but usually would include:
  - Hourly monitoring of the flap using clinical parameters for the skin paddle or implantable Doppler probe for buried flaps
  - Monitoring for development of hematoma at the recipient site

- Monitoring for development of hematoma or lymphorrhea at the donor site. The latter can usually resolve conservatively with prolonged drain use
- Prevention of thromboembolic problems using mechanical and chemical prophylaxis
- The patient being kept NPO overnight for emergent flap take back if required
- Early mobilization of patients on postoperative day (POD) 1
- Early use of compression wrapping by trained lymphedema therapists

- Patients are usually discharged on POD 3 or 4.
- Follow-up would include regular clinic visits for monitoring for wound complications and results of the VLNT. The latter is preferably done using the same techniques as preoperative assessment of lymphedema severity.

OUTCOMES

- The VLNT is like any free flap, requiring time for neovascularization and lymphangiogenesis. Typically, objective measurement results are not seen until 1 year postoperatively. Patients often report symptomatic improvement almost immediately postoperatively, especially in cases where scar tissue has been excised and vascularized flap is placed.
- As the technique of VLNT gains increasing popularity, the number of studies reporting on its results are growing, with reduction rates of 0% to 100%.[8,9,11–15] It is difficult to directly compare outcomes because there is a wide range of donor and recipient sites, as well as severity of lymphedema.
  - In a 20-year follow-up of 1500 cases of VLNT, Becker et al. reported a response rate of 98%, with 40% of patients with stage I and II extremity lymphedema achieving a 100% reduction rate.[8]
  - In a study of 13 cases in which the supraclavicular VLNT was used for lymphedematous limbs by Akita et al., there was an improvement in lower extremity lymphedema index of 27% and a 54% improvement in lymphatic function.[11]
  - In a study of seven patients receiving submental VLNT to the lower extremity with a mean follow-up of 9 months, Cheng et al. reported significant reduction in the volume of the lymphedematous limb of 23% above the knee, 22% below the knee, and 27% above the ankle, with reduction in episodes of cellulitis.[7]
  - In a study on 29 patients receiving simultaneous inguinal lymph node transfer with abdominal-based breast reconstruction with a mean follow-up of 11 months, Nguyen et al. reported a 79% symptomatic improvement and mean volume differential improvement of 10% at 12 months after reconstruction.[9]

COMPLICATIONS

- Complications of vascularized lymph node transfer
  - Lymphedema of donor site
  - Donor site pain
  - Lymphorrhea
  - Wound infection
  - Flap failure
  - Hematoma
  - Recurrence of lymphedema
- Complications of long-standing lymphedema
  - Infection
  - Sensory disturbance
  - Pain
  - Reduction in mobility
  - Reduced quality of life
  - Stewart-Treves syndrome (lymphangiosarcoma)

REFERENCES

1. Narushima M, Yamamoto T, Ogata F, et al. Indocyanine green lymphography findings in limb lymphedema. *J Reconstr Microsurg.* 2015;32(01):072-079.
2. Dayan J, Dayan E, Kagen A, et al. The use of magnetic resonance angiography in vascularized groin lymph node transfer: an anatomic study. *J Reconstr Microsurg.* 2014;30(01):041-046.
3. Sapountzis S, Ciudad P, Lim SY, et al. Modified Charles procedure and lymph node flap transfer for advanced lower extremity lymphedema. *Microsurgery.* 2014;34(6):439-447.
4. Chang DW, Suami H, Skoracki R. A Prospective analysis of 100 consecutive lymphovenous bypass cases for treatment of extremity lymphedema. *Plast Reconstr Surg.* 2013;132(5):1305-1314.
5. Dayan JH, Dayan E, Smith ML. Reverse lymphatic mapping. *Plast Reconstr Surg.* 2015;135(1):277-285.
6. Raju A, Chang DW. Vascularized lymph node transfer for treatment of lymphedema. *Ann Surg.* 2015;261(5):1013-1023.
7. Cheng M-H, Huang J-J, Nguyen DH, et al. A novel approach to the treatment of lower extremity lymphedema by transferring a vascularized submental lymph node flap to the ankle. *Gynecol Oncol.* 2012;126(1):93-98.
8. Becker C, Vasile JV, Levine JL, et al. Microlymphatic surgery for the treatment of iatrogenic lymphedema. *Clin Plast Surg.* 2012;39(4):385-398.
9. Nguyen AT, Chang EI, Suami H, Chang DW. An algorithmic approach to simultaneous vascularized lymph node transfer with microvascular breast reconstruction. *Ann Surg Oncol.* 2015;22(9):2919-2924.
10. Nguyen AT, Suami H. Laparoscopic free omental lymphatic flap for the treatment of lymphedema. *Plast Reconstr Surg.* 2015;136(1):114-118.
11. Akita S, Mitsukawa N, Kuriyama M, et al. Comparison of vascularized supraclavicular lymph node transfer and lymphaticovenular anastomosis for advanced stage lower extremity lymphedema. *Ann Plast Surg.* 2015;74(5):1-7.
12. Cheng M-H, Chen S-C, Henry SL, et al. Vascularized groin lymph node flap transfer for postmastectomy upper limb lymphedema. *Plast Reconstr Surg.* 2013;131(6):1286-1298.
13. Lin C-H, Ali R, Chen S-C, et al. Vascularized groin lymph node transfer using the wrist as a recipient site for management of postmastectomy upper extremity lymphedema. *Plast Reconstr Surg.* 2009;123(4):1265-1275. doi:10.1097/PRS.0b013e31819e6529.
14. Sapountzis S, Nicoli F, Chilgar R, Ciudad P. Evidence-based analysis of lymph node transfer in postmastectomy upper extremity lymphedema. *Arch Plast Surg.* 2013;40(4):450.
15. Sapountzis S, Singhal D, Rashid A, et al. Lymph node flap based on the right transverse cervical artery as a donor site for lymph node transfer. *Ann Plast Surg.* 2014;73(4):398-401.

Fasciocutaneous Debulking of Extremity Lymphedema: The Charles Procedure

Clifford C. Sheckter and Peter Johannet

DEFINITION

- Lymphedema is the accumulation of interstitial fluid and fibroadiposity in subcutaneous tissues as a result of dysfunction in the lymphatic system.
  - Compared with generalized edema, lymphedema by definition is caused by poor lymphatic outflow (compared to increased capillary leak).[1]
- The disease is generally described in terms of primary vs secondary (ie, acquired) causes.[1]
  - Primary lymphedema: congenital (less than 2 years), praecox (first to third decade of life), and tarda (greater than fourth decade of life).
  - Secondary lymphedema: malignancy, iatrogenic/surgery (most common in developed world), obesity, trauma, and infection/filariasis (most common worldwide).
- Although nonoperative treatment is the mainstay, each case should be evaluated individually. Surgical options including radical excision can offer significant improvement.

ANATOMY

- Lymphedema can occur anywhere in the body where lymphatics are present; however, the disease tends to be most problematic within the extremities and genitals.
- In the extremities, the lymphatic system courses within the soft tissue between the dermis and muscle fascia, and thus, the disease is confined to this area. Anatomic knowledge of the subcutaneous tissues and its contents is crucial for surgical treatment given many nerves run within or adjacent to muscle fascia.
  - Lower extremity considerations:
    - Common peroneal nerve at fibular head
    - Sural nerve at posterior calf

PATIENT HISTORY AND PHYSICAL FINDINGS

- Generalized edema due to any underlying medical disorder (heart failure, renal failure, cirrhosis) or medication should be ruled out, given these causes are often reversible with proper medical management.
- Other limb-enlarging disorders should be considered including chronic venous insufficiency, deep venous thrombosis, congenital musculoskeletal limb discrepancy disorders, myxedema, and neoplasia.
- For lymphedema, determine primary vs secondary lymphedema based on the timing of onset, travel history (endemic filariasis), family history, and any personal history of injury, surgery, or radiation.

- Two-thirds of cases involve a single extremity; however, bilateral lymphedema is possible depending on the nature of injury (eg, pelvic lymph node dissection).[2]
- Examination of affected limb reveals supple tissue that often "pits" when gently pressed. Long-standing lymphedema causes skin changes including thickening of the dermis and thickening of the epidermis (hyperkeratosis).
  - The classic *Stemmer* sign is considered positive when the examiner is unable to pinch the skin on the affected side at the dorsum of second toe or second finger. The unaffected side will easily tent when gently pinched.[3]
- Measuring the affected limb is important both in terms of comparison to the normal side (if present) and assessing for improvement with anticipated therapy.
  - Volumetric measurements are the standard and can be achieved through either estimated circumference measurements or water displacement testing.
    - Circumference measurements, while easily accessible, can be plagued by poor interrater reliability.[4]
    - Water displacement testing, whereby the affected limb is submerged into large containers, is highly precise, albeit cumbersome. Volume in excess of 200 cc (compared to normal side) is considered diagnostic.[4]

IMAGING

- In general, imaging is not necessary for diagnosis with a convincing history and physical exam. If there is uncertainty in diagnosis, tailored imaging can assist in excluding/confirming lymphedema. For surgical planning, some surgeons advocate for ultrasound to ensure competency of the deep venous systems.
  - Ultrasound can evaluate for deep venous thrombosis.
  - Computed tomography can evaluate for masses, lipodystrophy, venous thrombosis, and lymphedema with high sensitivity.
  - Lymphoscintigraphy can help confirm the diagnosis through demonstrating both quantitative and qualitative impairment in trace.
  - Indocyanine green lymphangiography can assist in delineating drainage patterns and is more often employed in the preoperative planning of lymphovenous anastomosis or vascularized lymph node transfer.

SURGICAL MANAGEMENT

- There are limited prospective studies comparing the different treatments of lymphedema, particularly surgical approaches. There is no defined period of waiting or algorithm for performing the different procedures.

- In general, nonoperative therapy is considered first line,[1] largely consisting of concentric extremity compression wrapping with or without mechanical compression. Surgery is usually reserved for those patients with the following characteristics:
  - Failed compression therapy
  - Recurrent soft tissue infection and/or cellulitis
  - Quality of life limitations such as pain, limited mobility, and psychosocial distress
- Operations are classified into two categories: physiologic and ablative.
  - Physiologic procedures involve three techniques
    - Creating new lymphatic anastomoses (lympholymphatic bypass).
    - Diverting lymphatic drainage into the venous system (lymphovenous bypass).
    - Autotransplanting lymph nodes from another part of the body (vascularized lymph node transfer). These techniques have their own chapter for further discussion on technique.
  - Ablative techniques involve directly removing tissue from the affected extremity and fall into two operations:
    - Liposuction
    - Direct excision
- Direct excision is further characterized based on reconstruction modality: skin graft vs flap.
  - Originally described by Sir Richard Henry Havelock Charles in the early 20th century from his proceedings in India, the surgery attributed to Charles involves radical debridement of all soft tissue superficial to skeletal muscle with placement of skin grafts from the excised tissue onto the limb muscle.[5]
  - Staged excision: the lower extremity is excised in at least two operations staged 3 months apart. Thick tissue flaps are elevated 1 to 2 cm in thickness and then underlying soft tissue is excised down to muscle fascia. Flap skin edges are closed in a single dermal layer using permanent suture (eg, 3-0 nylon). This procedure shares eponyms including Homans, Sistrunk, and Thompson procedure.
- Though effective in terms of reducing limb volume, the Charles procedure unequivocally yields a poor cosmetic result, which some patients are willing to accept given the burden of lymphedema (**FIG 1**).
  - Although the authors do not perform physiologic techniques for lymphedema, it is reasonable to attempt these procedures first, given the lower morbidity.

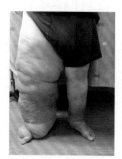

FIG 1 • Preoperative photo of a lower extremity with severe lymphedema.

- More recent advances in lymphovenous anastomosis and vascularized lymph node transfer have shown some successes in reducing limb circumference, yet for patients with significant soft tissue redundancy, surgical excision still plays a significant role.
- Reports of combined lymph node transfer with a Charles procedure have been described.[6,7]

Preoperative Planning

- Volumetric measurements should be obtained as mentioned above. This allows for postoperative comparisons to demonstrate effectiveness.
- Ultrasound can be useful in assessing the deep venous system to ensure competency.

Positioning

- Majority of cases will only involve a single lower limb; however, even if multiple extremities are involved, only one extremity should be excised at any given time the significant morbidity of the procedure.
- The patient is positioned in supine with the leg prepped circumferentially and free. A sterile tourniquet will assist in accessing more proximal upper leg in the event this tissue is involved.

Approach

- This is an elective procedure and should only occur when the patient is free of infection (ie, cellulitis) and healthy. If soft tissue infection exists, there is higher likelihood of graft failure.
- General anesthesia due to pain and inability to use local anesthesia due to large surface area.
- Consider regional anesthesia blocks and even an epidural if feasible.

■ Radical Fasciocutaneous Debridement With Split-Thickness Skin Grafts (Charles Procedure)

- After the limb has been prepped and draped in sterile fashion, all tissues planned for excision are marked and delineated.
  - Skin graft harvest trajectories are planned based on surfaces of greatest convexity with longest length (avoid anterior and posterior harvest over knee and elbow).
  - Skin graft donor site evaluation:
    - Evaluate the quality of the skin over the involved tissue planned for excision.

- Lymphedema can cause hyperkeratotic skin, which is poor quality for skin grafting. In this event, split-thickness skin grafts may be harvested from a noninvolved area of the same leg (eg, upper thigh) or other sites such as contralateral leg, trunk, etc.
- The extremity is exsanguinated with Esmarch from distal to proximal, and the tourniquet is inflated at the proximal limb to 250 mm Hg.
- Split-thickness skin grafts are harvested with a dermatome device using the widest guard possible (usually 3–4 in.) with at least 0.012 to 0.015 in. of depth.

- Thicker grafts yield better long-term results.
- Sheet grafting (ie, nonmeshed) is the preferred method for cosmetic considerations, but this requires frequent graft rolling postoperatively, which may not be institutionally feasible.
- Minimal meshing (such as 1:1.5) or graft fenestration can assist in seroma evacuation and graft take. However, graft meshing and expansion are not advised due to increased risks of secondary contracture and poor cosmetic result.
- Soft tissues are then excised down to muscle fascia using electrocautery.
  - Surgeons have the choice of preserving a thin film of adipose tissue overlying the fascia or excising the muscle fascia in entirety (**TECH FIG 1**).
  - Either way, avoid skin grafting directly on muscle fascia as this interferes with graft take.
- It is important to work systematically in excision.
  - It is often easiest to excise from proximal to distal given blood will run proximally when the leg is elevated.
  - Avoid excising distal to the ankle or proximal to the inguinal crease.
  - Take care to tie off or clip the large external veins of the leg (greater and lesser saphenous).
  - Also be careful to preserve the sural nerve and common peroneal nerve.
- Obtain meticulous hemostasis to increase likelihood of graft take.

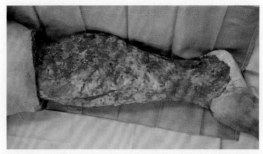

TECH FIG 1 • Lower leg following adipofascial excision. Note that a layer of adipose tissue is preserved over the muscle fascia.

- Epinephrine-soaked sponges can assist in blood loss (even with tourniquet).
- Skin grafts are either stapled or sutured in place depending on surgeon preference.
- Skin grafts are covered with nonadhesive dressing such as N-Terface followed by a silver product (eg, Acticoat Ag) to prevent infection. This is then wrapped with Kerlix gauze and elastic ace wrap.
  - A knee immobilizer is placed in extension.
- Of note, skin grafting can be delayed for 1 week if there is concern for problems in graft take (ie, concern for serous drainage or infection).
  - In this scenario, skin grafts are banked, and negative pressure wound therapy is applied to the circumferential wound.[8]

■ Staged Excision[9,10]

- Similar to the Charles procedure, the leg is prepped and draped circumferentially.
  - A vertical line is drawn on both the medial and lateral leg, dividing the leg into anterior and posterior halves.
- Skin is then incised vertically along the medial or lateral leg depending on which half is being excised.
- Adipodermal flaps are lifted in a suprafascial plane, preserving a cuff of adipose tissue (1–2 cm).
  - The elevation stops at the leg meridian.

- Soft tissues are then completely debulked from the adipofascial flap down to muscle.
- The anterior and posterior flaps are raised, and two drains are placed underneath.
  - The two flaps are secured to each other at midline using a single layer of 3-0 nylon sutures.
  - No deep sutures are used.
- Dressings are applied and the leg is wrapped circumferentially.

PEARLS AND PITFALLS

Hemostasis	■ When performing extremity adipofascial excision, use a sterile tourniquet, and limit runs to less than 2 hours. Let the tourniquet deflate to obtain hemostasis prior to placing skin grafts. Excise proximal to distal. Epinephrine 1:10 000 soaked sponges can assist in hemostasis.
Skin harvest	■ In general, it is easier to harvest the skin grafts prior to adipofascial excision given the difficulty in making a taught convex surface once the tissue is excised. ■ If excised donor leg skin is hyperkeratotic and poor quality, harvest skin grafts from contralateral leg or trunk.
Soft tissue excision	■ Leave a cuff of soft tissue around the ankle and knee (popliteal fossa, patella) to avoid exposing bone and vascular structures. ■ Be cautious when excising in the posterior calf and lateral upper lower leg to avoid the sural and common peroneal nerves.
Single vs staged	■ Consider staged excision in morbid patients who might not tolerate a complete leg debulking.
Cosmetic result	■ Appropriately set expectations with patients who these operations provide extremity debulking at the cost of poor appearance.

TECHNIQUES

POSTOPERATIVE CARE

- As with any skin graft procedure, patients should be immobilized for 4 or 5 days to allow for graft take. This will almost always involve a hospital inpatient admission, which can allow for physical/occupational therapy assistance for mobility, and intravenous pain medication.
  - All patients should be started on deep venous thrombosis prophylaxis such as subcutaneous heparin or low molecular weight heparin.
- Consider a 5-day course of intravenous antibiotics such as first-generation cephalosporin to prevent infection under the grafts.
- On postoperative day 5, all dressings are removed carefully with narcotic premedication. Wound care is targeted as needed to areas of healing difficulty.
- Prior to discharge, we recommend evaluation by occupational therapy and physical therapy for ambulation. Range-of-motion exercises are very important at the knee and elbow but are balanced against skin graft take. As soon as feasible, patients should be attempting full active range-of-motion exercises.
- Patients often require pressure garments for life to help prevent scar contractures. Lifelong follow-up with occupational therapy is advised.

OUTCOMES

- The largest series evaluating quality of life outcomes showed 63% satisfaction with limb-reducing surgery. 70% of all limb-reducing patients would opt for the surgery again.[11]
- A common problem with the Charles procedure is poor appearance.
  - This results from the absence of subcutaneous tissues (ie, leg looks much thinner than normal leg).
  - There can also be a large step off at the junction of normal tissue and excised tissue from lack of contour between these sites (**FIG 2**).
  - Additionally, the skin grafts can become hyperkeratotic.

COMPLICATIONS

- These patients are at elevated risk of deep venous thrombosis given postoperative mobility limitations, diverting all venous blood into the deep system, and the significant inflammation from extremity excision.
- Suboptimal skin graft take is the most common complication that often results from local hematomas and seroma. Meticulous hemostasis along with meshed grafts can reduce

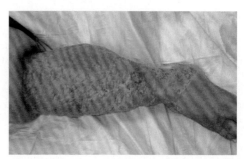

FIG 2 • Six months postoperatively with complete skin graft take. Note the hyperkeratotic appearance that is common following the Charles procedure.

this risk. Also, placing skin graft seems at lower tension points (avoiding joints) can ensure the highest graft take.
  - Amputation has been reported.[12]

REFERENCES

1. International Society of Lymphology. The diagnosis and treatment of peripheral lymphedema: 2013 Consensus Document of the International Society of Lymphology. *Lymphology.* 2013;46(1):1-11.
2. Tiwari A, Cheng K-S, Button M, et al. Differential diagnosis, investigation, and current treatment of lower limb lymphedema. *Arch Surg.* 2003;138(2):152-161.
3. Rockson SG. Diagnosis and management of lymphatic vascular disease. *J Am Coll Cardiol.* 2008;52(10):799-806.
4. Casley-Smith JR. Measuring and representing peripheral oedema and its alterations. *Lymphology.* 1994;27(2):56-70.
5. Farina R. Elephantiasis of the lower limbs; treatment by dermo-fibro-lipectomy followed by free skin grafting. *Plast Reconstr Surg.* 1946. 1951;8(6):430-442.
6. Yeo MS-W, Lim SY, Kiranantawat K, et al. A comparison of vascularized cervical lymph node transfer with and without modified Charles' procedure for the treatment of lower limb lymphedema. *Plast Reconstr Surg.* 2014;134(1):171e-172e.
7. Sapountzis S, Ciudad P, Lim SY, et al. Modified Charles procedure and lymph node flap transfer for advanced lower extremity lymphedema. *Microsurgery.* 2014;34(6):439-447.
8. van der Walt JC, Perks TJ, Zeeman BJ, et al. Modified Charles procedure using negative pressure dressings for primary lymphedema: a functional assessment. *Ann Plast Surg.* 2009;62(6):669-675.
9. Miller TA. A surgical approach to lymphedema. *Am J Surg.* 1977; 134(2):191-195.
10. Miller TA. Surgical management of lymphedema of the extremity. *Plast Reconstr Surg.* 1975;56(6):633-641.
11. Ogunbiyi SO, Modarai B, Smith A, Burnand KG; London Lymphoedema Consortium. Quality of life after surgical reduction for severe primary lymphoedema of the limbs and genitalia. *Br J Surg.* 2009;96(11):1274-1279.
12. Miller TA. Charles procedure for lymphedema: a warning. *Am J Surg.* 1980;139(2):290-292.

Liposuction for Treatment of Lymphedema

Dung Nguyen and Joseph Baylan

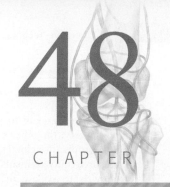

DEFINITION

- Lymphedema is lymphatic transport alteration/damage resulting in the accumulation of proteinaceous fluid in the interstitial compartment.
- Liposuction is the surgical removal of local excess fat from under the skin by vacuum suctioning using a cannula introduced through small skin incisions.
- Dry liposuction is performed without the use of local anesthetic or dilute epinephrine.
- Superwet liposuction uses a 1:1 mL ratio of infiltrate-to-aspirate for large volume aspirate removal, decrease blood loss, avoidance of lidocaine toxicity, and to minimize resultant fluid shifts.
- The pitting test refers to the amount of depression of the tissue (in millimeters) after the thumb is pressed as hard as possible on the extremity for 60 seconds.
- Tissue edema that harbors more fluid will have more pitting and tissue edema that is mainly hypertrophied fat or fibrous tissue shows little or no pitting.

ANATOMY

- Vital structures, such as neurovascular bundles and tendons that travel beneath the skin, can be injured during liposuction.
- The key anatomical areas to avoid during liposuction in the upper extremity are the axilla, antecubital region, and the wrist.
- In the lower extremity, liposuction at the femoral triangle, popliteal fossa, and ankles should be avoided.
- Subcutaneous fat is divided into superficial, intermediate, and deep layer. Distribution of each layer varies depending on anatomical location and liposuction is carried out in the intermediate and deep layer.
- Lymphatic capillaries are present in a subdermal plexus, which merge together into larger lymphatic vessels to form a complex network that carries lymph through the body. The lymph fluid enters a lymph node basin (ie, inguinal region, axilla) via several afferent lymph vessels where it is filtered and then transported toward the lymphatic ducts by efferent lymph vessels. Deep liposuction in the region of a lymph node basin can disrupt the lymphatic network and cause neurovascular injury.

PATHOGENESIS

- Long-term accumulation of lymph fluid causes chronic tissue inflammation that induces excess differentiation of fat precursors, fat hypertrophy, tissue fibrosis, and hyperkeratosis.

- Hypertrophied adipose tissue and tissue fibrosis are late signs of lymphedema.

PATIENT HISTORY AND PHYSICAL FINDINGS

- Candidates for liposuction are those with late stage II (spontaneously irreversible) to stage III lymphedema (lymphostatic elephantiasis).
- These patients have been treated and are refractory to complex decompressive physiotherapy (CDPT) and compression garments.
- Physical examination:
  - Presence of nonpitting edema on pitting test.
  - Intact skin without open wounds.
  - No erythema or signs of infection.
  - Negative Homans sign, defined as calf pain with extension of the foot.
- Treatment contract:
  - The success of the surgery relies on the patient being reliable and compliant with compression garment use 24/7 for life.
  - Patients who wish to proceed with surgery are asked to sign a treatment contract before surgery.

IMAGING

- Dual-energy x-ray absorptiometry (DXA) is used to estimate the excess fat, muscle, and bone tissue in the lymphedema limb.
- From the DXA scan, measurements are made in grams and transferred to volumes by density, which is useful in estimating the amount of excess fat to remove in patients scheduled for liposuction.

SURGICAL MANAGEMENT

- Preoperative preparation:
  - Optimize nonsurgical therapy to reduce residual pitting edema in the tissue as much as possible prior to surgery.
  - Patients who have history of deep vein thrombosis (DVT) should get a baseline venous duplex study.
  - Appropriate preoperative evaluation of cardiopulmonary status is always indicated prior to any surgical procedure.
- The patient must be aware of potential complications to include bleeding, infection, pain, numbness and tingling, contour irregularity, and wound healing problems.

- Garments:
  - Two sets of garments are made to match the size of the normal limb (Juzo, class II 30–40 mm Hg): one set is given to the surgeon to put on the patient immediately after surgery; the other set, the patient will bring to the first postoperative clinic appointment.
  - Upper extremity garments include Juzo compression sleeve from wrist to axilla with shoulder strap and gauntlet.
- Lower extremity garments include Juzo open toe compression stocking with adjustable waistband, toe cap, and biker shorts for compression of the thigh and hip area.
- Donning device to aid in putting on and removing garments.
- These garments are not sterilizable in the United States.

Anesthesia

- General endotracheal anesthesia is preferred.
- Epidural or peripheral nerve blockade performed by a regional anesthesia team is optional for postoperative pain management.

Position

- The patient is placed in supine position, and the affected extremity is rested on a hand table or a leg raise, respectively (**TECH FIG 1**).
- During surgery, the extremity is raised with the help of an assistant to access the posterior surface of the limb.

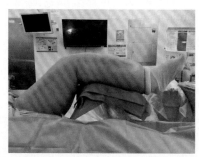

TECH FIG 1 • Positioning of affected extremity prior to suction-assisted lipectomy.

Equipment

- Sterile tourniquet.
- Liposuction set to include 3 and 4-mm cannulas.
- Suction-assisted or power-assisted liposuction machine.
- Wetting solution containing 20 mL of 1% lidocaine, 1 ampule of 1:1000 (1 mg/mL) epinephrine and 8 mL of sodium bicarbonate (8.4 mEq/L) in 1 L of lactated ringers.

Details of Procedure

- Preoperative antibiotic should be given prior to incision.
- Piperacillin-tazobactam (Zosyn) is preferred for broad-spectrum antibacterial coverage, particularly in patients with diabetes or significant comorbidities.
- After general endotracheal anesthesia is established, the entire affected extremity is prepped and draped circumferentially in the usual sterile fashion.

Superwet Liposuction

- Begin with superwet liposuction of the upper arm or thigh. Wetting solution is used in the proximal limb to minimize bleeding because tourniquet is not possible in this location.
- The amount of tumescent infused is the same as the expected amount of lipoaspirate removed. This is determined preoperatively by DXA scan.
- Using a no. 11 blade, 5 to 8 stab incisions, 3 mm in length, are made circumferentially in the proximal half of the arm or thigh.

- Wetting solution is injected in 1:1 infiltrate: aspirate ratio into the subcutaneous tissues of the upper arm or thigh using an infiltrating cannula. Wetting solution is infused until skin turgor is present at the desired location.
- After 10 to 15 minutes, liposuction is performed in the proximal extremity circumferentially.
- We prefer a 4-mm liposuction cannula for large volume liposuction and a 3-mm liposuction cannula for fine tuning and contouring with suction set at a medium setting.
- Start with the limb at rest on the table and begin liposuction of the anterior, medial, and lateral surfaces first.
- The limb is then raised and held by an assistant or placed on a leg raise (for a lower extremity) to allow liposuction of the posterior limb.
- Liposuction should be performed in segments to ensure maximal volume reduction at each location.
- Avoid liposuction of the axilla or the femoral triangle, respectively, to avoid inadvertent neurovascular injury.
- The end point is achieved when no fat is seen in the suction tubing and the skin is loose and hanging (**TECH FIG 2**).

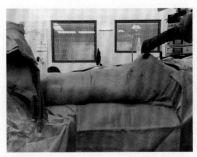

TECH FIG 2 • Tumescent liposuction is performed in the proximal thigh.

Dry Liposuction

- Dry liposuction is used for the remainder of the limb to avoid bleeding and excessive swelling of the tissue. This is beneficial in the immediate postoperative period for easier placement of the compression garment. It also facilitates quicker recovery as there is less postoperative edema.
- Place a sterile tourniquet on the proximal extremity with an Esmarch used to exsanguinate the limb.
- The tourniquet should be inflated to 175 mm Hg in the arm and 275 mm Hg in the leg.
- 10 to 20 skin stab incisions, 3 mm in length, are then made along the length of the extremity using a no. 11 blade to gain access for circumferential liposuction.
- Using a combination of 3 and 4 mm cannulas, gentle circumferential liposuction of the limb down to the wrist or ankle is performed to remove the excess fibrofatty deposits.

- Liposuction near the wrist and ankle should be done cautiously and with the smaller cannula to prevent excessive tissue trauma.

Irrigation

- All incision sites are irrigated with bacitracin solution (50 000 units/L) and cleaned.
- Apply antibiotic ointment to skin.
- With large volume of fat and lipoaspirate removed, there will be a noticeable reduction in the limb size and increased skin laxity in the extremity after liposuction is completed (**TECH FIG 3**).

Compression Garment Application

- The most challenging part of the operation is application of a clean custom compression garment, which is made preoperatively using the unaffected extremity as a sizer for the garment.
- We have found the most effective method is to be starting at the great toe and having an assistant lift the extremity while pulling force is being applied proximally to allow for the garment to span from the toes to the proximal thigh.
- Use of a donning device is also helpful to get the garment pass the hand or foot. The incisions are left open to drain through the sleeve.
- The tourniquet is then released once the garment is pulled to the level of the proximal thigh and secured.
- The entire extremity is additionally lightly wrapped with 6-in. Bias wrap to absorb the drainage.
- Total tourniquet time should be 120 minutes or less.
- There is typically minimal blood loss.

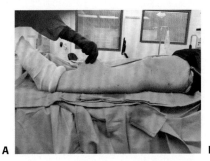
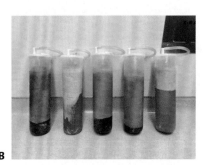

TECH FIG 3 • Liposuction is performed in segments. There is noticeable excess of skin envelope of the thigh and leg with reduction of large adipose volume. **A.** Dry liposuction is performed below the midthigh under tourniquet. **B.** Large volume of fibrofatty tissue is removed.

PEARLS AND PITFALLS

Patient selection	▪ The ideal patient is one who has isolated nonpitting edema and can be compliant with 24/7 postoperative compression garment.
Approach	▪ Use a systematic approach to liposuction by complete liposuction of each section of the extremity at a time. ▪ Avoid liposuction at the axilla, the femoral triangle, or at the joints.
Tourniquet time	▪ Allocate appropriate tourniquet time to each segment of the limb to avoid spending too much or inadequate time in one area. ▪ Avoid liposuction at the axilla, the femoral triangle, or at the joints.
Compression garment application	▪ Use a donning device to aid in garment placement.

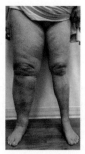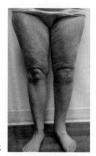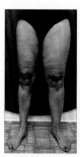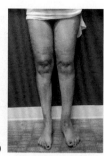

FIG 1 • **A.** 69-year-old female with 5 years history of right leg lymphedema status post hysterectomy, lymph node dissection, and postoperative radiation therapy. Preoperative DXA scan calculates 6150 mL of edema in the right leg. **B.** Results 1.5 years after liposuction of 6300 mL of fat from the right leg. **C.** 68-year-old female with 10 years history of left lower extremity lymphedema status post radical hysterectomy, pelvic lymph node dissection, and postoperative radiation therapy for cervical cancer. Preoperative DXA scan calculates 2583 mL of edema in the left leg. **D.** Results at 1 year after 3300 mL of fat tissue removed by liposuction.

POSTOPERATIVE CARE

- Due to the large amount of fluid (sometimes in excess of 10 L, depending on severity of lymphedema) removed from liposuction, overnight observation is indicated due to potential fluid shifts and for pain control.
- Patients are kept on an IV antibiotic for 24 hours and are discharged with a 2-week course of cephalexin (Keflex) or trimethoprim-sulfamethoxazole (Bactrim DS) for penicillin allergic patients.
- Prescription for oral narcotics is given for pain control.
- Patients are encouraged to ambulate regularly.
- Compression garment is to stay on 24/7 and may change the Bias wrap as needed when soiled.

FOLLOW-UP

- First postoperative appointment is on postoperative day 3, and the patient is asked to bring the second premade garment set to clinic to be changed by the surgeon.
- Patients are instructed to change their garment daily thereafter and to wear it 24/7.
- Subsequent visits are every 3 months in the initial 1 to 1.5 years with each visit adjustments to the garments are made as the edema improves.
- Once complete reduction is achieved, the patient is seen annually.

OUTCOME

- In patients who can remain compliant with 24/7 compression garment use, complete volume reduction can be achieved after 1.5 years and maintained long term (**FIG 1**).

COMPLICATIONS

- Blistering, particularly at the ankles, for which Mepilex may be used to protect areas of sensitive skin as needed
- Infection
- Contour irregularity
- DVT
- Paresthesias

REFERENCES

1. Bernas M. Assessment and risk reduction in lymphedema. *Semin Oncol Nurs.* 2013;29(1):12-19.
2. Brorson H. From lymph to fat: complete reduction of lymphoedema. *Phlebology.* 2010;25(suppl 1):52-63.
3. Chang CJ, Cormier JN. Lymphedema interventions: exercise, surgery, and compression devices. *Semin Oncol Nurs.* 2013;29(1):28-40.
4. Damstra RJ, Voesten HG, Klinkert P, Brorson, H. Circumferential suction-assisted lipectomy for lymphoedema after surgery for breast cancer. *Br J Surg.* 2009;96(8):859-864.
5. Greene AK, Maclellan RA. Operative treatment of lymphedema using suction-assisted lipectomy. *Ann Plast Surg.* 2016;77(3):337-340.
6. Maclellan RA, Greene AK. Lymphedema. *Semin Pediatr Surg.* 2014;23(4):191-197.

Acute Management: Tangential Excision and Skin Grafting

49

CHAPTER

Yvonne L. Karanas

DEFINITION

- Tangential excision of a wound is defined as the sequential removal of eschar in thin layers until healthy tissue is reached. Punctate bleeding of the underlying wound bed signals the presence of viable tissue and the end point of excision.
    - Tangential excision can be applied to any eschar of the skin in order to minimize the amount of tissue removed and preserve underlying viable tissue. It is most commonly used in burn surgery.
    - This procedure was first described by Janecovic in the 1970s and has been adopted worldwide by burn and plastic surgeons.[1]
- A split-thickness skin graft is a piece of skin removed from the body for the purpose of covering a wound in another location. The outer portion of the skin composed of the epidermis and some portion of the dermis is "split" from the remaining underlying dermis. Enough dermis is left in the "donor site" for re-epithelialization.
- A full-thickness skin graft is a piece of skin containing the "full thickness" of the epidermis and the dermis. Like a split-thickness graft, this piece of skin is removed from the patient and then transplanted to another site for wound closure or to add additional skin after contracture release. Unlike a split-thickness skin graft, no dermis is left behind so the wound must be closed primarily.
- Allograft is broadly defined as a tissue graft from another human being. In burn care and surgery, it refers to human cadaver skin used to provide temporary wound coverage.
- TBSA is Total Body Surface Area and refers to the amount of skin on the body that is burned.

ANATOMY

- Burns and traumatic injuries can result in partial-thickness and full-thickness injuries. These terms refer to the depth of the injury into the skin.
- Partial-thickness injuries involve the epidermis and some portion of the dermis.
- Full-thickness injuries involve the epidermis and the entire dermis and can even include the subcutaneous fat.

PATHOGENESIS

- Full- or partial-thickness skin necrosis may occur with trauma, burn injury, and severe soft tissue infections.
- There are approximately 486 000 burn injuries per year in the United States with 40 000 requiring hospitalization.[2]
- Worldwide, the magnitude of the problem is even greater.

NATURAL HISTORY

- Burns or traumatic injuries may initially appear as superficial injuries, but with time (72–96 hours), they may progress to full-thickness injuries.
- Judicious early debridement and serial wound care preserve all viable tissue while preventing wound infection.
- When the wound evolution is complete, areas of full-thickness and partial-thickness burns should be clearly delineated. Definitive surgical treatment may then be performed as needed.

PATIENT HISTORY AND PHYSICAL FINDINGS

- Full-thickness injuries may present as white, yellow, or brown leathery, insensate areas that lack capillary refill. With time, they will progress to a black eschar (**FIG 1**).
- Partial-thickness injuries may be superficial with pink, moist, sensate tissue that has capillary refill.
    - Deep partial-thickness burns may be cherry red in color, lack capillary refill, have decreased sensation, and may be dry. These burns are often described as "indeterminate thickness" as it is often unclear initially whether they will require surgical treatment or not.
    - Burns and traumatic injuries may result in wounds that are a combination of different depths of injury (**FIG 2**).

NONOPERATIVE MANAGEMENT

- Partial-thickness burns may be managed with wound care alone.
- In general full-thickness skin, necrosis requires surgical treatment. It may be managed conservatively in select situations, for example, small wounds that are less than 1% TBSA on the torso. A large burn is commonly defined as a burn greater than 20% TBSA.

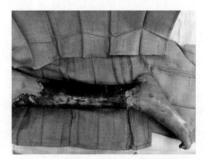

FIG 1 • Lower extremity full-thickness necrosis from a severe soft tissue infection.

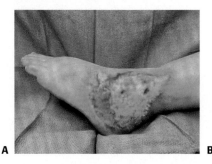
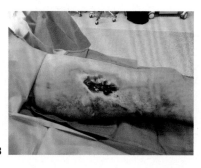

FIG 2 • A. Contact ankle burn with second-degree and third-degree components in a paraplegic patient. **B.** Flame burn to the thigh with mainly third-degree burns and small patches of second-degree burns.

- Wound care may be performed once or twice daily with silver sulfadiazine to soften and debride the eschar and prevent infection. Eventually the eschar will separate from the underlying wound bed; however, this process may take weeks or even months and lead to poor scarring and contractures.
- For large wounds, an expectant management strategy carries a high risk of wound infection.
- Surgical treatment remains the standard of care for large full-thickness wounds.

SURGICAL MANAGEMENT

Preoperative Planning

- Equipment for Tangential Excision
  - Watson Knives (**FIG 3A**)
  - Weck/Goulian Knives (**FIG 3B**)
  - Epinephrine solution
- Equipment for Skin Grafting
  - Dermatome electric or air powered
    - Guards of different widths (**FIG 3C**)
  - Mineral Oil
  - Tumescent solution: I L crystalloid, 1 cc (1:1000) epinephrine, 0.25% Marcaine (30 cc)
  - Klein Infiltration Pump—allows for high-volume infusion of tumescent solution in a rapid fashion

- Tangential excision is performed using a variety of knives designed for this purpose, or a dermatome may be used.
- The choice of instrument is based on the location of the wound and the size and thickness of the eschar. Small burns or burns in delicate areas such as the hands, face, or feet are excised with a Weck knife. Larger, thicker burns on the extremities or trunk are excised with a Watson knife. The depth of the excision can be set by adjusting the guard on the Weck knife or on the Watson knife itself.
- The Weck knife has three guards that can be placed over the blade to control for the depth of excision: 0.012, 0.010, and 0.008 in. The selection of the thickness of the excision is based on the surgeon's perception of the depth of the wound and the thickness of the skin in that region. The narrower guards of the Weck knife are used for less deep burns and areas of thin skin such as the dorsum of the hand, foot, or nose (**FIG 3D**).
- The Watson knife can be adjusted manually for thinner or thicker excisions. The knife is opened to its widest for large deep back burns, whereas more superficial leg burns would be treated with the knife only partially opened.
- Skin grafts are harvested using a dermatome which can be electric or air powered.
- A mesher is used to place holes in the skin, so that it can be stretched to cover a larger surface area (**FIG 3E**).

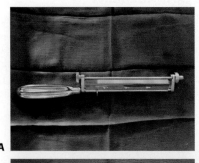
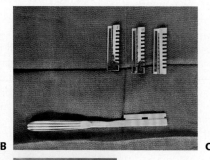
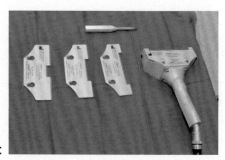
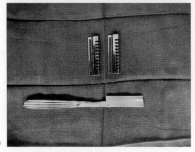
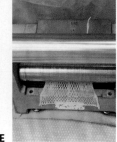

FIG 3 • A. Watson Knife. **B.** Weck knife with guards. **C.** Dermatome with 1″, 2″, 3″, 4″ guards. **D.** Weck knife with guard loaded on blade. **E.** Skin being meshed in a 2:1 fashion.

Positioning

- The patient is positioned to access the eschar and available donor sites. If necessary, the patient may be repositioned during the operation. For most lower-extremity wounds, the patient can be placed in the supine position.

- A plan to keep the patient warm during surgery should be formulated prior to the OR and implemented on arrival. Common strategies to maintain the patient's temperature include warming the room and all IV fluids, covering all nonoperative body parts with warm blankets and placing a heating pad or warming blanket under the patient.

■ Tangential Excision

- Direct the blade of the knife at the skin in approximately a 30 degree angle to engage the eschar in the blade.
- Decrease the angle so that the blade is parallel to the skin through the remainder of the excision.
- Gentle pressure is applied as the blade is moved back and forth to slice off the eschar at a uniform depth. The motion of the blade is akin to playing the violin where the bow is slid back and forth across the strings.[3]
- Excise the most dependent portion of the eschar first, so that the bleeding will not obscure the remaining areas that require excision.
- This process should be repeated until the entire wound has healthy tissue present with punctate bleeding.
- Each area should be tangentially excised until a viable wound bed is obtained before moving to the next area. This will minimize blood loss and ensure that entire wound bed is adequately excised.
- After initial excision, the entire wound bed should be assessed to assure punctate bleeding is present throughout. If immediate skin grafting is planned, any areas of questionable viability should be excised again in the same method until the surgeon is satisfied with the appearance of the wound bed. If allograft is planned for areas of questionable viability, then these wounds can be left to see if they will survive. These areas can then be re-excised at the next surgical session as needed (**TECH FIG 1**).
- Epinephrine-soaked sponges are used for hemostasis followed by electrocautery to any bleeding that has not subsided.

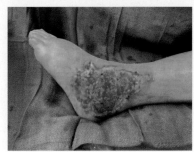

TECH FIG 1 • Contact ankle burn after tangential excision and hemostasis.

- In the extremities, tourniquet control can be used while performing tangential excision.
  - A sterile tourniquet can be applied to the normal skin or even injured tissue proximally on the extremity.
  - The extremity is elevated and the brachial or popliteal artery compressed prior to inflation of the tourniquet. In general, exsanguination is not performed as the wounds may be contaminated or infected.
  - Excision then proceeds as outlined above. Given the inflated tourniquet, bleeding is not the end point of excision. The surgeon must become adept in assessing the underlying wound bed in the absence of bleeding. The dermal tissue should be glistening white and the fat a moist light yellow without hemorrhage. All thrombosed blood vessels should be excised. Once excision is completed, the tourniquet is deflated and the wound bed reassessed. Areas that do not bleed should be re-excised as outlined above.

■ Skin Grafting

- Split-thickness skin grafts are harvested using a dermatome.
- In general, 0.012-in. thickness is the standard setting for harvesting a split-thickness skin graft.
  - Thinner grafts may be used for large burns or when wound contraction is desired as is the case for fingertip injuries or plantar heel wounds.
  - Thicker grafts can be harvested for areas of functional importance and where graft contracture should be minimized.
  - The hands, face, feet, and genitalia are a few examples where thicker split-thickness grafts or full-thickness grafts would be utilized.
- Harvesting a skin graft is ideal when the donor surface is flat.
  - This can be achieved both by positioning the patient and manipulating the tissue with pressure and traction.

- For these reasons, the thighs are the preferred donor site for harvesting a skin graft.
- Local anesthetic can be injected prior to skin graft harvest for postoperative pain control.
- Other areas can be made smooth and flat by "tumescing" the underlying tissue similar to the technique used for liposuction.
  - This involves inflating or swelling the subcutaneous tissues with liquid.
  - A solution consisting of lactated ringers, local anesthetic, and epinephrine is injected into the subcutaneous tissue of the area of the planned harvest.
  - The amount of solution required is assessed for adequate "tumescence" by manual palpation to see if it is indurated and filled with fluid such that it is smooth and all bony prominences are now obscured.
  - Care must be taken to ensure the injection is subcutaneous and not within the deeper tissues.

TECHNIQUES

- Tumescence is commonly performed over the back and chest where the ribs are palpable and the anterior lower extremities where the tibia is prominent.
  - If injected too deeply in the extremities, compartment syndrome could ensue.
- The tumescent solution also aids with hemostasis from the epinephrine effect and postoperative pain control from the local anesthetic.
- Mineral oil is applied to the skin and dermatome immediately prior to harvesting to allow the dermatome to slide more easily along the skin.
- Once the donor site has been prepared, the dermatome is turned on and applied to the skin at approximately a 45-degree angle.
- Light to moderate pressure is applied and the skin engaged by the dermatome.
- Once the graft is visible in the dermatome, the angle of harvest can be decreased to roughly 30 degrees.
- Under physician control, gentle forward pressure is applied to the dermatome along the entire length of the skin being harvested.
- The dermatome is then disengaged from the skin by angling it up akin to a "plane taking off from the tarmac." The motor is engaged until the dermatome is off of the skin.
- After the skin grafts are harvested, topical epinephrine-soaked sponges can be applied to the donor site wound bed for hemostasis.
- Grafts can be kept on the technician's table in moist saline soaked gauze until the surgeon is ready to apply them.
- The grafts can be applied as sheet grafts or meshed grafts. Sheet grafts contract less than meshed grafts, and their appearance is better. Grafts can be meshed 1:1 up to 9:1 as needed. Narrow mesh allows for fluid egress while minimizing the mesh appearance of the healed graft. Wider meshing allows for coverage of large wounds with minimal amounts of intact skin. The wider the graft is meshed, the longer the time to healing and the more wound contracture there will be. Widely meshed grafts can be difficult to work with as it may be challenging to identify the dermal side of the graft.
- Grafts should be placed with the dermal side in contact with the underlying wound bed. The surgeon should try to avoid having seams or joining areas over joints.

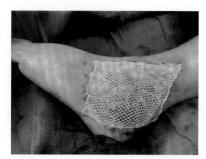

TECH FIG 2 • Meshed skin graft secured in place with staples.

- For the lower extremity, there are two techniques that facilitate grafting.
  - The first is to wrap the grafts circumferentially around the leg so that the seam is on the anterior surface of the leg.
  - The second is to place one long strip vertically on the posterior side of the leg.
- The remaining grafts can then be placed on the anterior, medial, and lateral sides.
- Both of these techniques minimize the amount of stapling or suturing that needs to be done to the posterior surface of the leg. Technically, this makes the surgery easier and allows it to proceed more expeditiously.
- The grafts can be secured with surgical staples (**TECH FIG 2**), sutures, and tissue glue or Steri-Strips/Hypafix (Smith & Nephew, London, UK) dressing tape.
  - Skin staples are the traditional method of fixation for large grafts.
  - Smaller grafts can be sutured in place obviating the need and pain of staple removal.
  - In recent years, Artiss fibrin sealant (Baxter, Westlake Village, CA) has become available and can be used to adhere grafts to the underlying wound bed.
    - Artiss is used in conjunction with staples, but these can be removed at the completion of grafting and when the Artiss has dried or alternatively a few critical staples may be left in place to be removed later.
  - Steri strips or other adhesive tapes can also be used on grafts that border the normal skin.

PEARLS AND PITFALLS

Technique	• If the Watson, Weck/Goulian blade is held in a too vertical position, it will incise the skin like a standard knife and can injure underlying structures. • Care should be taken over the Achilles tendon, malleoli, and the patella as overzealous excision will quickly result in tendon and bone exposure.
Tumescent technique	• Care must be taken to ensure the injection is subcutaneous and not within the deeper tissues. • If injected too deeply in the extremities, compartment syndrome could ensue.
Excision	• Adequate excision is the key to a successful outcome. It is critical that the surgeon ensure that all nonviable tissue has been excised prior to skin grafting.

POSTOPERATIVE CARE

- For larger grafts or in larger wounds, the grafts are covered with nonadherent gauze and silver impregnated dressings for antimicrobial protection. In the contaminated wound, the dressings are left in place for 72 hours, and then daily dressing changes are instituted. Early changing of bandages in these high-risk wounds helps identify infections and promote aggressive treatment to salvage skin grafts. Pseudomonas infection is a common culprit in these scenarios and can be treated effectively with mafenide solution-containing dressings. Smaller or less contaminated burns can be left in the postoperative dressing for 5 to 7 days, and then wound care can begin with any moisture-containing products. We commonly use Xeroform and Bacitracin. There is currently no conclusive data to support the use of systemic antibiotics after a skin graft procedure is performed.

- The vacuum-assisted closure (VAC) device can also be used to secure skin grafts during the early postoperative period. The VAC is placed in the operating room and left on for 5 to 7 days postoperatively depending on the surgeon's comfort with the cleanliness of the wound. After removal, standard daily dressing changes are instituted. The VAC is extremely helpful in getting grafts to adhere to a wound bed that has concavities or irregularities. The VAC provides excellent fixation of the grafts so that movement of the extremity will not shear the grafts. This feature makes it an excellent choice for children who may not be compliant with immobilization instructions. In addition, the VAC provides a less painful wound environment often giving patients a break from the daily pain of wound care. In order to place the VAC, there must be a 1- to 2-in. border of the normal skin around the wound for tape placement (**FIG 4**).

- Grafts that cross joints should be immobilized with splints to prevent shearing of the grafts.

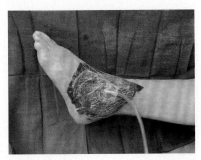

FIG 4 • VAC dressing in place.

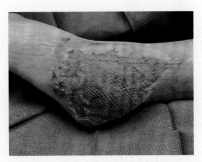

FIG 5 • Six days after excision and grafting. The graft is pink and adherent.

- Bolsters can be used to present movement of the graft and promote adherence of grafts in convex and irregular wound beds.
- Physical therapy with ambulation and range of motion is instituted on postoperative day 5 when the grafts should be adherent. For larger wounds and grafts, compression garments are worn once the wound is healed.

OUTCOMES

- With experience, skin graft take should consistently be above 80% (**FIG 5**). Long-term outcomes from skin grafting depend on the severity of the injury, length of time to healing, and patient participation in therapy. Hypertrophic scarring, contractures, pigment changes, itching, and pain are long-term sequelae of the disease process and the treatment. Often, surgical release of contracture is necessary to regain full function after tangential excision and skin grafting.

COMPLICATIONS

- Graft loss (partial or total) remains the main complication.
- Causes:
  - Inadequate excision of the underlying wound bed
  - Hematoma
  - Seroma
  - Graft shear
  - Infection
- Contracture

REFERENCES

1. Janzekovic Z. A new concept in the early excision and immediate grafting of burns. *J Trauma*. 1970;10:1103-1108.
2. Burn Incidence and Treatment in the United States: 2016. http://ameriburn.org/resources_factsheet.php
3. Mosier MJ, Gibran NS. Surgical excision of the burn wound. *Clin Plast Surg*. 2009;36(4):617-625.

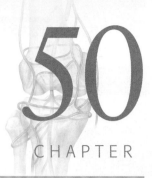

50
CHAPTER

Reconstruction of Contractures: Z-Plasty, Skin Grafting, and Flaps

Xiangxia Liu

DEFINITION

- Scar contracture is the result of tightening of the skin during and after the wound healing process.
- The continuous and progressive contraction of the scar will cause the impairment of appearance and significant dysfunction of the affected area.
- In the lower extremities, especially around the knee and ankle joint, the contracture scar can cause significant restriction in movement and, therefore, should be treated as soon as possible.
- There are many surgical interventions to treat scar contracture, including Z-plasty technique for mild scar contracture, skin grafting for a larger area of skin defects after the releasing of the contraction, and a skin flap, especially around the knee and ankle joint area or when there are any bone, tendon, nerve, and blood vessel exposure.

ANATOMY

- The scar contractures in the lower extremities usually only affect the superficial fascia layer. Sometimes there will be

exposed bone, tendons, nerves, and vessels after scar resection or revision.
- Lateral femoral circumflex artery (LFCA) arises from the deep femoral artery; it goes deep to the rectus femoris muscle and divides into three branches: the ascending, transverse, and descending branch. The Anterolateral thigh flap (ALT) is designed base on the perforator of the descending branch of LFCA (**FIG 1A**).
- Pedicled reverse-flow ALT flap is a useful tool to repair the defects around the knee joint. The descending branch of LFCA will communicate with the arteries around the knee joint, which perfuses the pedicled reverse-flow ALT flap (**FIG 1B**).
- Perforator flaps based on the peroneal artery or posterior tibial artery (**FIG 1C**) are powerful tools to repair the defects around the ankle joint and the heel (**FIG 1D**).

PATIENT HISTORY AND PHYSICAL FINDINGS

- Patient history and physical examinations will help us to determine whether a simple Z-plasty can release the contracture or skin grafting or a flap is needed (**FIG 2**).

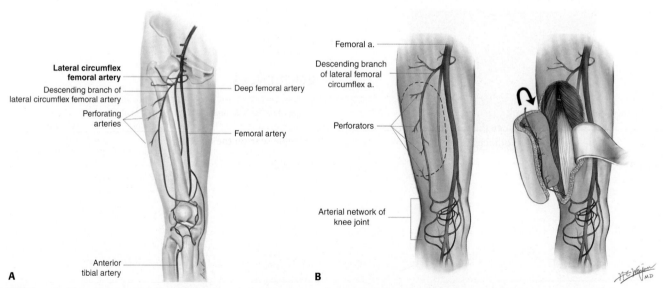

FIG 1 • A. Arising from the produnda femoral trunk, the lateral circumflex femoral artery (LCFA) gives three branches: ascending, transverse, and descending branch. The descending branch of LCFA travels deep with the space between the rectus femoris muscle and the vastus lateralis muscle. As traveling distally, it distributes the perforators, in most cases musculocutaneous perforators to the flap. **B.** The distal communicating artery between the descending branch of LFCA and the lateral superior geniculate artery is the anatomic basis for the reversed ALT flap.

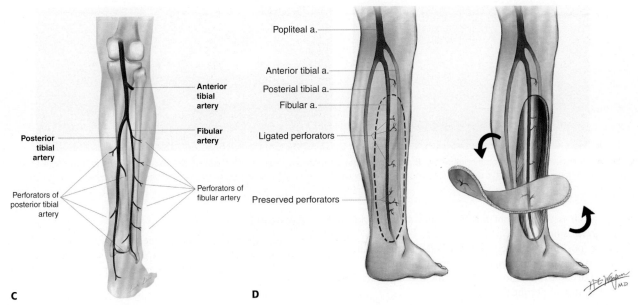

C   **D**

FIG 1 (Continued) • **C.** Through its course in the leg, the posterior tibial artery usually gives two to four major septocutaneous perforators; these perforators arise from between the soleus and the flexor digitorum longus muscle or between the flexor digitorum longus muscle and the medial aspect of tibial bone. The distance between the lowest perforator and the medial malleolus ranges from 3.5 to 8.2 cm.[1] **D.** The perforators of peroneal/fibular artery arise from between the soleus and the peroneus longus/brevis muscle. They are usually located within 2 cm from posterior border of fibular bone and are closer to the fibular bone proximally than distally.

IMAGING

- Preoperative radiography can help to distinguish simple and complex scar contracture, especially if an underlying skeletal abnormality is suspected.
- CT and MRI scanning play an important role in the evaluation of skin cancer.
  - An MRI can well identify the relationship among the tumor, calcaneus bone, and Achilles tendon in the case of Marjolin ulcer, an aggressive squamous cell carcinoma presenting in an area of chronic inflammatory scar tissue (**FIG 3**).

SURGICAL MANAGEMENT

Indications

- Z-plasty is designed to elongate a less contracted linear scar or to break a scar tension line.
- Skin grafting is an option when the primary closure is impossible and there is a lack of adjacent tissue for coverage.

- Flap should be applied when there is an exposure of the bone, nerve, blood vessel, and other tissues, which are unsuitable for skin graft.

Preoperative Planning

- Prepare the donor site for skin grafting.
- Use Doppler ultrasonography to confirm the perforator before the operation.
- Pathological study of the chronic ulcer in the scar area before the surgery is important.

Positioning

- The patient is placed supine on the operating room table with the entire lower extremity prepared into the field.
- The ipsilateral or contralateral thigh is prepared into the field in the event that a split-thickness skin graft is needed.
  - The scalp is another option for harvesting thin split-thickness skin grafts if the patients do not want to leave a visible scar on the donor site.

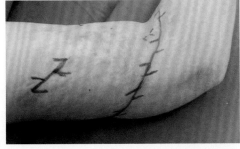 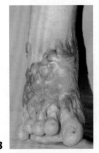 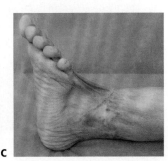

A   **B**   **C**

FIG 2 • **A.** For a superficial nonhypertrophic scar on right arm with minimal contracture, the simple technique of Z-plasty will release the contracture scar and break the tension line. **B.** For this patient, skin grafting is needed to replace the unwanted hypertrophic scar on the dorsum of the right foot and to release the dorsal contracture of the second, third, and fourth toes. **C.** Both the Z-plasty and skin grafting are needed to fully release the contracture bands of the left ankle and foot.

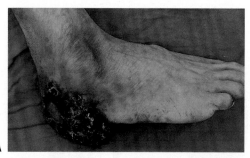
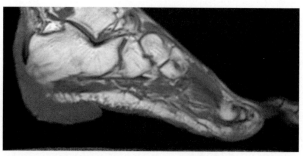

FIG 3 • **A.** Cauliflowerlike tumor on the right heel. **B.** MRI shows the tumor has a close relationship with the calcaneus bone and the Achilles tendon. A flap would be needed to cover this defect after tumor resection because there will be an exposure of both the bone and tendon.

- The groin is prepared in the event that a full-thickness skin graft is needed.
- A prone position will be helpful when the procedure is related to the posterior aspect of lower extremity.
- A lateral decubitus position will facilitate the exploration of the perforator of peroneal artery.

Approach

- Make the incision on the medial margin of ALT flap first as this will facilitate the exploration of perforators in the medial thigh in case that there is no perforator available in the lateral side.

TECHNIQUES

■ Z-Plasty

- Draw the center line on the part of the scar with the most contracture.
- Make a paired and paralleled limb line on each side of the center line (**TECH FIG 1A**).
  - Try to set the angle around 60 degrees between the center line and limb lines.
- Cut the skin along the designed lines.

- Release the subcutaneous bands.
- Elevate the flap superficial to the deep fascia (**TECH FIG 1B**).
- Transpose the paired skin flaps (**TECH FIG 1C**).
- Trim the dog ears and overly abundant subcutaneous tissues.
- Place several sutures in dermal layer of the key areas.
- Close the wound accordingly.

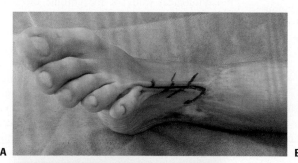
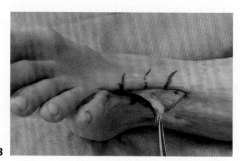
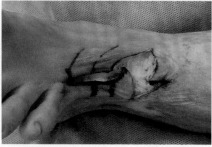

TECH FIG 1 • **A.** Multiple Z-plasties marked on a contracture band. **B.** The flap is elevated superficial to the deep fascia. **C.** The paired Z-plasty flaps are transposed initially.

■ Skin Grafting

Preparation of the Recipient Site

- Release the contracture bands of the scar (**TECH FIG 2A**).
- Make multiple zigzag incisions along the cutting edge of the wound to lessen the tension of the scar (**TECH FIG 2B,C**).
- Remove the scar tissues in the wound.
  - Control bleeding with bipolar electrocautery.
- Make a template of the defect.

Harvesting the Skin Grafts

- Use the tumescent fluid to flatten the surface of donor site and reduce bleeding.
- Use a power-driven (**TECH FIG 3A**) or freehand dermatome to harvest the split-thickness skin grafts from the thigh or scalp.
  - Choose the width and the thickness of the harvested grafts by adjusting the dermatome (**TECH FIG 3B,C**).
    - A simple way to assess the thickness is by passing a no.15 blade between the guard and the blade.
  - Install and lock a new disposable blade.
  - Make a 30- to 45-degree angle between the handle and the surface of the skin (**TECH FIG 3D**).
- Apply gentle downward pressure, and advance the machine slowly during the harvesting (**TECH FIG 3E**).
- Assess the thickness of the cut during harvesting by observing the grafts through the guard and the wound of donor site.

- Angle the machine upward, and lift off from the donor site when the harvest is complete.
- Cover the donor site with petroleum jelly gauze (**TECH FIG 3F**) or Melgisorb (Mölnlycke Health Care, Gothenburg, Sweden) combined with Mepilex (Mölnlycke Health Care, Gothenburg, Sweden).
- Put the grafts on petroleum jelly gauze with the dermal side facing up (**TECH FIG 3G**). A graft tends to fold over on itself, and this will help to keep it extended.

Placing and Securing the Grafts

- Place the grafts on the wound.
  - Keep the dermal side downward, and attach to the wound directly. The dermis has a shiny appearance and sticky sensation.
- Tailor the grafts to the wound and staple the key area.
  - Adding a suture at the tip of a small full-thickness skin graft and holding it against the index finger can help to trim the grafts with scissor (**TECH FIG 4A,B**).
- Secure the grafts with suture, surgical staple, or fibrin glue (**TECH FIG 4C**), flushing beneath the grafts with normal saline before dressing.
- Place a petroleum jelly gauze directly on the grafts (**TECH FIG 4D**), and top that with a single layer of moistened gauze.
- Next, apply a circumferential wrap/tie-over bolster/negative pressure technique (**TECH FIG 4E**).
- A splint is applied to immobilize the extremity.

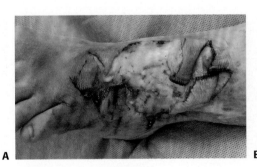

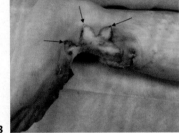

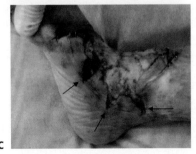

TECH FIG 2 • A. The contracture band is completely released. **B,C.** Zigzag incisions (*arrows*) are made along the cutting edge of the wound to minimize the scar contracture later on.

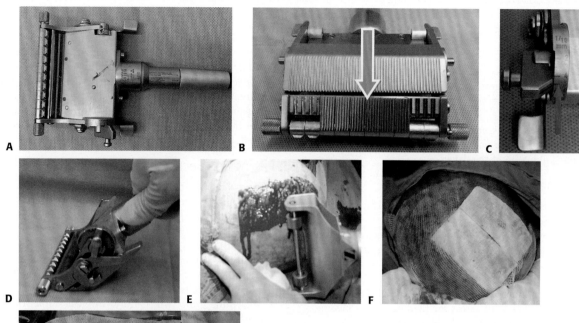

TECH FIG 3 • A. Aesculap model dermatome. **B.** Width is adjustable with 10 individual 8.0-mm cutting flaps. **C.** Cutting thickness varies from 0.2 to 1.2 mm in lockable 0.1 mm increments. The thickness reading indicates the maximal thickness the surgeon can harvest; grafts may be thinner depending on the pressure applied on the handle. **D.** The device is held at 30- to 45-degree angle between the handle and the surface of the skin. **E.** Split-thickness skin grafts being harvested from scalp. **F.** The donor site is covered with petroleum gauze. **G.** The harvested skin grafts are placed on the petroleum jelly gauze with dermal side facing up, which will facilitate placement in the wound.

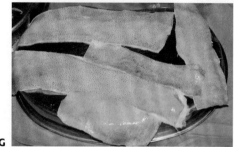

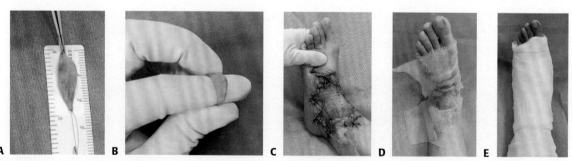

TECH FIG 4 • A. A stitch is placed in the tip of the graft. **B.** Placing the graft on the dorsal of index finger and holding with thumb and middle finger helps with trimming. **C.** Graft in place and secured with staples. **D.** Petroleum jelly gauze is placed on the graft. **E.** Wrapped before splinting.

■ Skin Grafting Combined with Acellular Allodermal Matrix

- The recipient site is prepared by excising the scar as previously described.

- Acellular allodermal matrix is used to cover the defect (**TECH FIG 5A,B**).
- Split-thickness skin grafts are harvested and placed as described (**TECH FIG 5C**).

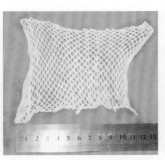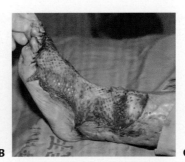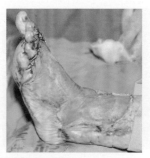

TECH FIG 5 • **A.** Premeshed acellular allodermal matrix. **B.** Placement of the matrix. **C.** Placement of split-thickness skin graft.

■ Flaps

Using an Expanded Flap to Repair a Contracture Scar

- Release the contracture scar.
- Harvest the expanded flap (**TECH FIG 6A,B**).
- Transpose and inset the expanded flap (**TECH FIG 6C**).
- Close the recipient and donor sites (**TECH FIG 6D**).

Using a Flap and Skin Graft

- In this patient, a pedicled reverse-flow ALT flap was used to reconstruct an ulcer of the scar in the knee area.
- The lesion is excised (**TECH FIG 7A,B**).
- The ALT (ALT) flap is designed, including the pivot point (**TECH FIG 7C**).
- The flap is elevated, rotated, and inset (**TECH FIG 7D–G**).
- Split-thickness skin graft is used to cover the donor site, and the recipient and donor sites are closed (**TECH FIG 7H**).

Using a Skin Flap to Repair a Heel Wound

- In this patient, lateral lower leg skin flap based on the perforator of peroneal vessel was used to repair a Marjolin ulcer on the heel.

Stage 1: Tumor Resection

- A 2 cm margin is marked.
- Dissection plan is under the deep fascia.
- The periosteum of calcaneus under the tumor is resected (**TECH FIG 8**).
- The wound is packed with iodine gauze.
- The second stage of reconstructive surgery is delayed until the negative margin is confirmed by the final pathology report.

Stage 2: Wound Repair

- Perforator investigation
  - Mark the head of the fibula, lateral malleolus, and fibula bone.

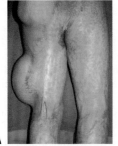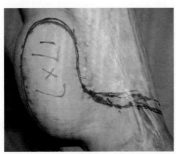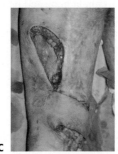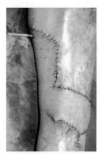

TECH FIG 6 • **A.** Scar contracture of the popliteal fossa with tissue expander placed on the lateral aspect of the thigh. **B.** Inferior-based flap design. **C,D.** Contracture scar excised and flap transposed.

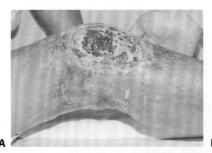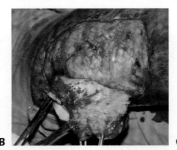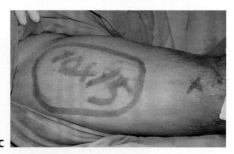

TECH FIG 7 • **A.** Chronic ulcerative scar on the anterior aspect of the right knee with limited knee extension function. **B.** Excise the lesion completely. **C.** Design of the ALT flap and the marking of pivotal point.

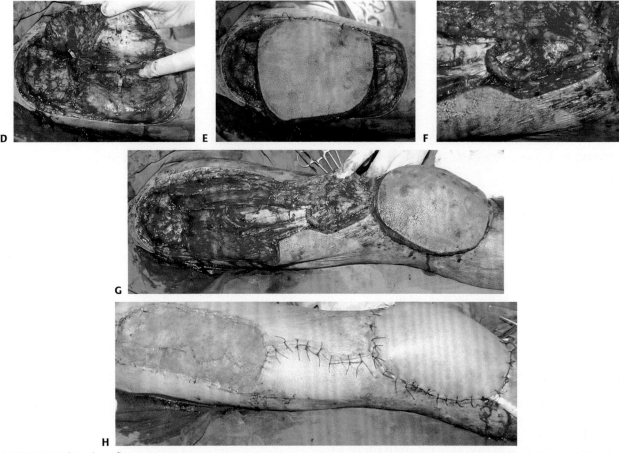

TECH FIG 7 (Continued) • **D.** Flap monitor is used during the surgery. **E.** The ALT flap is incised and elevated. **F.** The perforator. **G.** The flap is rotated into place to repair the defect. **H.** Skin graft is used to cover the donor site, and both sites are closed.

- Make an incision at the posterior margin of the flap, usually 3-5 cm posterior to fibula bone and between 6 and 15 cm above the lateral malleolus.
- Dissect under the deep fascia, from posterior to anterior toward the fibula.
- Identify any perforators coming out from the septum (**TECH FIG 9A,B**).
- Flap elevation and coverage
  - The incision is complete all around the flap.
  - Elevate the flap under the deep fascia.
  - Microclamp the perforators that are going to be ligated.
  - Release the tourniquet and observe the flap perfusion.
    - If flap perfusion is good, all the perforators, other than the selected one, are ligated.
    - If flap perfusion is not satisfactory, wait for about 15 minutes.

- If perfusion is still not good, an adjacent perforator should be reopened and the perfusion reassessed until a satisfactory vascularity of the flap is guaranteed.
- Rotate the flap and cover the wound (**TECH FIG 9C**).
- Donor site closure with skin grafting
  - Temporarily staple the flap to the margin of the wound, and measure the defect of donor site and the uncovered one.
  - Use power-driven dermatome to harvest the split-thickness skin grafts from the thigh.
  - Tailor the skin grafts to the wound and staple it (**TECH FIG 9D**).
  - Soft bulky dressing is put on the flap.
  - The distant part of the flap is exposed without dressing for flap monitoring.

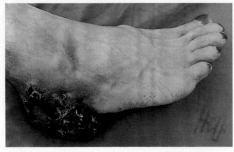

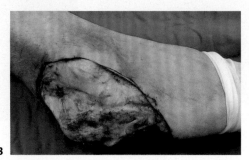

TECH FIG 8 • **A.** Cauliflowerlike tumor on the right heel. **B.** The defect after the excision surgery.

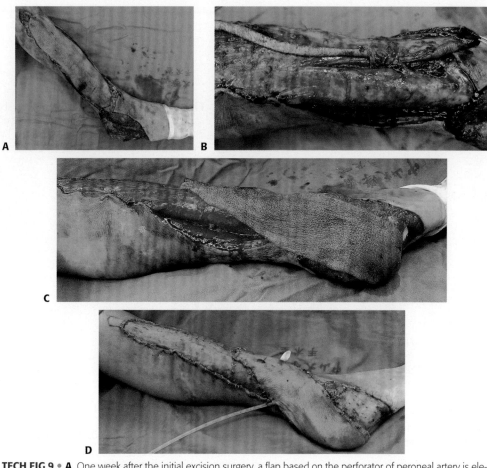

TECH FIG 9 • A. One week after the initial excision surgery, a flap based on the perforator of peroneal artery is elevated. The blue dot shows the location of the perforator. **B.** The perforator is seen arising between the soleus and peroneus brevis muscle. **C.** Flap rotation to cover the area of the Archilles tendon and calcaneus bone exposure. **D.** Donor site is covered by split-thickness skin graft. No active suction drainage is placed around the perforator.

PEARLS AND PITFALLS

Z-plasty	■ Flap angle of 60 degrees will get maximal elongation (**FIG 4**).
	■ The angles should set up to be a little more than 60 degrees when there is a severe contracture of the scar line because as the contracture scar is released, the angles tend to go sharper than designed.
	■ Place the lateral limbs parallel to the line in which the new central line will lie.
	■ Always cut the center line before cutting the limb.
	■ In scarred tissues, raise a thick flap that includes a layer of subcutaneous tissue to ensure adequate blood supply.
	■ In multiple Z-plasty, the designed flaps may not always interdigitate to each other perfectly.
Skin grafting	■ Make sure the defect is suitable for skin grafting before harvesting the graft.
	■ Kirschner wire fixation can help in patients with severe contracture deformity (**FIG 5**).
	■ The formula for tumescent fluid: 500 mL lactated Ringer solution plus 1 mL/1 mg epinephrine.
	■ Harvest 5%–10% more grafts than the template because the graft always tends to shrink.
	■ Always keep the grafts moist.
	■ It is important to keep the dermal side downward and attach to the wound directly. False orientation will lead to a complete necrosis of the grafts.
	■ Inadequate wound preparation always contributes to the failure of skin grafting.
Flaps	■ Locate the perforators by using ultrasound Doppler preoperatively to help dissection during the surgery.
	■ Always explore the perforator under tourniquet control before elevating the flap.
	■ Modify the design of the flap based on the perforators discovered during surgery.
	■ Although the perforators that are identified by ultrasound preoperatively may be good, sometimes better ones will be uncovered during the dissection.
	■ Placing a drain near the perforator that can compress the vessel or putting excessive compression over the pedicle of the flap will jeopardize the blood supply of the whole flap.

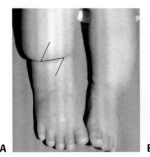
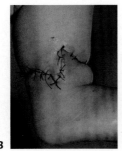
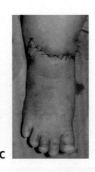

FIG 4 • A. The angle of a Z-plasty should be about 60 degrees, as shown on this congenital constriction ring of right lower leg. Black = center line; blue = limb lines. **B,C.** Immediately after Z-plasty, the constriction ring had been excised.

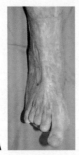
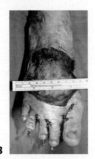

FIG 5 • A. Dorsal contracture of the second, third, and fourth toe of the right foot. **B.** Placement of K-wire fixation before the placement of acellular dermal matrix and split-thickness skin graft.

POSTOPERATIVE CARE

- A soft dressing is applied to the wound of Z-plasty. There is no need to restrict the mobility of patients with simple Z-plasty reconstruction.
- Dressing is applied to provide compression over the skin graft site.
  - Tie-over bolster technique or negative pressure wound therapy may be helpful to increase the take rate of the grafts.
  - The lower leg and foot cast or splint should be applied if the skin graft site is near to the knee or ankle.
  - The cast or splint can be removed after about 2 weeks. If the tie-over bolster technique was applied, remove the bolster carefully to avoid the shear injury to the grafts.
- After the flap surgery, mark the location of flap's pedicle where the perforators enter the flap and avoid pressure over it.

- Postoperative flap monitoring is vital for the reconstruction.
- Capillary refill time is still a secure and practical way to monitor the flap.
- A cast or splint on the surgical site would be helpful if there is a skin grafting at the same time.
- The postoperative scar care, such as pressure garments and silicone gel, should be applied to all patients for a better functional and aesthetic result.

OUTCOMES

- Outcome photos for the cases in this chapter are shown in **FIG 6.**

COMPLICATIONS

- Potential causes of skin graft loss

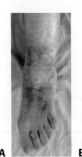
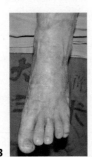
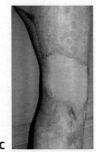
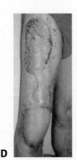
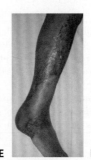
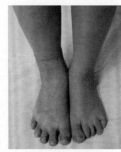

FIG 6 • Case outcomes. **A.** Two-year follow-up of split-thickness skin grafting in the patient in **TECH FIG 4**. **B.** One-year follow-up of skin graft combined with acellular dermal matrix in the patient in **TECH FIG 5**. **C.** Six-month follow-up of expanded thigh flap to repair a contracture scar in the patient in **TECH FIG 6**. **D.** One-year follow-up of an ALT flap in the patient in **TECH FIG 7** shows a pliable flap and full extension of the knee. **E.** Three-month follow-up of the patient in **TECH FIG 9**, who underwent skin flap repair of a Marjolin ulcer on the heel. **F.** Ten-year follow-up of the patient in **FIG 4**, who underwent Z-plasty for a congenital constriction ring.

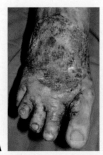 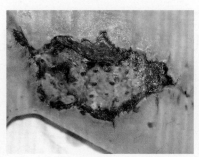 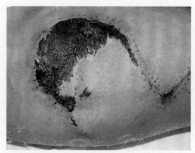

FIG 7 • A. Epidermolysis of skin graft. **B.** Partial necrosis of skin graft caused by hematoma underneath. **C.** The distal part of an expanded flap became necrotic.

- ▪ Infection
- ▪ Hematoma/seroma
- ▪ Poor vascularization
- ▪ Irradiation
- ▪ Other complications
  - ▪ Epidermolysis of skin graft (**FIG 7A**)
  - ▪ Partial necrosis of the skin grafts (**FIG 7B**)
  - ▪ Partial necrosis of an expanded flap (**FIG 7C**)

ACKNOWLEDGMENTS

The author thanks Drs. Xunxun Lin and Wenjun He for their help in preparation of **FIG 1**.

REFERENCE

1. Hung LK, Lao J, Ho PC. Free posterior tibial perforator flap: anatomy and a report of 6 cases. *Microsurgery.* 1996;17:503-511.

51
CHAPTER

Soft Tissue Reconstruction With Propeller Flaps

Adam Jacoby, John T. Stranix, and Pierre Saadeh

DEFINITION

- Propeller flaps represent one of the most recent technical advances in perforator flap dissection.
- Propeller flaps are especially useful alternatives to microvascular free tissue transfer when reconstructing distal lower extremity defects.
- The perforator propeller flap can provide soft tissue coverage on all parts of the body despite its original and most common use for lower extremity defects. Its adipocutaneous composition and ability to be rotated up to 180 degrees provide an excellent source of thin pliable tissue along with a faster and relatively simpler dissection compared with free flap harvest.
- To be considered a "propeller," the flap must rotate between 90 and 180 degrees around its perforating vessels.

ANATOMY

- Propeller flaps can be classified based on pedicle anatomy, either the type of pedicle supplying the flap or the pedicle position.
    - Island propeller flaps are skeletonized along the perforator vessels and allow up to 180 degree rotation with relative protection from pedicle kinking.
    - Nonskeletonized propeller flaps can be either skin- or muscle-based pedicled flaps where the dominant perforator is not skeletonized. Although operative times are shorter and there is less risk of perforator injury from dissection with nonskeletonized flaps, pedicle kinking is more likely—especially when rotated greater than 90 degrees (**FIG 1**).
- Propeller flaps can also be classified as a central axis propeller (pedicle in the middle of the flap) or an eccentric axis propeller (at its periphery).
- The arterial supply to the lower extremity is provided by the posterior tibial, anterior tibial, peroneal, descending genicular, and popliteal arteries with its venous supply largely mimicking the arterial network.
- Perforators of the lower extremity form five vascular territories, separated by four organized rows of perforators originating within the intermuscular septa of the leg (**FIG 2**). Anterior tibial artery perforators are most often the smallest caliber.

PATIENT HISTORY AND PHYSICAL FINDINGS

- Lower extremity defects are often caused by trauma, burns, or tumor extirpation. The defect size, depth, and location must be evaluated in addition to the surrounding skin quality. Additionally, exposed hardware (in the presence of orthopedic injuries), the bone, and the tendon must be taken into consideration when planning a durable reconstruction.

- If the patient has severe peripheral vascular disease or insulin-dependent diabetes, atherosclerotic disease may prevent adequate inflow to the flap.
- If the defect is from tumor ablation, the patient may undergo perioperative chemotherapy or therapeutic irradiation.

IMAGING

- While computer tomographic (CTA) or conventional angiography is not required for surgical planning, CTA may demonstrate the presence and location of larger caliber perforators, which can aid in flap design.

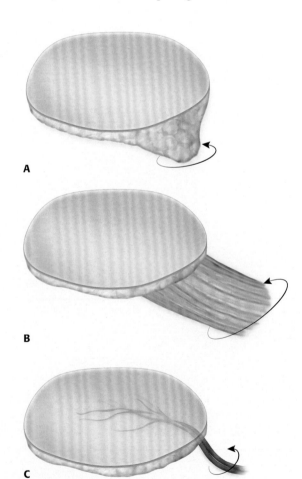

FIG 1 • Diagram of different pedicle dissections in propeller flap harvest; **A.** subcutaneous propeller flap, muscle-based propeller flap **(B)**, and "true" skeletonized propeller flap **(C)**. Note the relative bulkiness of the subcutaneous and muscular pedicles, placing them at higher risk for pedicle kinking with greater than 90 degrees of rotation.

SURGICAL MANAGEMENT

Preoperative Planning

- Unless contraindicated, general anesthesia with endotracheal intubation is preferred for these cases as the meticulous perforator dissection benefits from muscular paralysis intraoperatively. We routinely utilize preoperative Doppler detection of perforators for flap planning; however, it is not always necessary.
  - Although we find the use of a Doppler to be helpful, perforator detection may be confounded by superficial feeding blood vessels. In the setting of normal lower extremity arterial anatomy, intermuscular perforators are reliably found during intraoperative dissection, making preoperative Doppler identification a useful adjunct rather than a requirement.
- If a Doppler is used, the length and width of the flap can be designed as follows:
  - The distance between the marked perforator and most distal aspect of the planned defect is measured; this distance is then transposed proximally, and 1 to 2 cm is added to determine the total length of the flap.
  - Half a centimeter is added to the anticipated defect width (to allow for contraction of the flap) to determine flap width (**FIG 3**).

Positioning

- Location of the anticipated defect and dominant perforator dictate operative positioning as propeller flaps are useful in head-to-toe reconstruction.
- For propeller flaps supplied by the posterior tibial artery system, supine positioning is used with the hip in abduction and leg externally rotated. Propeller flaps based off the peroneal system also require supine positioning, but a "bump" is placed under the ipsilateral hip. The hip and knee are then flexed and internally rotated.
- For all flaps below the hip, a circumferential prep of the entire extremity is used routinely to ensure full visualization and allow intraoperative repositioning as needed. This also facilitates split-thickness skin graft harvest if required for donor site coverage.
- For gluteal, sacral, or lumbar flaps, the patient is placed in prone position. The patient is sterilely prepped and draped widely—typically from the midthoracic region to the upper thighs.

Approach

- When designing a propeller flap, it must be kept in mind that a skeletonized perforator can be rotated maximally 180 degrees around itself, whereas subcutaneous and muscle pedicled propeller flaps only allow for 90 degree rotation without kinking (see **FIG 1**).
- As mentioned above, though preoperative Doppler use may help identify perforator locations, for skeletonized perforator flaps, the target perforator is only chosen after a suprafascial or subfascial dissection allows for visual inspection and confirms palpable pulsatility. An exploratory incision must be planned for adequate perforator exposure and examination which should not violate bail-out local flaps or an adjacent propeller flap supplied by a different perforator.
- Predicted preoperative flap outlines (based off on-table Doppler examinations) often change after intraoperative dissection locates the dominant perforator.

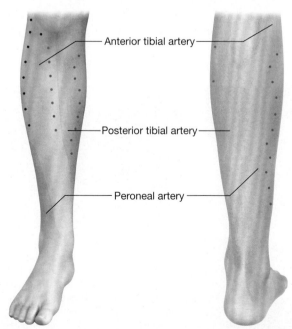

FIG 2 • Schematic of lower extremity vascular territories and their feeding vessels. ATA: anterior tibial artery, PTA: posterior tibial artery, PA: peroneal artery. Small dots represent location of reliably found septocutaneous perforators within each angiosome.

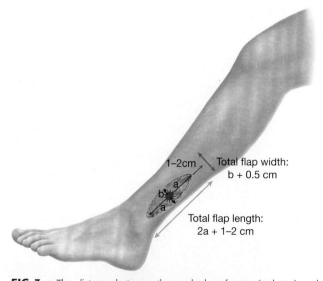

FIG 3 • The distance between the marked perforator (red star) and most distal aspect of the planned defect is measured (distance *a*). This distance is then transposed proximally, and 1 to 2 cm is added to determine the total length of the flap (length = 2*a* + 1–2 cm). Half a centimeter is added to the anticipated defect width (to allow for contraction of the flap) to determine flap width (*b* + 0.5 cm).

■ Maximum size has yet to be described, but there are case reports of a 22 × 8 cm peroneal artery perforator propeller flap[1,2] and a 19 × 13 cm posterior tibial artery propeller flap[1] based off one perforator. Perforators off the anterior tibial artery are generally the smallest caliber in the lower extremity and require smaller flap designs accordingly.

■ Skin grafting may be required for donor site coverage; however, in our experience, primary closure is often achievable when defects are lesser than 6 cm in greatest width.

■ Although primary donor site closure is ideal, it should not be done under excessive tension that could potentially compromise the flap or lead to wound breakdown. A small skin graft is preferable to either of those potential consequences.

■ Islandized Propeller Flap

■ The defect with its appropriate margins is first defined (**TECH FIG 1A**).

■ A Doppler is then used to locate dominant perforators (most often originating from the intermuscular septa).

■ The length between the perforator and most distal aspect of this defect is transposed proximally (1 cm is usually added) to determine total length of the flap whereas 0.5 cm is added to the defect width to calculate flap width (**TECH FIG 1B**).

■ If the defect is below the hip, a thigh tourniquet may be applied. The leg is elevated for 1 minute prior to tourniquet inflation, but not completely exsanguinated in order to assist with visual identification of perforators.

■ After completion of the flap design, a no. 15 blade is used to incise only one edge of the planned flap.

■ Using loupe magnification and microsurgical dissection technique, exploration of perforators is then carried out in either the supra- or subfascial plane.

■ We recommend using 3.5× loupe magnification for optimal perforator visualization in addition to a subfascial approach as we find this dissection plane is often faster and safer.

■ In either the supra- or subfascial plane, perforators are identified. The ideal perforator is large, associated with two venae comitantes, and has a strong palpable pulse (**TECH FIG 1C**).

■ The tourniquet is released, allowing assessment of the vessel's pulsatility.

■ Spasm may prevent a pulse from being palpable; it can take up to 10 to 20 minutes after tourniquet deflation for pulse appearance.

■ To protect against vasospasm, papaverine or 4% lidocaine is used liberally on preserved perforators.

■ If two or more perforators have characteristics capable of flap sustainability, they can be alternatively clamped after the tourniquet is released to determine the optimal source vessel.

■ Once the ideal perforator is located, the perforator foramen is then enlarged to allow for 2 cm clearance of fascial strands and muscular side branches (to prevent pedicle kinking during rotation) (**TECH FIG 1D**).

■ After complete skeletonization, the flap design is adjusted to optimize the perforator location for rotation into the defect. The remaining edges of the flap are then incised, and dissection is carried out in the same plane until the flap is fully elevated and isolated on the single perforator.

■ The flap can be rotated up to 180 degrees (see **TECH FIG 1D**) clockwise or counter clockwise (whichever direction provides greatest coverage with the least amount of pedicle kinking).

■ After rotation around the pedicle is complete, the edges of the flap are evaluated for healthy bleeding, and the distal flap is inspected for any signs of venous congestion.

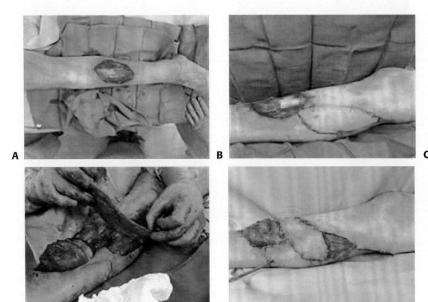

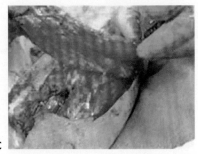

TECH FIG 1 ● A. Defect with exposed tibia. **B.** The flap is marked adjacent to the defect. **C.** Subfascial dissection reveals a dominant perforator. **D.** The pedicle is appropriately skeletonized around the dominant perforator and rotated 180 degrees. **E.** Flap inset and closure can often be achieved without skin grafts and closed suction drains unless the donor site is too large to be closed primarily as seen above.

TECHNIQUES

- Satisfied with flap viability, inset occurs in the following sequence:
  - Secure the flap in place with two to four deep (fascial) sutures (often 3-0 PDS), equally spaced along the perimeter of the flap.
  - If a closed suction drain is necessary, it is positioned away from the vascular pedicle.
- Superficial, interrupted, skin sutures (3-0 nylon) complete the flap's inset.
- Loose inset is preferable as postoperative swelling may cause venous congestion and/or ischemia.
- If the donor is not amenable to tension-free primary closure, a skin graft is harvested for coverage (**TECH FIG 1E**).

■ Nonskeletonized Propeller Flaps

- The design and execution of a nonskeletonized propeller flap is similar to its islandized counterpart, and the initial steps are similar, but the dissection is significantly faster; the differences in planning and techniques will be outlined here.
- The defect is first defined (either by tumor ablation or adequate wound debridement) and converted into a circular shape (**TECH FIG 2A**).
- A Doppler is then used to locate dominant perforators within 360 degrees of the defect.
- Note that when planning these nonskeletonized flaps, tissue can only be rotated a maximum of 90 degrees to avoid pedicle kinking (see **TECH FIG 2C**).
- Once the ideal perforator is located, the flap can then be designed. Depending upon the degree of rotation, flap length must be greater than defect width as the effective length of a flap becomes shorter with increasing rotation (**TECH FIG 2B,C**).

- A subfascial plane is again preferred for dissection. After rotation around the pedicle is complete, the edges of the flap are evaluated for healthy bleeding, and the distal flap is inspected for any signs of venous congestion.
- Satisfied with flap viability, inset occurs in the following sequence:
  - Secure the flap in place with two to four deep (fascial) sutures (often 3-0 PDS), equally spaced along the perimeter of the flap.
  - If a closed suction drain is necessary, it is positioned away from the vascular pedicle.
  - Superficial, interrupted, skin sutures (3-0 nylon) complete the flap's inset.
- Loose inset is preferable as postoperative swelling may cause venous congestion and/or ischemia.
- If the donor is not amenable to tension-free primary closure, a skin graft is harvested for coverage (**TECH FIG 2D**).

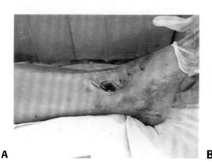
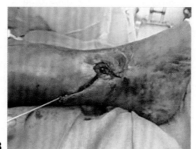
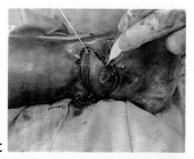
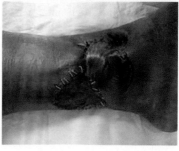

TECH FIG 2 • A. Defect and surrounding indurated tissue around the medial malleolus. **B.** The defect is created and the anterior flap is raised; the perforators perfusing the flap are left in the subcutaneous tissue and not skeletonized, making a relatively easy and fast dissection. **C.** When the dominant perforator is not skeletonized, maximum rotation is 90 degrees. **D.** If the defect is too large for primary closure, a skin graft may be used.

PEARLS AND PITFALLS

Incision placement	■ Incisions should not violate adjacent bail-out options or alternative flaps. ■ Initial exploratory incision should be as wide as possible so multiple perforators can be evaluated.
Perforator choice	■ Visual and manual inspection is key to determining the optimal perforator. ■ When possible, the chosen perforator should be at least 2 cm away from the most proximal aspect of the defect. ■ Venae comitantes are at high risk of kinking during rotation and fascial attachments must be cleared liberally. ■ Perforators from the anterior tibial artery are usually the smallest in the leg and allow for the smallest flap dimensions.
Flap inset	■ After dissection of the flap is complete and only attached by the skeletonized perforator, the tourniquet should be released to assess viability and perfusion. ■ Vasodilators (lidocaine, papaverine) should be used liberally. ■ Before inset, the flap should be rotated clockwise and counterclockwise to determine which way causes less kinking. ■ Excessively tight closure can result in vascular compromise with subsequent partial or complete flap loss.
Contraindications	■ Poorly controlled diabetes ■ Peripheral vascular disease ■ Peroneal artery and its perforators are most likely to be resistant to atherosclerotic disease and can still be used in diabetic and peripheral vascular disease patients.

POSTOPERATIVE CARE

■ Patients should rest with the reconstructed extremity or body part elevated above heart level where possible.

■ A gentle ACE wrap can be applied to lessen postoperative edema but should not be too tight to cause ischemia; a small window should be cut in the dressing (especially over the most distal aspect of the flap) to monitor perfusion and congestion.

■ An orthotic boot or plaster posterior slab can be applied to maintain optimal positioning for pressure offloading.

■ Skin sutures can be removed 10 to 14 days after surgery.

■ If a skin graft is placed over the donor site, a VAC dressing bolster should be applied over the skin graft and removed 5 to 7 days postoperatively.

OUTCOMES

■ Complication rates of propeller perforator flap are close that of free flaps.[3–5]

■ Most flap loss is related to venous congestion from pedicle kinking.[4,5]

■ In the case of flap loss, outcomes are usually better than free flap loss as most often only the superficial portion of the propeller flap becomes necrotic, leaving vital structures covered by deep portions of the flap.[2,4]

■ If congestion or ischemia is suspected, flap can be deinset and derotated, or a venous microsurgical anastomosis can be performed if feasible.

COMPLICATIONS

■ Distal tip necrosis
■ Pedicle kinking
■ Venous congestion
■ Flap loss
■ Contour deformities, scarring
■ Hematoma
■ Infection

REFERENCES

1. Ayestaray B, Ogawa R, Ono S, Hyakusoku H. Propeller flaps: classification and clinical applications. *Ann Chir Plast Esthet.* 2011;56:90-98.
2. Georgescu AV. Propeller perforator flaps in distal lower leg: evolution and clinical applications. *Arch Plast Surg.* 2012;39:94-105.
3. Hallock GG. The propeller flap version of the adductor muscle perforator flap for coverage of ischial or trochanteric pressure sores. *Ann Plast Surg.* 2006;56(5):540-542.
4. Hyakusoku H, Yamamoto Y, Fumiiri M. The propeller flap method. *Br J Plast Surg.* 1991;44:53-54.
5. Teo TC. Perforator local flaps in lower limb reconstruction. *Cir Plast Iberolatinoam.* 2006;4:15-16.

Index